Contents

Building Brains

Building Brains: An Introduction to Neural Development

**David Price, Andrew Jarman, John Mason
and Peter Kind**

WILEY-BLACKWELL

A John Wiley & Sons, Ltd., Publication

Library of Congress Cataloging-in-Publication Data

Building brains : an introduction to neural development / David Price ... [et al.].
    p. ; cm.
  Includes index.
  ISBN 978-0-470-71230-6 (cloth) – ISBN 978-0-470-71229-0 (pbk.)
 1. Developmental neurobiology. 2. Nervous system–Growth. I. Price, David J., 1957 Nov. 20-
 [DNLM: 1. Neurons–physiology. 2. Nervous System–anatomy & histology.
 3. Neurogenesis. WL 102.5]
  QP363.5.B85 2011 00724880 ʌ
  612.8–dc22

                                                          2010053724

A catalogue record for this book is available from the British Library.

This book is published in the following electronic formats: ePDF: 978-0-470-97963-1; Wiley Online Library: 978-0-470-97962-4; ePub: 978-0-470-97988-4

Set in 10/12pt OUP Swift-Regular by Thomson Digital, Noida, India.
Printed in Singapore by Ho Printing Singapore Pte Ltd

First Impression   2011

Preface

A few years ago we started teaching a new course at the University of Edinburgh aiming to stimulate undergraduates in the middle years of their studies to think about the challenges and excitement of trying to understand how nervous systems are built. We did not set out to cover all possible topics equally. Instead, we selected areas that we thought provided the best understood or the most intriguing examples of how developmental events are controlled by genetic instructions combined with information from other cells and from the developing organism's environment. We used examples taken from all stages of neural development from its earliest beginnings in the embryo to its refinement as a mature functioning structure. We selected research on vertebrates and invertebrates to illustrate key findings that provide the greatest insight into developmental mechanisms and that can be extrapolated to many or even all species of animal. One of our main reasons for writing this book was to gather together the material that we teach into a single text that might appeal to students taking similar courses elsewhere.

We also teach a variety of other students about these topics: some are in their final undergraduate year, some are in the middle year of a medical degree and some are taking courses that are components of a postgraduate degree. Although these students are at more advanced levels, many of them have received little or no training in one or more of several crucial subjects such as embryology, neuroscience, genetics and molecular biology. Increasingly, many students enter developmental neurobiology with backgrounds in mathematics, physics or computer science. We have, therefore, to teach our topics without assuming a great level of biological knowledge, and so another of our reasons for writing this book was to provide an accessible but rigorous introduction to mechanisms of neural development for students with little or no prior knowledge in this or related fields.

A third reason for writing this book was to provide students with many memorable, colourful illustrations of developmental mechanisms and the experiments that have led to their discovery. Neural development is a highly visual branch of biology: experiments are often made on structures that can be seen without great technical difficulty. The real problem with neural development, as pointed out by one of our students, is the need to understand genetics, molecular biology, biochemistry and physiology, and then apply it all in four dimensions. In this book we have tried to tackle this admittedly daunting task by depicting the essential three-dimensional anatomy of developing embryos early in the book, and then using this information to help orient the reader throughout the remaining chapters.

Most of all, we hope that the reader will find our book clear and interesting, and we hope that it succeeds in conveying some of the enthusiasm we feel for this subject. If the reader is inspired to go deeper, for example by reading one of the more detailed books on neural development that are available (some suggestions are made at the end), then one of our major aims is achieved.

We thank the many people who helped us. A number of reviewers, some anonymous, made very constructive comments: in particular, we thank Patricia Gaspar, Frank Sengpiel, Ian Thompson, Tom Pratt, Alex Crocker-Buque, Valentin Nagerl and David Willshaw. We thank our undergraduate students who gave us invaluable feedback. We thank Gillian Kidd, Julie Robinson, Anna Price and Natasha Price for help with the illustrations; Gillian's expert work on the cover illustration is greatly appreciated. We thank Siân Jarman for her help and insight and Nicky McGirr and our publishers for their patience and support.

Finally, we would like to hear what you think works well and what could be improved so talk to us on the Building Brains page on Facebook.

David Price
Andrew Jarman
John Mason
Peter Kind
August 2010

Conventions and Commonly used Abbreviations

Naming conventions for genes and proteins

The conventions for naming genes and their protein products are complicated and vary from species to species. We have taken the following pragmatic approach. We hope that in most (if not all) places where a gene or protein name is used, the context will provide all the information that the reader needs, but just in case . . .

Genes
In many cases this will be roman non-italic if the gene is named after its protein (e.g. the follistatin gene). Cases where the gene was named before the protein are usually italicized, for example *reeler*.

Gene abbreviations
These are italicized and have an initial capital, for example *Pax6, Hoxb4*. This is the convention for the mouse. Frog, chick and zebrafish have a variety of conventions for gene abbreviations, but here we have mostly followed the mouse.

Names of gene families do not necessarily follow these rules, and we follow the prevailing conventions in each field, for example Hox genes and SMAD genes, but *Sox* genes.

Species-specic exceptions

Human
The same as above, except gene abbreviations are italic, all capitals, for example *PAX6*.

Drosophila
Genes and gene abbreviations are italicized.
If mutation of the gene is recessive, for example *hedgehog* (*hh*), then all the letters are lower case.
If mutation is dominant (e.g. *Krüppel* (*Kr*)) – or if the gene is secondarily named after the protein (e.g. *Dscam*) – then the initial letter is a capital.

C. elegans
Gene abbreviations are lower-case italic and include a hyphen, for example *ced-7*.

Proteins (all species)

Proteins are generally in lower-case roman, for example follistatin and reelin, but may have an initial capital letter in cases that might otherwise be ambiguous or odd in a sentence, for example Dishevelled, Sonic hedgehog.

Proteins named after a gene abbreviation are given the gene name in roman letters, all capitals, for example PAX6, SOX1, HOXB4 and SMADs.

Commonly used abbreviations

We have tried to minimize the use of abbreviations. We have defined abbreviations where they are first used and in some cases repeatedly in multiple locations where we thought it would be helpful to remind the reader. Here is a list of some of the more commonly used abbreviations.

AMPA	α-amino-3-hydroxyl-5-methyl-4-isoxazole-propionate
AP	anteroposterior
BDNF	brain-derived neurotrophic factor
bHLH	basic helix–loop–helix
BMP	bone morphogenetic protein
BrdU	bromodeoxyuridine
CAM	cell adhesion molecule
cDNA	complementary DNA
CNS	central nervous system
CP	cortical plate
CR cells	Cajal–Retzius cells
CSPG	chondroitin sulphate proteoglycan
DiI	1,1'-dioctadecyl-3,3,3',3'-tetramethylindocarbocyanine perchlorate
dLGN	dorsal lateral geniculate nucleus
DNA	deoxyribonucleic acid
DV	dorsoventral
ECM	extracellular matrix
EGL	external granule layer
EPSP	excitatory postsynaptic potential
ES cells	embryonic stem cells
FGF	fibroblast growth factor
G protein	guanine nucleotide binding protein
GABA	γ-amino butyric acid
GAP	GTPase activating protein
GDNF	glial cell derived neurotrophic factor
GEF	guanine-nucleotide exchange factor
GFP	green fluorescent protein
GMC	ganglion mother cell
HES	hairy/enhancer of split
HSN	hermaphrodite specific neuron
HSPG	heparan sulphate proteoglycan
IPSP	inhibitory postsynaptic potential
ISO	isthmic organizer

LGE	lateral ganglionic eminence
LTD	long-term depression
LTP	long-term potentiation
MAP	microtubule-associated protein
MAPK	mitogen-activated protein kinase
MD	monocular deprivation
mEPSP	miniature excitatory postsynaptic potential
mIPSP	miniature inhibitory postsynaptic potential
ML	mediolateral
mRNA	messenger RNA
MZ	mantle zone
NCAM	neural cell adhesion molecule
NGF	nerve growth factor
NMDA	N-methyl-D-aspartic acid
NMJ	neuromuscular junction
OD	ocular dominance
PIP3	phosphatidylinositol (3,4,5)-trisphosphate
PKA	protein kinase A
pMN	progenitor domain of the motor neurons
PNS	peripheral nervous system
PSD	postsynaptic density
r1–8	rhombomeres 1–8
RA	retinoic acid
RGC	retinal ganglion cell
RNA	ribonucleic acid
SOP	sense organ precursor
SVZ	subventricular zone
TCA	thalamocortical axon
TTX	tetrodotoxin
UAS	upstream activating sequence
Vp0	progenitor domain of the V0 interneurons
VZ	ventricular zone
ZLI	zona limitans intrathalamica

Significance of bold and blue bold terms

All terms that are shown using a blue bold typeface are defined in the margin close to their appearance in the text and also in the Glossary section at the end of the book. All terms that are shown using bold lettering are defined in the Glossary. The terms are not shown as bold every time they appear, just the first time or in other places where their emphasis might be helpful. The Glossary also contains some additional terms that are not given a bold type face in the text but whose definition might be helpful.

Models and Methods for Studying Neural Development

1

1.1 What is neural development?

Neural development is the process by which the nervous system grows from its first beginnings in the embryo to its completion as a mature functioning system. The mature nervous system contains two classes of specialized and closely interacting cells: **neurons** and **glia**. Neurons transmit signals to, from and within the brain: their axons transmit electrical signals and they communicate with other cells via **synapses**. There are many types of neuron with specialized shapes and functions, with cell bodies that vary in diameter from only a few micrometers to around 100 micrometers and with axons whose lengths vary from a few micrometers to more than 1 meter. There are also different types of glial cell. The interactions between neurons and glia are very precise and they allow the nervous system to function efficiently. Fig. 1.1 shows a beautiful example of the complex structures created by interacting neurons and glia, in this case a microscopic view of a labelled node of Ranvier, which allows rapid signalling in the nervous system.

The great molecular, structural and functional diversity of neurons and glia are acquired in an organized way through processes that build on differences between the relatively small numbers of cells in the early embryo. As more and more cells are generated in a growing organism, new cells diversify in specific ways as a result of interactions with pre-existing cells, continually adding to the organism's complexity in a highly regulated manner. The development of an organism is a bit like human history, during which growth in population size and sophistication have emerged hand-in-hand, each stage building on what went before – with one obvious difference that development repeats over and over again in the same way in each species. To understand how organisms develop we need to know how cells in each part of the embryo develop in specific and reproducible ways as a result of their own internal mechanisms interacting with an expanding array of stimuli from outside the cell. Many laboratories around the world are researching this area.

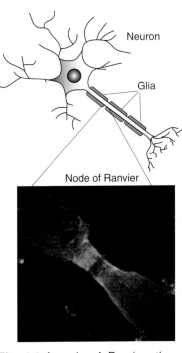

Fig. 1.1 A node of Ranvier: these highly organized structures, formed as a result of interactions between axons and glia, are essential for speeding up the transmission of electrical signals along axons. In this single fibre from the mouse spinal cord, sodium channels (blue) are sandwiched between the regions where axons and glia form junctions (called axoglial junctions) (green), which are, in turn, flanked by potassium channels (red). This picture is courtesy of Peter Brophy and Anne Desmazieres, University of Edinburgh, UK.

Building Brains: An Introduction to Neural Development, First Edition.
David Price, Andrew Jarman, John Mason and Peter Kind.
© 2011 John Wiley & Sons, Ltd. Published 2011 by John Wiley & Sons, Ltd.

1.2 Why research neural development?

1.2.1 The uncertainty of current understanding

One reason for researching neural development is that we still know relatively little about it. In this book we shall try to explain some of the main events that occur during neural development and, in particular, the mechanisms by which those events are brought about, in so far as we understand them. It is important, however, to appreciate that much of what we present, particularly our understanding of molecular mechanisms, is best thought of as continually evolving hypotheses rather than established facts. The biologist Konrad Lorenz once stated that 'truth in science can be defined as the working hypothesis best suited to open the way to the next better one'; this is highly appropriate in developmental neurobiology.

Some of our understanding is incomplete or may be shown by future experiments to be inaccurate. We have tried to highlight issues of particular uncertainty or controversy and to indicate where the limits of our knowledge are, since it is at least as important and interesting to acknowledge what we don't know as it is to learn what we do know. Much of the excitement of developmental neurobiology arises from the mystery that surrounds Nature's remarkable ability to create efficiently and reproducibly neural structures of great power.

One reason that we still know relatively little about the mechanisms of neural development is the sheer size and complexity of the finished product in higher animals. During the development of the human brain, for example, about 100 000 000 000 cells are generated with about 100 000 000 000 000 connections between them; if this number of connections is hard to visualize then consider that it might roughly equal the number of grains of sand on a small beach. Although cells and connections with similar properties can be grouped together, there is still great variation in their molecular make-ups, morphologies and functions throughout the nervous system. In reading this book you will see that many of our hypotheses about neural development are formulated at the level of tissues or populations of cells rather than individual cells and their connections, particularly in higher mammals. Only in very simple organisms containing a few hundred neurons (e.g. in some worms) do we fully understand where each cell of the adult nervous system comes from and even then we don't know for sure what mechanisms determine how each cell and its connections develop. We still have a long way to go to gain a profound understanding of the molecular and cellular rules that govern the emergence of cells of the right types in the right numbers at the right places with the right connections between them functioning in the right ways.

1.2.2 Implications for human health

Just because we don't know much about a subject is not sufficient reason to want to invest time and resources in researching it

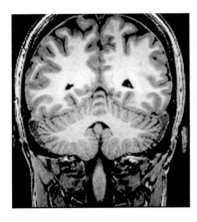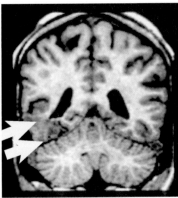

Fig. 1.2 Schizophrenia, autism and epilepsy are neurological disorders affecting about 2–5% of people. Based on epidemiological and neuro- biological evidence, schizophrenia is now believed to be a neurodevelop- mental disorder with a large heritable component. Many possible suscep- tibility genes have been identified, but how abnormalities of these genes cause the symptoms of the disease is unknown. Similarly, autism and related autism spectrum disorders are highly heritable and many of the known ge- netic causes seem to regulate the for- mation of synapses. Malformations of cerebral cortical development are among the commonest causes of epi- lepsy. Some are large defects that would be obvious to the naked eye whereas others would only be seen at a microscopic level. They are a conse- quence of a disruption of the normal steps of cortical formation, for exam- ple defective migration, and can be environmental or genetic in origin. A large number of malformations of cor- tical development have been de- scribed, each with characteristic pathological and clinical features. An example of a large congenital defect causing epilepsy is shown in the scan of a patient's brain on the right (between the arrows): for comparison, a scan of the brain of a normal person is shown on the left. This picture is courtesy of Professor John S. Duncan and the National Society for Epilepsy MRI Unit, UK.

further. However, there are many practical reasons for wanting to know more about the ways in which the nervous system develops. A better understanding should help us to tackle currently in- curable diseases of the nervous system. Many congenital diseases affect neural development[1] but their causes are often unknown; some examples of such diseases will be given later in this and in subsequent chapters. Numerous relatively common psychiatric and neurological diseases, such as schizophrenia, autism and epilepsy (Fig. 1.2), are now thought to have a developmental origin, but the mechanisms are poorly understood. Knowledge of how cancers form should be helped by a better understanding of normal devel- opment; the uncontrolled growth of cancer cells is often attributed to abnormalities of the same molecules and mechanisms that control growth during normal development. Turning to possible treatments, it has been suggested that brains suffering from neurodegenerative diseases might be repaired by implanting new cells into the nervous system. Such an approach would re- quire that implanted cells recapitulate a developmental pro- gramme allowing their survival and functional integration into the nervous system and its circuitry. How this might be achieved is currently unclear.

1.2.3 Implications for future technologies

Another, perhaps unexpected, motivation for understanding how the brain develops comes from the drive to revolutionize computer tech- nology. The application of current manufacturing methods to build much more complex computers than exist at present will need to over- come exponential increases in the production cost of ever smaller and faster circuits. In contrast, evolution has produced brains of enormous computing power that self-construct with great efficiency. Can lessons learned from studying the way the brain constructs itself be used to invent new, more efficient ways of generating computers by having them self-construct? Maybe this sounds like science fiction, but

---

[1] For a comprehensive list and images of the numerous developmental and genetic diseases that affect humans, see www.gfmer.ch/genetic_diseases_v2/index.php [20 November 2010].

international organizations are taking it seriously enough to put large amounts of money into research aimed at establishing whether it might be possible.

1.3 Major breakthroughs that have contributed to understanding developmental mechanisms

The twentieth century saw breakthroughs that have added greatly to our knowledge of how the nervous system develops. Most notable were the discovery of the structure of DNA and the development of methods for manipulating the functions of genes. We assume that the reader is familiar with the structure and function of DNA; methods for manipulating gene function will be outlined later in this chapter.

Another critically important advance in the twentieth century was the realization that, although animal species differ hugely in size and structure, the mechanisms by which their development is controlled are remarkably highly conserved. Many of the genes that control the development of relatively simple invertebrates have clear **homologues** in higher mammals, including primates. This means that by studying the mechanisms controlling the development of simple experimentally tractable organisms we can learn much of relevance to human development, which cannot be studied extensively for practical and ethical reasons.

A small handful of animal species, referred to as **model organisms**, are used in most developmental neurobiological research because each has clear advantages for certain types of research. The following sections describe the best-studied of these and their advantages; there are many others that have been used less frequently.

homologue a gene or structure that is similar in different species since it was derived from their common ancestor during evolution.

1.4 Invertebrate model organisms

1.4.1 Fly

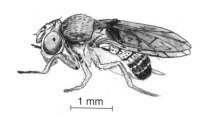

1 mm

One of the most famous invertebrate model organisms for developmental genetics is the fruit fly, **Drosophila melanogaster** (left), a small insect often found around rotting fruit. *Drosophila* has a life cycle of only 2 weeks and is cheap and easy to breed in large numbers. The eggs can be collected easily and embryogenesis takes only 24 hours. Much of the research that has been done with this organism started when scientists established lines of mutant flies with abnormal **phenotypes** (Fig. 1.3). The analysis of these mutant lines led to the discovery of the genes that were mutated in each case. By finding the genetic defects that caused the abnormal phenotypes, researchers gained knowledge of the functions of critical genes.

Working from phenotype to gene is often referred to as **forward genetics**. Box 1.1 illustrates in more detail how lines of *Drosophila* with abnormal phenotypes can be generated in a so-called forward genetic screen. *Drosophila* contain 13 000–14 000 genes many of which are

phenotype the observable characteristics of an organism, such as its physical appearance or behaviour.

named, sometimes fancifully, after the phenotype that results from their mutation; in comparison, the human genome contains around 20 000–25 000 genes. Remarkably, about 50% of fly protein sequences have mammalian homologues. *Drosophila* is being used increasingly as a model organism in which to study human disease[2]: 75% of human disease-associated genes have fly homologues. The importance of research on this organism was recognized in 1995 by the award of a Nobel Prize to Ed Lewis, Christiane Nusslein-Volhard and Eric Wieschaus for their discoveries on the genetic control of early embryonic development.[3]

As well as being ideal for forward genetics, *Drosophila* can also be used for the opposite type of approach, called **reverse genetics**, in which one starts with an interesting-looking gene and manipulates its activity so as to learn about its function. It is possible to activate specific genes in *Drosophila* using a method called the GAL4/UAS system. Box 1.2 outlines how the GAL4/UAS system works.[4] It allows specific genes to be activated in a spatially and temporally controlled manner and it can be used in a variety of ways. For example, genes normally found in the *Drosophila* genome can be activated by the experimenter to discover what they do (called a **gain-of-function** approach). Alternatively, the method can be used to activate genetic inhibitors manufactured by the experimenter to produce molecules that block the actions of a specific *Drosophila* gene (called a **loss-of-function** approach). How such blocking molecules work is discussed in more detail below (see Fig. 1.4).

1.4.2 Worm

Another invertebrate model organism even simpler than *Drosophila* whose analysis has contributed greatly to understanding mechanisms of neural development is the nematode worm, **Caenorhabditis elegans** (*C. elegans*, right), which lives in the soil and feeds on bacteria and fungi. It is easy to maintain in the laboratory and viable organisms can be stored frozen. Its development is completed rapidly within 2–3 days, it is transparent and its anatomy is known in precise detail: for example, all of its neurons and the connections between them are known. Furthermore, its development is highly stereotypical and, from **zygote** to adult worm, we know all the cell divisions that occur to generate a particular differentiated cell (i.e. we know the full details of each cell's **lineage**). Detailed knowledge of cell lineage is unusual and valuable; in most model species indirect methods must be used to deduce lineages and knowledge is usually far from complete. Further discussion of cell lineage can be found in Box 1.3.

In *C. elegans*, for any cell at any point in normal development it is possible to know what that cell will do and what it will become, that is

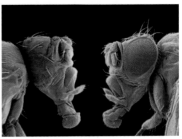

Fig. 1.3 Two fruit flies face each other: the fly on the right is a normal (wild-type) fly, the one on the left is a mutant. In the mutant, a gene that is essential for the formation of eyes is defective. Flies lacking this gene don't develop eyes. The gene in question, *Pax6*, can be found in virtually all animals: in humans, flies, molluscs and even very simple worms. The *Pax6* gene is also called *eyeless* in *Drosophila*, since *Drosophila* genes are often named after their mutant phenotype: thus, somewhat confusingly, the *eyeless* gene is *required* to make the eye. This striking image is reproduced here with permission and is the copyright of Jürgen Berger and Ralf Dahm, Max Planck Institute for Developmental Biology, Tübingen, Germany (www.ralf-dahm.com).

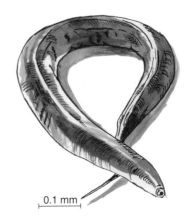

0.1 mm

zygote a fertilized cell that gives rise to an embryo.

[2] www.nature.com/ng/journal/v39/n5/full/ng0507-589.html [20 November 2010].
[3] www.nobel.se/medicine/laureates/1995/illpres/index.html [20 November 2010].
[4] See also Brand, A.H. and Perrimon, N. (1993) Targeted gene expression as a means of altering cell fates and generating dominant phenotypes. *Development*, **118**, 401–415.

Box 1.1   Forward genetics: working from phenotype to gene

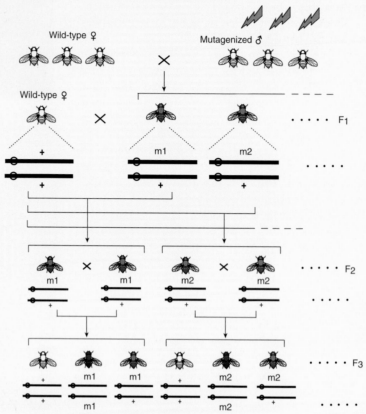

This diagram in Box 1.1 shows an example of a strategy in *Drosophila* to mutate randomly a large number of genes and then screen for those mutations that produce abnormal phenotypes in the offspring. This allows the experimenter to go on in further work to identify genes that are important for the normal generation of the structures that are rendered defective. Mutations are usually induced by feeding male flies the potent mutagen ethyl methane sulphonate or by X-ray irradiation (top right). This induces mutations in the male germ cells. These mutagenized males are crossed to wild-type females (top left) to generate an F_1 population containing a large number of flies many of which will be heterozygous for a random mutation (m1, m2, . . .). At this stage, the experimenter will only know of flies carrying **dominant** mutations that generate phenotypes in the heterozygotes. Each F_1 fly is crossed to wild-type females (second row) to generate populations of F_2 flies (third row). Sibling mating between the members of each of these populations will generate populations of F_3 flies (final row) some of which will be homozygous for each mutation, allowing phenotypes due to **recessive** mutations to be identified. In this way, the experimenter can establish many lines of *Drosophila* carrying dominant or recessive mutations that generate phenotypes of interest.[5] Similar approaches can be taken in other species. Amongst mammals, the mouse is the species of choice and many lines carrying naturally-occurring mutations or mutations induced by chemicals or radiation have been established (Section 1.5.4). Once phenotypes of interest have been identified by these screens, the process of identifying the genes whose mutation causes them begins. Descriptions of how this is done can be found elsewhere.[6]

---

[5] The reader should also be aware that this is a simplified description of only one type of screen and for a more comprehensive review we suggest St Johnston, D. (2002) The art and design of genetic screens: *Drosophila melanogaster*. *Nature Reviews Genetics*, **3**, 176–188.

[6] For example, Kile, B.T. and Hilton, D.J. (2005) The art and design of genetic screens: mouse. *Nature Reviews Genetics*, **6**, 557–567.

Box 1.2 Reverse genetics: working from gene to phenotype

The GAL4/UAS system is used by many researchers to study the function of genes in *Drosophila* (it has also been used in other species such as frogs and fish). The system has two parts, each contained in a different line of organisms. The two parts are brought together by crossing the two lines, resulting in a line in which a specific gene is activated in a specific set of cells.

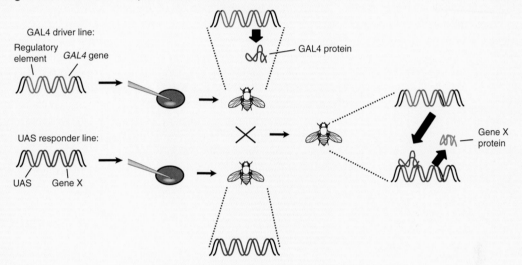

(1) To make the first line, the experimenter generates a length of DNA with three components: (i) the sequence of the gene (X) to be activated, (ii) a sequence that will activate the gene (called the Upstream Activation Sequence, or UAS) provided it is bound by a protein called GAL4 and (iii) a sequence called a P-element (not shown) that allows the whole piece of DNA to enter the genome when it is injected into an embryo. In this way, the experimenter generates a line of **transgenic** organisms (called a responder line) carrying this part of the system. However, gene X will not be activated in this line since GAL4, which the UAS needs if it is to activate gene X, is a yeast protein that would not normally be there. Thus, the second part of the GAL4/UAS system is designed to deliver GAL4 to cells where the experimenter wants the gene of interest (X) to be activated.

(2) For the second line, the experimenter generates another line of transgenic organisms (called the driver line) in which GAL4 is activated selectively in the cells where the experimenter eventually wants the gene of interest (X) to be activated. To do this, the experimenter makes a piece of DNA containing: (i) the *GAL4* gene, (ii) sequences that will activate the *GAL4* gene in the desired pattern (called regulatory elements) and (iii) a P-element (not shown) to carry the DNA into the genome. Making this piece of DNA requires the experimenter to select a regulatory element that will activate the *GAL4* gene in the desired pattern. This selection would be based on prior knowledge from research on the regulatory elements that normally activate specific genes in specific patterns. How genes are controlled by regulatory elements is described in Chapter 3.

Once these two lines have been generated, they are crossed to achieve activation of the gene of interest (X) in the desired pattern. This might seem a long-winded way of doing things: for example, why not put the gene to be activated (X) directly under the control of sequences that will activate it in the desired pattern? There are several reasons for this; a main one is that large numbers of GAL4 driver lines have already been made and, in practice, the experimenter should only need to make the responder. Once the responder line is made it can then be crossed to a large variety of existing GAL4 driver lines, increasing the flexibility of the experiment.

transgenic describes an organism whose genetic material has been modified.

Box 1.3 Cell lineage

Cell lineage is a term used to describe the sequence of cell divisions that have given rise to any particular cell in an organism. To describe the lineage of a cell, therefore, we must observe directly, or infer by more indirect means, the divisions that have generated it. Direct observation is feasible in simple organisms. The first cell lineage studies were done by Charles Whitman in 1870 on leech embryos; since then, direct observations have been used to follow cell lineages in other invertebrate species such as *C. elegans* and *Drosophila*. In some situations in the analysis of invertebrate lineages, and in most situations in the analysis of vertebrate lineages, it is not possible to observe lineages directly. In such cases, the use of molecular markers carried through the generations from a cell to its descendents can help define cell lineages; suitable markers include dyes or reporter molecules (for example green fluorescent protein, see Box 1.4) whose genes are incorporated into the genome of selected cells. The latter have the advantage that they are not diluted with each round of division. In simple organisms such as leech (see below) and *C. elegans*, patterns of cell division are very similar or identical from individual to individual, and the lineages of the cells that are generated in this way are described as invariant. In the complex nervous systems of higher organisms it is hard to know the extent to which lineages are invariant. It is likely that lineages in higher organisms show greater variation because, as we shall see in later chapters, the fates of their cells rely heavily on signalling between cells and this process is inherently susceptible to variation from individual to individual.

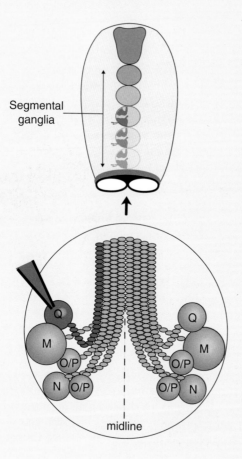

Segmental
ganglia

midline

Bottom: early leech embryo developing from bilateral sets of teloblasts, five on each side named M, N, O/P, O/P and Q. Dye injection (red) into a teloblast labels the cells generated by that teloblast (small red cells making a bandlet). Top: front end cut off from a mature leech showing dye labelled cells descended from the injected teloblast in the segmental ganglia on the injected side.

its **fate**. Against this background of precise morphological knowledge, it is relatively straightforward to study gene function by forward or reverse genetic methods, that is by generating mutant worm strains or by interfering with the actions of specific genes (for example, using RNA interference methods, Fig. 1.4). Since one of the sexes of *C. elegans* is **hermaphrodite** (the other is male), mutant worms that are severely defective and would be unable to mate can still be bred via self-fertilization. In 2002, Sydney Brenner, Robert Horvitz and John Sulston were awarded a Nobel Prize for work on the genetics of *C. elegans* development.[7] Since many of the genes in *C. elegans* have functional counterparts in humans and whole biochemical pathways are often conserved, research on this relatively simple organism has given us a major insight into our own development (for example, in work on naturally occurring cell death described in Chapter 11).

hermaphrodite an organism with both male and female sexual characteristics and organs.

1.4.3 Other invertebrates

Other invertebrates have been used as model organisms for research on neural development, including sea urchins (used since the 1800s because their embryos are easily viewed under the microscope), leeches (Box 1.3) and sea squirts (which, despite their appearance, are most closely related to vertebrates). These species have provided invaluable insights and have significant advantages for some studies. Sea squirts, for example, will be discussed again in the context of neural induction in Chapter 3.

1.5 Vertebrate model organisms

1.5.1 Frog

Among vertebrate model organisms, the frog, in particular the African clawed frog **Xenopus laevis** (right), provided some of the earliest and most important insights into mechanisms of embryogenesis, including the initial formation of the nervous system. Starting in the late 1800s, German scientists exploited the relatively large robust frog eggs and embryos in experiments aimed at understanding how specific groups of cells instruct others to develop in particular ways. In this work the scientists studied the extent to which specific groups of cells are committed to the fates they are normally instructed to follow. At the heart of this work was the question: could the normal developmental fates of cells be altered by experimental manipulation? The experiments involved microsurgery on the embryos, which are easily accessible since they develop outside the body. In some experiments, portions of embryos were grafted from one region into another, to discover how they develop at the new site and their effects on their new neighbours. In other experiments, cells were cultured in isolation. One scientist, Hans Spemann, had his great contribution to the field of experimental

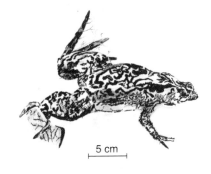

5 cm

---

[7] http://nobelprize.org/nobel_prizes/medicine/laureates/2002/horvitz-lecture.html [20 November 2010].

embryology through research on *Xenopus* recognized by the award of a Nobel Prize in 1935;[8] the discoveries that were made will be discussed further in Chapter 3.

Unfortunately, *Xenopus laevis* is not ideal for forward genetics because it takes many months for females to reach maturity, which would make the breeding required to establish mutant lines difficult, and they have four copies of many genes (allotetraploid), complicating the study of inheritance. The feasibility is greater with *Xenopus tropicalis* which matures more quickly and is **diploid**. In reverse genetic experiments, the size, accessibility and robustness of *Xenopus* eggs and embryos does make them favourable targets for the injection of molecules designed to raise or lower levels of specific gene products. The levels of a specific protein can be raised by injecting mRNA molecules; the levels of specific proteins can be lowered by injecting molecules that interfere with the function of specific mRNAs (this is sometimes called a knockdown, Fig. 1.4).

diploid an organism with a pair of each type of chromosome.

1.5.2 Chick

Chick (*Gallus gallus*) embryos are favoured model organisms because of the ease with which eggs can be obtained and stored. The embryo has a short incubation time – the nervous system is well developed after only a few days – and is very accessible, allowing easy observation of embryogenesis. Since the early 1900s experimenters used fine surgical methods (micromanipulation) to transplant pieces of live embryos from one place to another (a process known as grafting) to find out how the transplanted parts respond (discussed further in Chapter 3). More recently, chick embryos have proved useful models for testing the functions of developmentally important genes using mRNA-mediated reverse genetic methods (Fig. 1.4).

1.5.3 Zebrafish

In the past decades the small freshwater zebrafish (*Danio rerio*, left), native to India, has become another very popular vertebrate model organism. Since its eggs are fertilized and its embryos develop externally, they are accessible for experimental manipulation. Its embryos develop rapidly and are translucent allowing morphogenesis to be recorded relatively easily as it unfolds under the microscope (Fig. 1.5) using stains such as **green fluorescent protein** and its variants that are compatible with life (see Box 1.4). Not only are reverse genetic approaches being exploited successfully in zebrafish, but the species is also proving suitable for large-scale forward genetic screens in which mutagens are used to create lines of fish carrying phenotypic abnormalities (along the lines shown in Box 1.1).

1 cm

---

[8] www.nobelprize.org/nobel_prizes/medicine/laureates/1935/spemann-lecture.html [20 November 2010].

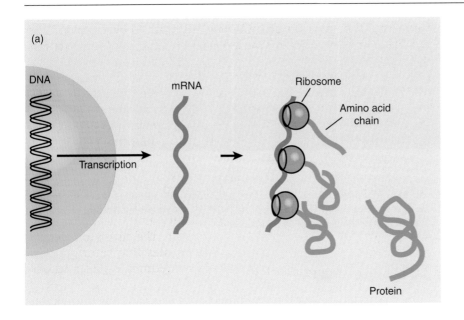

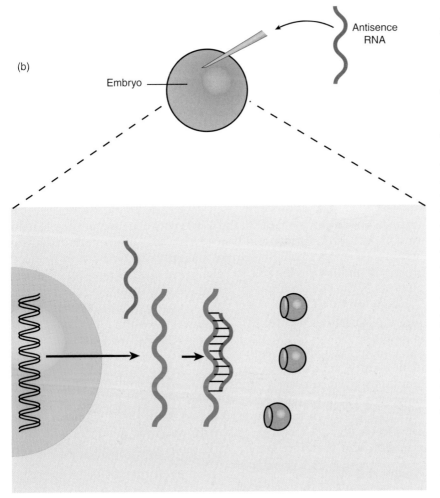

Fig. 1.4 Reverse genetics RNA interference can be used to block gene function experimentally. (a) Inside normal cells, genes are transcribed to make single-stranded messenger RNA (mRNA) that is translated by ribosomes to generate specific proteins. (b) To block gene function, **antisense RNA** molecules with sequences complementary to the sense sequences of specific mRNAs are introduced into cells where they interact with their target mRNAs and block their translation. Many types of antisense molecule have been developed. They fall into two broad groups: after binding to target mRNA, some cause its enzymatic degradation whereas others can block its translation. For example, antisense molecules called morpholinos, which have been exploited very successfully in studies of *Xenopus* development, are examples of the latter. As well as being experimental tools, antisense molecules have therapeutic potential for treatment of human diseases. The development of antisense methods to regulate gene function experimentally or therapeutically was followed by the discovery of a wide range of small RNA molecules called microRNAs that are generated naturally by cells and act as physiological antisense molecules (see Section 3.8.4 in Chapter 3).

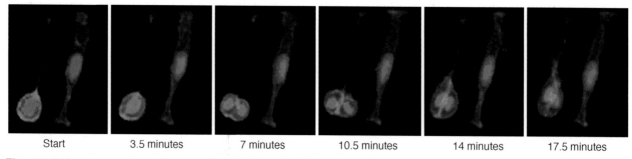

| Start | 3.5 minutes | 7 minutes | 10.5 minutes | 14 minutes | 17.5 minutes |

Fig. 1.5 A time-lapse series of images of labelled neural cells in a live zebrafish embryo showing one dividing while the other remains quiescent, made by Paula Alexandre in Jon Clarke's laboratory, King's College London, UK. Green is green fluorescent protein (GFP) that is being used to label cell membranes. Red is red fluorescent protein (RFP), a different fluorescent protein that is being used here to show nuclei (see Box 1.4 for details of these fluorescent molecules).

1.5.4 Mouse

Among mammalian species, the mouse (*Mus musculus*) has tremendous advantages for molecular genetics. Originally, Gregor Mendel studied inheritance in mice, but this was stopped by the religious hierarchy in Austria who considered it inappropriate for a monk to share a room with copulating animals! The topic was re-examined at the start of the twentieth century in France by Lucien Cuénot, who confirmed Mendel's predictions from plants. Many inbred strains and lines selected for particular phenotypes now exist and are maintained for experimental research by large breeding facilities around the world, such as the Jackson Laboratories in the USA.[9] For many lines the genes and their variants responsible for the phenotypes have been identified (an example of forward genetics). These lines are often the results of screening for abnormal phenotypes among populations of laboratory mice in which mutations have occurred spontaneously or been induced randomly with mutagens (e.g. the chemical N-ethyl-N-nitrosourea, or ENU).[10]

A huge breakthrough came in the 1980s with the discovery by Martin Evans, Matthew Kaufman and Gail Martin that **stem cells** from the early mouse embryo could be grown in culture and when reintroduced into mouse embryos were able to generate at least most if not all of the cell types in the body, a property known as **pluripotency** (Fig. 1.6).

The genomes of these stem cells, known as **embryonic stem cells** (or **ES cells**), can be manipulated by adding DNA sequences, for example encoding specific proteins, or mutating genes by replacing endogenous DNA sequences with mutated sequences by **homologous recombination** (Fig. 1.7). The modified ES cells can then be injected into early mouse embryos to generate **chimeras**: a chimera is an individual created when cells of different genotypes come together to form an embryo (Box 1.5). In these chimeras, some of the cells derived from ES cells with modified genomes will form germ cells and therefore genetic alterations made in the ES cells can

stem cell a relatively unspecialized cell that can divide repeatedly to regenerate itself (self-renewal) and give rise to more specialized cells, such as neurons or glia.

homologous recombination a phenomenon in which nucleotide sequences are exchanged between two similar or identical strands of DNA.

---

[9] http://www.jax.org/ [20 November 2010].
[10] For more details of these screening methods in mice, see Kile, B.T. and Hilton, D.J. (2005) The art and design of genetic screens: mouse. *Nature Reviews Genetics*, **6**, 557–567.

Box 1.4 Green fluorescent protein (GFP)

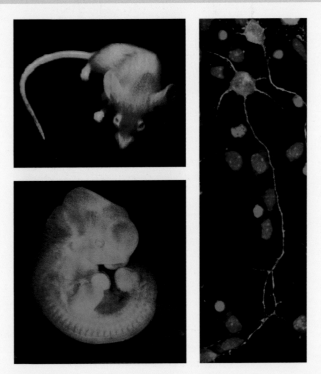

GFP in living cells fluoresces bright green when illuminated with blue light. It was first isolated from jellyfish. Its gene can be introduced into organisms in a variety of ways, so as to label either all their cells (e.g. the mouse pictured top left, or a mouse embryo pictured bottom left) or only some of their cells (e.g. pictured right: red is a non-specific stain for all nuclei). Whether all cells are labelled or only some specific cells are labelled depends on what regulatory sequence the experimenter chooses to activate the GFP gene. GFP can also be joined to specific proteins to visualize their subcellular location. Labelling cells with GFP can be used in numerous ways, for example to follow cell lineages (Box 1.3) or to study where and when regulatory elements activate their genes. We will describe many examples of the use of GFP throughout the book. Martin Chalfie, Osamu Shimomura and Roger Y. Tsien were awarded the Nobel Prize in chemistry in 2008 for their discovery and development of GFP.[11] Variations of GFP that fluoresce with other colours are now available, allowing more than one label to be used simultaneously (Fig. 1.5). Photographs of GFP-labelled embryo and cells are courtesy of Tom Pratt, University of Edinburgh, UK; photograph of GFP-labelled adult mouse reprinted from Hadjantonakis, A-K., Gertsenstein, M., Ikawa, M., Okabe, M. and Nagy, A. (1998) Generating green fluorescent mice by germline transmission of green fluorescent ES cells. *Mechanisms of Development* **76**, 79–90 with permission from Elsevier.

be transmitted through the germ line to subsequent generations (Fig. 1.7). In this way, hundreds of lines of **transgenic** mice with specific additional DNA sequences (known as knock-in mice) or with loss-of-function mutations in specific genes (known as knock-out mice) have been established and studied. The generation of knock-out mice is an excellent example of reverse genetics. It was particularly effective in advancing an understanding of the mechanisms of neural development since the homologues of many developmentally important

[11] http://nobelprize.org/nobel_prizes/chemistry/laureates/2008/chalfie-lecture.html [20 November 2010].

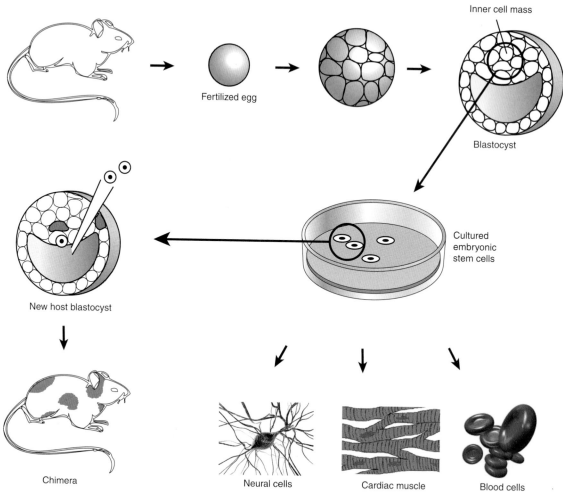

Fig. 1.6 Mouse embryonic stem (ES) cells are derived from the inner cell mass of a mouse blastocyst (here from a line of mice with a white coat). The inner cell mass is transferred into culture medium in a plastic laboratory culture dish. The cells from the inner cell mass divide and spread over the surface of the dish to become ES cells. ES cells can be differentiated into many cell types in culture, including neurons, heart muscle cells and blood cells. They can be injected into new blastocysts, here from a line of mice with brown fur (although the blastocyst cells are shaded brown to help make the diagram clear, in reality they would be no different in colour to those from the blastocyst of mice with white fur). The injected blastocysts are implanted into the uterus to generate chimeric (Box 1.5) offspring comprising a mixture of cells derived from the ES cells and the host blastocyst (the chimeric mice would have a mixture of brown and white fur).

genes discovered initially in *Drosophila* could be targeted and shown to play critical roles in development of the mammalian central nervous system. Work developing the methods that made this possible was recognized in 2007 by the award of a Nobel Prize to Mario Capecchi, Martin Evans and Oliver Smithies.[12]

Although the nervous system of mice is very much smaller than that of humans, it does share many of the same major structures carrying out similar functions. The mouse is, therefore, a popular choice of model organism for researchers wishing to investigate the molecular

---

[12] http://nobelprize.org/nobel_prizes/medicine/laureates/2007/evans-lecture.html [20 November 2010].

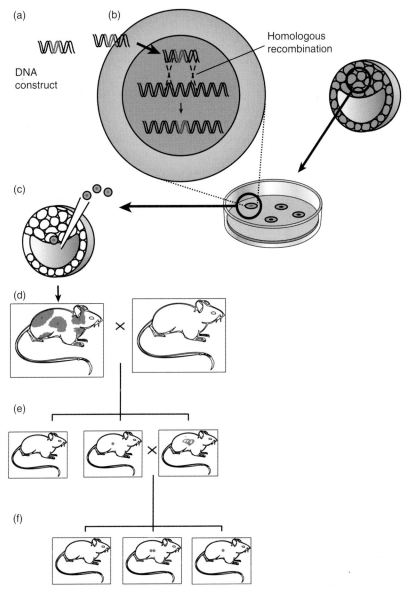

Fig. 1.7 Reverse genetics: generation of transgenic mice. This method allows the experimenter to manipulate specific genes in a mammalian species so as to learn about their functions. For example, a normal gene might be replaced with a non-functional version to generate a knock-out. To do this, the genome of embryonic stem cells (see Fig. 1.6) is manipulated in culture. (a) The experimenter constructs DNA molecules that have (i) stretches at each end identical to sequences in and/or around the gene that is to be mutated and (ii) a central portion whose incorporation into the target gene will prevent its function (red). (b) To enable the embryonic stem cells to take up these DNA molecules, they are put into the solution around the embryonic stem cells and a current is passed through the cells (this is called electroporation). In some cells the flanking sequences swap places with the identical sequences in the genome (a chance event called homologous recombination, indicated in (b) by the two × symbols), carrying the central portion into the genome to prevent the function of the target gene. (c) The mutated embryonic stem cells are then injected into blastocysts to generate chimeras (d) in which some of the animal's cells are mutant, including some germ cells. (e) Since some germ cells in these chimeras should be mutant, subsequent breeding with normal mice will generate offspring in which all cells are heterozygous for the mutation as well as other mice that are normal. (f) A second round of breeding between heterozygotes will generate some mice that are homozygous for the mutation (double red dot), some that are heterozygous for it (single red dot) and some that are normal. Many variations of this method are possible: for example, DNA containing an entire gene controlled by appropriate regulatory elements might be added to the genome so as to overproduce a specific protein in a specific part of the animal.

Box 1.5   Chimeras and mosaics

Chimeras and mosaics are animals that have more than one genetically-distinct population of cells. The terms mean different things but are sometimes used incorrectly. *Chimeras* arise when cells originating from different fertilized eggs come together to create a single embryo. Chimeras can be created by ES cell injections (Figs 1.6 and 1.7) or in other ways, for example by pushing two very early embryos together so that they fuse. In *mosaic* organisms the genetically-distinct cell types all arise from a single fertilized egg. For example, normal female mammals are mosaic. They have two X chromosomes but, early in embryogenesis, one X chromosome is functionally inactivated, a process called X chromosome inactivation. This inactivation occurs randomly: in roughly half of a female's cells, the paternal X chromosome is inactive and in the other half the maternal X chromosome is inactive. This has important biological and medical implications, particularly for X-linked genetic diseases such as Fragile X Syndrome (see Chapter 10).

mechanisms of development of neural structures found in humans. Similarities between mice and humans extend to the DNA level: a large multinational study reported in 2002 that 99% of mouse genes have homologues in humans and 96% of genes in the two species are arranged on the chromosomes in the same order. This degree of similarity is remarkable. While it does help justify the use of mouse as a model in which to learn more about human development, it also raises an intriguing unanswered question: what in our DNA makes us so different from mice?

1.5.5 Humans

We cannot experiment on humans, nor can we manipulate human embryos during nervous system development. However, it is important to recognize that major contributions to developmental neurobiology have been made by identifying genes whose disruption in humans is associated with disease. Studies in human genetics have now been complemented by the sequencing of the entire human genome. The identification of numerous genes that are critical for normal developmental processes has been achieved by analysing the genome of patients with genetic disease. Examples will be given in later chapters. How this type of research is done is outside the scope of this book.[13] In overview, however, this approach can be seen as an excellent example of forward genetics, working from phenotype to gene.

1.5.6 Other vertebrates

Other mammalian species that have proved useful for studying specific aspects of development, for example cerebral cortical development, include the rat, guinea pig, hamster, ferret, cat and monkey. None have the advantages of the mouse for molecular genetics but they do have advantages for some types of study. For example, ferrets are born more immature than many other mammalian species commonly used in research, allowing easier access to the

---

[13] We suggest Part 3 of *Human Molecular Genetics* by T. Strachan and A. P. Read (Garland Science, 2004) for a detailed account.

developing nervous system at an earlier stage. Cats have relatively high resolution binocular vision and have been subjects of research on the development of the visual system for many decades; the success of research in this area was recognized by the award of a Nobel Prize to David Hubel and Torsten Wiesel in 1981[14] (see also Box 9.5 in Chapter 9). Monkeys have the advantage of being closely related to humans and they have been used particularly to study the development of neural connections and function. Work using these species will be discussed mainly in the book's final chapters (especially Chapters 9 and 12).

1.6 Observation and experiment: methods for studying neural development

Biological research often progresses through the following stages: (i) naturally-occurring phenomena are observed; (ii) experiments are designed to test hypotheses about the mechanisms responsible for the phenomena; (iii) the experiments are carried out; (iv) hypotheses are refined, dependent upon the outcome of the experiments. To discover the mechanisms responsible for a phenomenon, it is often necessary to challenge the biological system by altering some aspect of it and assessing the effects. In studying neural development, for example, a commonly used approach is to remove a specific gene's function by making a line of knock-out mice to discover whether that gene is *necessary* for the developmental phenomenon in question. Alternatively, one might cause a gene to become active in the wrong place so as to discover whether, in those cells, its activity is *sufficient* to cause the developmental phenomenon or whether other factors are important. These and other similar approaches are critically dependent on methods for manipulating developing cells and their environment. In this chapter we have described how several model organisms offer advantages for experimental interventions that alter gene function, protein production and cellular environments (e.g. by transplanting cells).

In addition, experimental biology relies on methods for observing biological phenomena and for assessing the effects of experimental manipulations. As technology has advanced scientists have been able to employ an ever increasing range of sophisticated molecular, cellular, anatomical and functional methods to observe when and where specific genes act during development, to observe cells as they proliferate, grow, migrate, differentiate and die, and to observe cells functioning physiologically. Many such observational methods will be explained at appropriate places throughout the rest of this book.

Finally, there is the important issue of deciding which experiments are most likely to give insights into the mechanisms of development. An approach that can help greatly with this involves the use of formal computational models of developing systems. The design of formal models to test hypotheses relating to specific biological questions is now

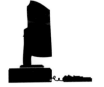

---

[14] http://nobelprize.org/nobel_prizes/medicine/laureates/1981/wiesel-lecture.html [20 November 2010].

common to many areas of biology. Such models are formulated as a set of mathematical equations that represent the actions of the cellular or subcellular elements and their interactions in the biological system under consideration. Solution of the equations, which often uses computer simulation, specifies how (according to the model) the systems under consideration will behave under given conditions. This allows theoretical predictions to be made that can then be tested experimentally.

All biological research is based on the development of hypotheses but often these hypotheses are expressed in informal terms, using words or diagrams to represent the idea. Formal models are simply an extreme version of this same process in which the use of mathematics forces the designer to make a logically consistent hypothesis. One advantage of this approach is that it can generate theoretical reasons against hypotheses that might seem perfectly plausible at a less formal level. Another advantage is that formal models can involve a larger number of interacting elements than can be accommodated easily in informal models. Formal models do have potential problems, of course. They have to make assumptions concerning the underlying biology they are designed to model and in some cases the assumptions they are based on are questionable, or the model might be too simple. In the worst case it might not be possible to test the conclusions from a formal model. The development of formal models is not always possible – it depends on the system and the experimental questions being asked – but where their application is feasible they can provide an invaluable guide to experimental research. This will be discussed again particularly in Chapter 9.

1.7 Summary

- Understanding how nervous systems develop remains a major challenge for research with implications for human health and future technologies.
- Most modern developmental neurobiology seeks to understand the molecular mechanisms controlling key developmental events. The development of methods for manipulating the functions of genes has had a massive impact in this field.
- A small handful of animal species, referred to as model organisms, are used in most developmental neurobiological research because each has clear advantages for certain types of research. Such organisms include flies, worms, frogs, fish, chicks, mice and humans.
- To understand the molecular genetics of development two broad approaches are used: (i) forward genetics, where one seeks to find the genes responsible for a particular aspect of an organism's phenotype; (ii) reverse genetics, where one starts with a gene and manipulates its expression to discover its functions.
- A major breakthrough in understanding mammalian neural development was the application of transgenic methods for manipulating the genome of mice.
- Some areas of developmental neurobiology are amenable to the application of computational modelling approaches to test hypotheses theoretically prior to the use of experimental methods.

The Anatomy of Developing Nervous Systems

2

An understanding of the mechanisms of neural development is built on a knowledge of the anatomy of developing nervous systems. There is a vast amount of literature describing the three-dimensional geometry of developing neural structures from a plethora of species and here we shall give only the briefest of accounts containing essential details required to follow later chapters. The focus is on the model organisms described in Chapter 1.

Nervous systems develop both peripheral and central components. The periphery extracts information from around and within the body. It passes neural signals to the centre, where neural information is processed and memories are stored. Decisions made centrally are signalled back to the periphery to make the body respond. The most complex nervous systems are found in vertebrates, in which the brain and spinal cord make up the **central nervous system**, or **CNS**, and all the neurons that reside or extend axons outside the CNS make up the **peripheral nervous system**, or **PNS**.

2.1 The nervous system develops from the embryonic neuroectoderm

One feature common to the embryos of animals is their early organization into three primary tissues called the germ layers (from the Latin word *germen*, meaning seed or bud). These layers are shown on the drawing of a frog embryo cut in half on the right: (i) an outer layer called the **ectoderm** (yellow and orange); (ii) a middle layer called the **mesoderm** (purple); (iii) an inner layer called the **endoderm** (grey). Ectodermal derivatives include the epidermis (or skin) and the nervous system, which is derived from the **neuroectoderm** (i.e. the *neurogenic* region of the *ectoderm*, shown in orange). The neuroectoderm is sometimes called the neuroepithelium since it comprises cells on the surface of the embryo that are part of the **epithelium**. The colour scheme on the right is used throughout this chapter (and where it would be useful in later ones) to help the reader recognize the germ

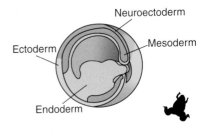

epithelium a tissue that lines the external and internal surfaces, including internal cavities and organs and other free open surfaces of the body, of all animals and their immature developing forms.

Building Brains: An Introduction to Neural Development, First Edition.
David Price, Andrew Jarman, John Mason and Peter Kind.
© 2011 John Wiley & Sons, Ltd. Published 2011 by John Wiley & Sons, Ltd.

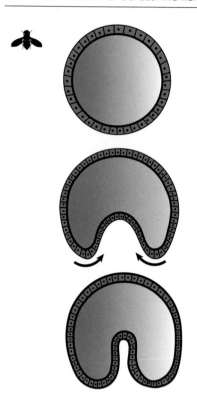

layers and their derivatives. Mesodermal derivatives include muscles and skeleton and endodermal derivatives include gut and associated organs. There is great variation from species to species in the shapes of the three germ layers but their presence and relative positions remain conserved.

Formation of the germ layers follows the repeated division of a fertilized egg to generate a collection of cells that are then rearranged to generate the germ layers. This rearrangement is called **gastrulation**. Gastrulation involves the movement of cells from the outer surface of the embryo to its inside. While this feature of gastrulation is common to the embryos of different species, the exact three-dimensional anatomy of gastrulating embryos varies greatly between different species, as will be seen from the examples in this chapter. The sequence shown on the left illustrates gastrulation in cross sections through a *Drosophila* embryo. We do not know for sure what mechanisms make cells move into the embryo but it is likely that changes in the shapes of cells generate mechanical forces that are important. In the diagram on the left, some of the cells at the bottom of the embryo become narrower along their outer edge, as if pulled by a drawstring, effectively pinching this surface. The cells caught in the pinch move inwards. Such changes in shape are brought about by contractile proteins in cells (the types of protein that do this are described throughout Chapters 6 to 8). Other forces from outside these cells pulling them into the embryo might also be important.

2.2 Anatomical terms used to describe locations in embryos

The aim of this chapter is to describe the major stages of development of the nervous systems of the model organisms described in Chapter 1. Before doing so, we need to explain some terms used to describe how the different parts of developing organisms are located relative to each other; these same terms are also applied to adult organisms. The terms front, back, top, bottom and sides are avoided since they are likely to be used inconsistently in different species (e.g. along the top of a fish we might expect to find its spinal cord whereas at the top of a person we might expect to find a head). The end of the embryo where the head forms is referred to as **anterior**, and its opposite end is **posterior**. Anterior is also described as **rostral** (which means 'pertaining to a beak'); posterior is also described as **caudal**, (which means 'pertaining to a tail'). The axis running through the embryo from anterior to posterior is referred to as the anteroposterior or rostrocaudal axis. Perpendicular to this axis is the dorsoventral axis, running from the embryo's **dorsal** side (i.e. its back, where the spinal cord develops in vertebrates) to its **ventral** side (meaning the side towards the chest). The third axis (mediolateral) runs perpendicular to the other two from **medial** (towards the midline) to **lateral** (away from the midline). These axes are indicated for an adult organism and an embryo in the drawings on the left.

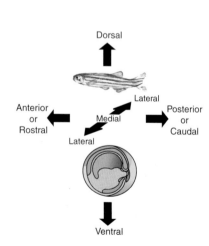

2.3 Development of the neuroectoderm of invertebrates

2.3.1 C. elegans

The embryo's first cleavage generates a large cell (called the AB **blastomere**) and a smaller cell (called the P_1 cell). The AB blastomere gives rise to ectodermal cells that spread to form the outer wall of the embryo, originally called the hypodermis but now sometimes called the **epidermis**, and the nervous system. The nervous system arises almost entirely from the AB blastomere. Gastrulation in *C. elegans* is not as spectacular as in other species in which cells move over much greater distances, but has the equally important result of internalizing cells that form endoderm and mesoderm. These cells come from the P_1 cell and generate internal structures of the embryo, including the muscles, gut and gonads. These events are summarized in Fig. 2.1(a).

To generate the nervous system, some of the ectodermal cells situated ventrally **migrate** inside the embryo (red arrows Fig. 2.1(b)) where they differentiate to form neurons (Fig. 2.1(c)). A fully developed *C. elegans* has 302 neurons with about 7000 synapses and 56 glial cells. Many of its neurons are organized into dorsal and ventral nerve cords running along the length of the worm. *C. elegans* has no real brain, but dense collections, or ganglia, of sensory neurons and interneurons are present in the anterior of the organism. There are also smaller ganglia in the tail. The nerve cords link these anterior and posterior ganglia; they contain motor neurons and receive sensory inputs. An excellent website (Wormatlas) contains more detailed information.[1]

2.3.2 Drosophila

The early stages of development involve an unusual process of nuclear replication without cell division. This results in the formation of a nuclear **syncytium**, the name given to a structure in which many nuclei share a common cytoplasm. This syncytial stage is important because it provides nuclei the opportunity to communicate without cell membranes getting in the way (discussed further in Chapter 4). As the time of gastrulation approaches, several hours after fertilization, dividing nuclei move out to the surface of the embryo and become surrounded by membranes, forming cells. The embryo is now a cellular **blastoderm**. Fig. 2.2 picks up from this point in development.

Gastrulation gets underway with the formation of a furrow along the embryo's ventral surface. Future mesodermal cells enter the interior (Fig. 2.2(a)). As this is happening, ectodermal cells that were initially positioned laterally along the two sides of the ventral part of the embryo now come together at the ventral midline (indicated by the arrows in Fig. 2.2(a)). These ventral ectodermal cells become the neuroectoderm, which goes on to form the fly's CNS. The formation of the CNS involves cells in the neuroectoderm enlarging and moving inside the embryo, a process called delamination, where they

blastomere any of the cells resulting from the first few cleavages of a fertilized egg during early embryonic development.

epidermis the outermost layers of cells covering the exterior body surface.

blastoderm the superficial layer of the early embryo in species whose eggs contain relatively large amounts of yolk; cell division occurs in this layer, which surrounds the yolk in insects but is a flat disc at one pole of the egg in birds.

---

[1] http://www.wormatlas.org/ [20 November 2010].

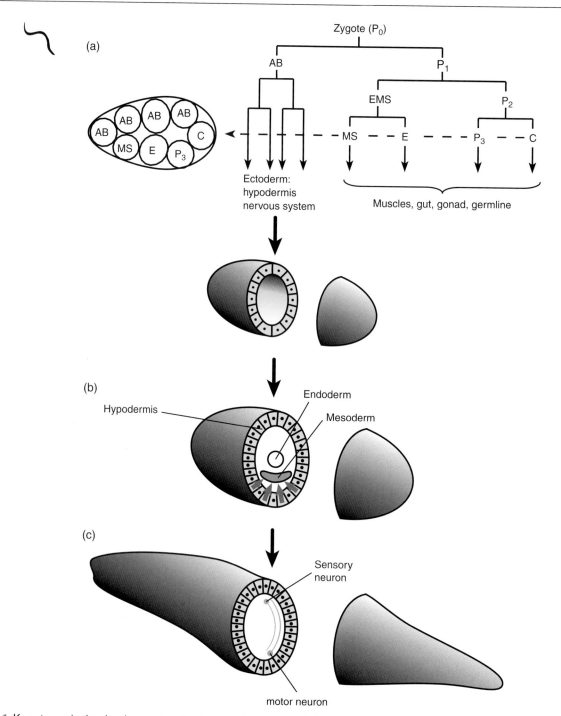

Fig. 2.1 Key stages in the development of *C. elegans*: development is highly stereotypical and the lineages of all the cells of *C. elegans* are known. (a) This diagram charts the first divisions of the embryo. The nervous system arises from the AB blastomere. Gastrulation is complete once derivatives of the AB blastomere have covered the internalized derivatives of the P_1 cell. (b) Arrows show the inward migration of AB-derived ectodermal cells on the ventral side of the embryo. (c) AB-derived ectodermal cells form sensory and motor neurons along the body: single examples of each are shown here.

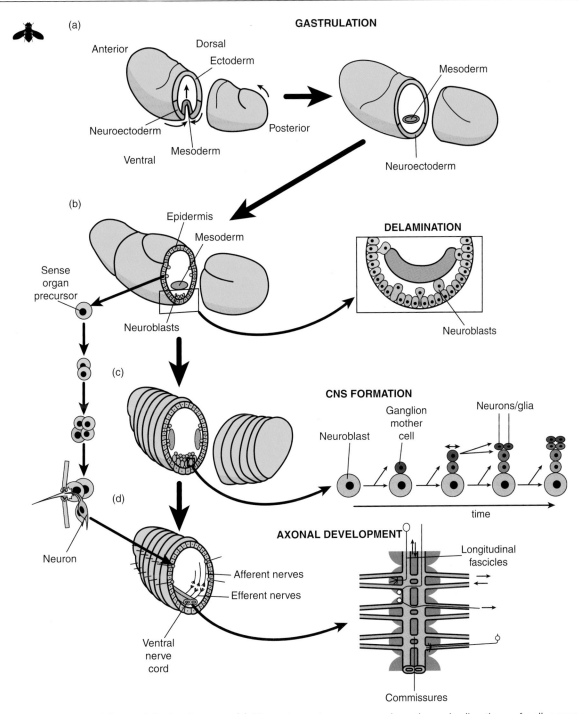

Fig. 2.2 Major stages of *Drosophila* development. (a) Blastoderm stage: arrows show the main directions of cell movements during gastrulation. The neuroectoderm (orange) is initially split into two domains along either side of the ventral part of the embryo and as the mesoderm involutes these domains coalesce ventrally. (b) Subsequently, some of the cells in this ventral neurogenic region move inside the embryo to become neuroblasts; this process is called delamination. Other cells in the lateral ectoderm delaminate to become sense organ precursors: the development of these cells is shown down the left between (b) and (d) (see also Section 2.6.1). (c) The neuroblasts divide to generate the neurons and glia of the *Drosophila's* CNS, many of which reside in the ventral nerve cord. This is achieved through the production of intermediate cells the ganglion mother cells (GMCs), which divide to generate pairs of neurons or glia. (d) Sensory nerves from developing sense organs converge on the ventral nerve cord, which generates motor nerves. Axons in the ventral nerve cord are organized into longitudinal fascicles linked by commissures.

form **neuroblasts** (Fig. 2.2(b)). Neuroblasts are dividing cells that generate neurons and glia.

The ectoderm becomes divided into reiterated units called **segments**. Within each segment, five waves of delamination eventually result in a stereotypic array of some 60 neuroblasts. Neuroblasts are progenitor cells that divide many times to form numerous intermediate cells called ganglion mother cells (GMCs) (Fig. 2.2(c)). Each GMC divides just once more to form neurons and glia. GMCs and their progeny pile up on the neuroblasts forming the bilaterally symmetrical **ventral nerve cord**.

Eventually, each segmental unit of the larval CNS (a ganglion) contains about 800 neurons, giving a late embryonic CNS consisting of about 100 000 neurons in total. A scaffold of axon bundles is generated on the inner (or dorsal) surface of the ventral nerve cord. Some bundles run in the anteroposterior direction and are called longitudinal **fascicles** while others run perpendicular to them and are called transverse **commissures** (Fig. 2.2(d)). The development of peripheral sensory organs depicted in Fig. 2.2 will be discussed again below, in Section 2.6. A second stage of neurogenesis occurs during **metamorphosis** in the pupa. This gives rise to a more complex adult nervous system with many more neurons.[2]

fascicle a bundle of nerve or muscle fibres.

commissure a bundle of axons (commissural axons) that extends across the midline to connect structures on either side of the nervous system. Commissures are important for coordinating neural activity on the two sides of the animal.

2.4 Development of the neuroectoderm of vertebrates and the process of neurulation

In mature vertebrates, a narrow cavity filled with cerebrospinal fluid called the central canal runs longitudinally through the middle of the spinal cord. It expands into several larger cavities called ventricles inside the brain (left). The fact that the mature central nervous system is hollow reflects its origin from a hollow structure in the embryo known as the **neural tube**. The process by which the neural tube is formed and acquires increasingly complex morphology is referred to as **neurulation**; it occurs through (i) rapid growth at rates that vary from region to region, (ii) cell movements and (iii) changes in cell shapes.

Neurulation is usually considered to be of two types, primary and secondary. **Primary neurulation** is the process by which a sheet of neuroectoderm called the **neural plate** rolls up as it grows to form the neural tube. This is schematized in Fig. 2.3, where the neuroectoderm (orange region situated dorsally) of a simplified vertebrate embryo (in this case a frog) is shown in isolation. The buckling that occurs as the neural plate rolls up is associated with changes in the shape of its cells: in general, they become more columnar but in some regions, such as along the centre of the neural plate, there are more complex shape changes. It is hard to tell whether changes in the shapes of cells are the cause or the effect of changes in the shape of the neural plate; the mechanics of neural tube closure remain poorly understood. **Secondary neurulation** achieves the same result as primary neurulation, that is a tube of neural tissue, but through a

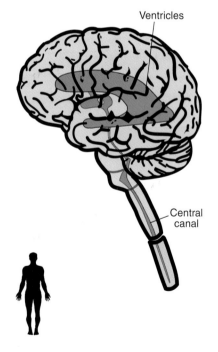

Ventricles

Central canal

[2] For details refer to Tissot, M. and Stocker, R. F. (2000) Metamorphosis in Drosophila and other insects: the fate of neurons throughout the stages. *Prog Neurobiol.*, **62**,89–111.

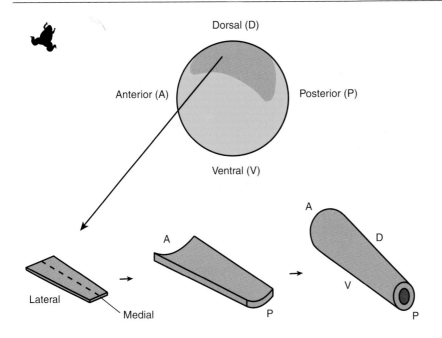

Fig. 2.3 Schematic of primary neurulation in a vertebrate: note how the lateral edges of the neural plate roll up and join dorsally, while cells that are medial in the neural plate end up ventrally. This establishes the dorso-ventral axis of the vertebrate neural tube.

different process that involves the hollowing out of an initially solid rod of tissue (see below, Section 2.5).

2.4.1 Frog

The first steps in development are illustrated in Fig. 2.4(a). As cell division progresses, the embryo's dorsal region, called the **animal cap**, becomes packed with many small cells. Cells in the opposite ventral region are fewer, larger and yolk-rich (this region is called the vegetal hemisphere). Prior to gastrulation, a fluid-filled cavity known as the blastocoel opens beneath the animal cap; the embryo is now called a **blastula**.

Fig. 2.4(b) illustrates gastrulation, which involves the inward movement of cells from the embryo's outer layer at a region called the **blastopore**. This involution of a layer of cells is like the deformation of the surface of a balloon when poked. The first cells to move in migrate anteriorly from the dorsal lip of the blastopore (which has important organizing functions, discussed in Chapters 3 and 4). Their movement displaces the blastocoel anteriorly (it eventually disappears). These cells form the endoderm which lines the primitive gut (called the archenteron), the mesoderm of the future head and a transient dorsal mesodermal structure, the **notochord**, which is essential for differentiation of the overlying neuroectoderm. During these events, cells derived from the animal pole spread to cover the embryo with ectoderm (a process called epiboly). The result is an embryo surrounded by ectoderm, with an inner primitive gut lined with endoderm and with mesoderm forming between them.

Fig. 2.4(c) illustrates subsequent major steps in neural development, including primary neurulation. The development of the **neural crest** along the dorsal aspect of the neural tube is discussed further

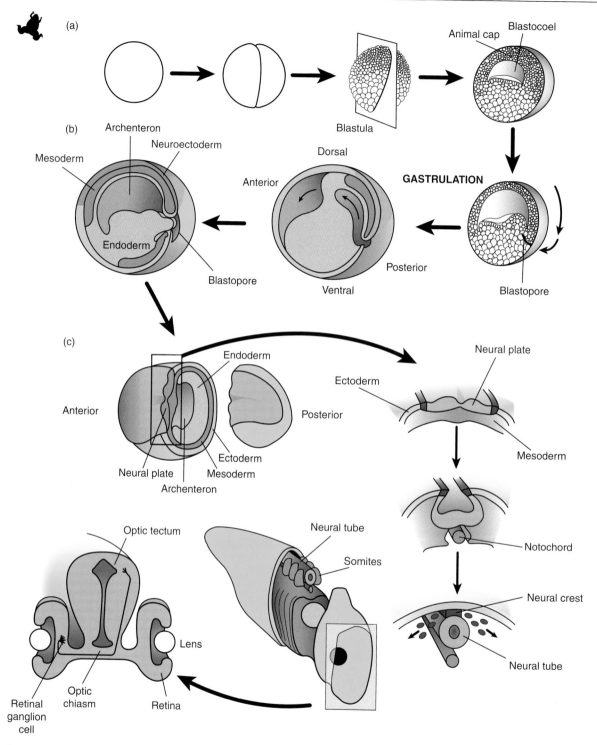

Fig. 2.4 The main stages of development of *Xenopus*: (a) formation of the blastula, (b) gastrulation and (c) development of the neural plate and neural tube (orange) through primary neurulation. In (c), the neural plate is first shown in a transected embryo tilted towards the viewer along its anteroposterior axis. Cells along the lateral edges of the neural plate (brown) form the neural crest: its cells migrate laterally throughout the body (see later in this chapter, Section 2.6). The final drawings show the tadpole stage: brain structures such as the retinae and optic tectum, which are major components of the visual system, develop from the neural tube anteriorly and become connected by axons, forming a favourite model for the study of axonal guidance (discussed further in Chapter 8).

below in the context of the formation of the peripheral nervous system (Section 2.6).

2.4.2 Chick

When the egg is laid the embryo is a disc of cells on the surface of the yolk. It comprises a central transparent area (the area pellucida) surrounded by an opaque ring (the area opaca) (Fig. 2.5(a)). The area pellucida is transparent because there is a fluid-filled cavity, initially cell-free, between the yolk and an overlying single-cell-thick layer of epithelial cells. The epithelial layer is called the **epiblast**. The area opaca is opaque because cells lie beneath the epiblast in contact with the yolk and there is no cavity. The epiblast generates the three germ layers of the embryo.

The posterior part of the area pellucida contains a crescent-shaped ridge of small cells called Koller's sickle (Fig. 2.5(a)). Fig. 2.5 (b) shows the remarkable events that occur in this region. As epiblast cells are produced they move posteriorly in the plane of the epiblast towards Koller's sickle, from where they move anteriorly along the midline forming a structure called the **primitive streak**. Formation of the primitive streak involves the ingression of epiblast cells into the interior of the embryo and results in the generation of the germ layers of the embryo, that is gastrulation (Fig. 2.5(c)). As the primitive streak lengthens from posterior to anterior, a bulge called **Hensen's node** appears at the anterior tip of the streak. Hensen's node is equivalent to the dorsal lip of the blastopore in *Xenopus* and has important organizing functions that will be discussed in Chapter 3.

Hensen's node contains cells that are precursors of the notochord. The notochord is a midline mesodermal structure that has been described above in the context of *Xenopus* development (Fig. 2.4(c)). It is long and thin and it forms by a process of cell movement called convergent-extension in which tissue elongation is achieved by the convergence and intercalation of adjacent cells in a sheet to form a narrower, longer strip of tissue, a principle illustrated on the right.

This process forms the entire length of the notochord anterior to the primitive streak. Hensen's node is sometimes described as retreating from the anterior end of the embryo, leaving behind the head process (cells that will eventually form the chick's head) and subsequently cells destined to become the notochord. This relative movement of Hensen's node is indicated by an arrow in the right-hand diagram in Fig. 2.5(c).

With the retreat of Hensen's node, structures begin to differentiate; since Hensen's node retreats from the anterior end of the embryo first, development in this region is ahead of that in more posterior regions. The process of neurulation is similar to that of other vertebrates and is not repeated in Fig. 2.5.

Fig. 2.5(d) shows later stages of development including (i) the elongation and bending of the neural tube, (ii) the formation of anterior swellings that become the **forebrain**, **midbrain** and **hindbrain** (further information on these regions of the brain will be found in the following section on mouse development), (iii) the division of the

epiblast the layer of cells in the early embryos of birds, reptiles and mammals that gives rise to the three germ layers at gastrulation.

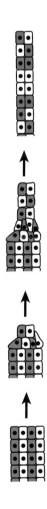

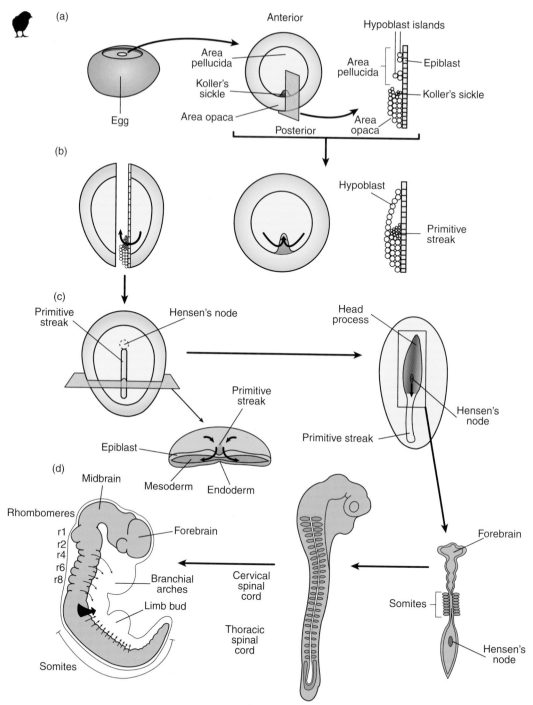

Fig. 2.5 Main stages of chick development. (a) A small portion of the shell of the hen's egg is removed to expose the early embryo (yellow), which is enlarged and viewed from above in the central drawing. A perpendicular section through the embryo's posterior part reveals the cells beneath the epiblast around Koller's sickle. (b) Arrows show the movement of cells in the epiblast posteriorly and then inside the embryo to form the primitive streak and, at its anterior end, Hensen's node. (c) Gastrulation involves the movement of epiblast cells inside the embryo and the formation of the three germ layers, shown in a slice through the embryo. This is similar in principle to gastrulation in *Xenopus* but takes place in a flatter embryo. Hensen's node retreats from the anterior end where the head process forms, elongating the neural plate as it moves. (d) Later stages show elongation of the nervous system, the formation of somites, the development of brain structures and the growth of nerves from the CNS (arrows). The branchial arches are a set of mesodermal structures on either side of the developing pharynx.

hindbrain into a series of anatomically distinguishable tissue blocks called **rhombomeres** (see Chapter 4, Section 4.3.4) and (iv) the formation of **somites**.

somites segmental masses of mesoderm lying on either side of the notochord and neural tube during the development of vertebrate embryos.

2.4.3 Mouse 🐁

Following fertilization, the embryo develops through the **blastocyst** stage (Fig. 2.6(a)) before implanting into the uterine wall and undergoing gastrulation (Fig. 2.6(b)). At implantation, the mouse blastocyst comprises three tissues: the epiblast, situated at one pole of the embryo, the primitive endoderm beneath it and the trophectoderm surrounding both tissues and the blastocoel cavity (which will disappear later).

blastocyst the mammalian embryo prior to gastrulation, comprising up to about 100 cells surrounding a fluid-filled cavity.

After implantation the epiblast expands and a central fluid-filled cavity opens in the middle of it. The epiblast organizes into an epithelium that surrounds this new cavity and is itself surrounded by primitive endoderm. The trophectoderm generates tissues such as the ectoplacental cone and extraembryonic ectoderm that go on to form placenta and membranes surrounding the embryo.

Whereas the chick epiblast is essentially a flat disc on the surface of the yolk, the mouse epiblast is a concave sheet on the inside of the embryo, but otherwise the process of gastrulation is similar in the two species. As in the developing chick embryo, gastrulation in the mouse embryo involves the movement of cells in the plane of the epiblast towards and through the primitive streak to form a new mesodermal layer between the outer endoderm and the inner ectoderm (shown in the right-hand drawing in Fig. 2.6(b)). The primitive streak elongates along the middle of the embryo in its anteroposterior axis (see Section 2.2 above for a reminder of the body axes). The node (which is equivalent to Hensen's node in chick) forms at the anterior end of the primitive streak (Fig. 2.6(c)). The notochord grows anteriorly from the node forming a narrow midline rod ending in the broader **prechordal mesoderm** under the future forebrain. The notochord comes to lie along the midline of the embryo beneath the part of the ectoderm that will form the nervous system, the neuroectoderm (Fig. 2.6(c)).

The process of primary neurulation begins in the overlying neuroectoderm with the formation and folding of the neural plate (Fig. 2.6(c)) to form the neural tube. The neural plate is broader anteriorly and the folds it generates (the cranial neural folds, Fig. 2.6(d)) are larger than those made posteriorly. When they fuse, the cranial neural folds produce anterior swellings of the neural tube (called vesicles) that will develop into the brain.

Cells along the dorsal neural tube give rise to the neural crest (Fig. 2.6(d) and see Section 2.6), which forms at the junction of the surface ectoderm and the neuroectoderm. Strips of mesoderm on either side of the developing neural tube generate the somites (Fig. 2.6(d)), whose derivatives include vertebrae, ribs and skeletal muscle.

Neural tube closure begins around the posterior boundary of the midbrain and spreads anteriorly and posteriorly from this point, as if a zip were being closed in both directions (Fig. 2.6(d)). While this is

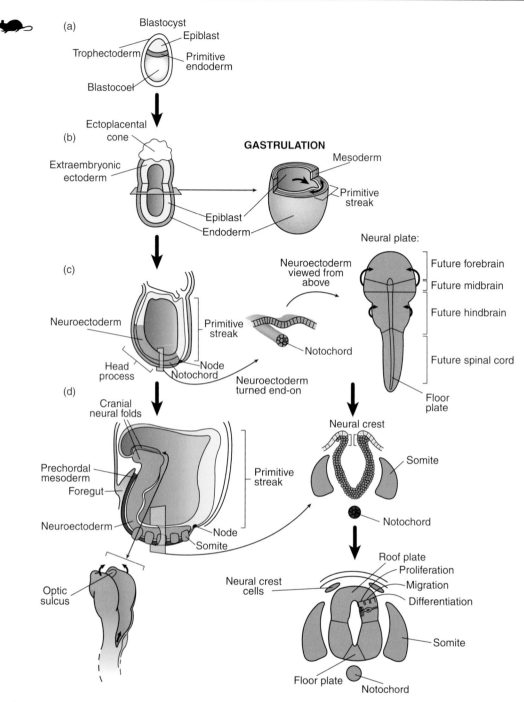

Fig. 2.6 Development of the mouse nervous system from (a) the blastocyst stage to (d) neural tube closure. (b) Cell movements at gastrulation, indicated by arrows, result in the formation of the primitive streak. To help understand this stage, imagine the flat chick embryo on the left in Figure 2.5(c) rolled up with its right- and left-hand edges joined and the primitive streak on the inside: essentially, this would give the diagram on the right in (b) here. (c) The notochord and the neuroectoderm form anterior to the node. Look at the diagram on the right in Figure 2.5(c): imagine looking at it along the surface of the page from its left-hand side, in which case the neuroectoderm (orange) would be to the left, the primitive streak to the right and the node in the middle, and if it is bent upwards at its ends it will have the equivalent layout of structures to those on the left of (c) and (d) here. The neural plate is divided into domains that will form the forebrain, midbrain and hindbrain before it folds as indicated by arrows. (d) The origin of the neural crest is shown. Growth of the neural tube is accomplished by proliferation on the side nearest the lumen, followed by migration to and differentiation on the other side. Further development continues in Figure 2.8.

underway, new closures occur further anteriorly and the closures spreading from these points meet to complete the formation of the neural tube. Photographs of neural tube closure are shown in Fig. 2.7. Analysis of the mechanisms regulating neural tube closure is very important for humans. Our neural tube closes in very similar ways and defects of these processes are relatively common, for example generating spina bifida (Box 2.1).

At the stage of neural tube closure, the embryo alters its shape dramatically. At the start of this phase, most of the anteroposterior axis of the closing neural tube is bent in a large curve with the convexity towards its ventral side: as shown in Fig. 2.6(d), it looks a bit like a snake rearing its head. Cell movements indicated by arrows in Fig. 2.8(a) cause it to turn. This process of turning results in its anteroposterior axis becoming concave along its ventral surface (Fig. 2.8(a)): effectively, the neural tube curls up into a shape retained until birth. The anterior part of the neural tube forms the forebrain (or **prosencephalon**), the midbrain (or **mesencephalon**) and the hindbrain (or **rhombencephalon**) (Fig. 2.8(a)). The **optic vesicles** form bilaterally and generate the retinae and optic nerves (development of the eye is outlined in more detail in Box 2.2). The posterior part of the neural tube forms the spinal cord.

Fig. 2.8(b) shows more details of the embryonic brain. The forebrain vesicle expands to form two bilateral **telencephalic** vesicles and a central **diencephalic** vesicle that becomes engulfed by the rapidly expanding telencephalic vesicles. The telencephalon is divided into dorsal and ventral components that differ anatomically and molecularly. Dorsal telencephalon generates the **cerebral cortex**, which includes the neocortex (the part of the cerebral cortex that has expanded massively in the evolution of higher mammals) and surrounding phylogenetically older cortical regions such as the **hippocampus**. Ventral telencephalon generates the **basal ganglia** (large groups of neurons lying under the cortex involved in the control of movement). The major derivative of the diencephalon is the **thalamus**, which transmits sensory input to the cerebral cortex.

Throughout the process of primary neurulation, most proliferation to generate new progenitors and/or neurons occurs on the inner side of the neural tube closest to its lumen (Figs 2.6(d) and 2.8(b)). Cells destined to become neurons migrate away from this proliferative zone towards the outside of the tube to differentiate into mature neurons. In the brain, the proliferative zone is known as the **ventricular zone**, since the lumen of the embryonic brain forms the ventricular system of the adult. In the cerebral cortex, the first cells to migrate and differentiate form a structure called the preplate, that is later split into a superficial layer called the marginal zone and a deep layer called the subplate by newly arriving neurons which form a rapidly thickening layer called the cortical plate (Fig. 2.8(b)). The marginal zone forms layer 1 of the cortex, the cortical plate forms layers 2 to 6, and the subplate is a transient structure that largely disappears after birth. These processes and structures will be discussed more in later chapters.

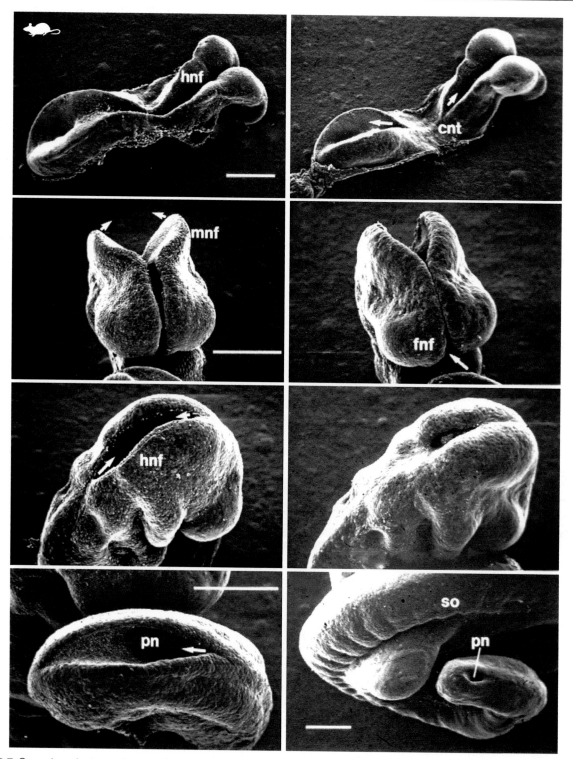

Fig. 2.7 Scanning electron micrographs of neural tube closure in mouse embryos: reprinted from Copp, A. J., Brook, F. A., Estibeiro, J. P., Shum, A. S. W. and Cockroft, D. L. (1990) The embryonic development of mammalian neural tube defects. *Prog. Neurobiol.*, **35**, 363–403 with permission from Elsevier. Abbreviations: hnf, mnf or fnf: hindbrain, midbrain or forebrain neural folds; cnt: caudal neural tube; pn, posterior neuropore; so, somite. Arrows indicate the directions of neural tube closure. Scale bars are 0.1–0.3 millimeter.

Box 2.1 Neural tube defects

Neural tube defects are congenital malformations of the CNS resulting from a failure of neurulation. There are many different types, the commonest of which are (i) anencephaly, in which the cranial neural folds do not fuse in the developing embryo and most or all of the brain is missing, and (ii) spina bifida, in which there is a failure of the neural tube to fuse at its caudal end resulting in either an open lesion on the spine, with significant damage to the nerves and spinal cord, or a closed lesion. These two defects have a prevalence of about one in 1000 births, with variations throughout the world; anencephaly results in death around birth whereas infants with spina bifida can survive with a variable degree of disability. Spina bifida cystica is a severe condition causing nerve damage and disability, in which the membranes of the spinal cord and, rarely, spinal nerves, protrude through openings in the spine resulting in a sac filled with cerebrospinal fluid on the back. Spina bifida occulta is a mild condition in which the spinal cord is normal and there are no openings to the back, although there may be a gap in the vertebral column and subtle motor and sensory problems can develop with age. Craniorachischisis is a relatively rare failure of closure involving the entire body axis. The causes of neural tube defects are genetic and environmental, but are poorly understood.[3]

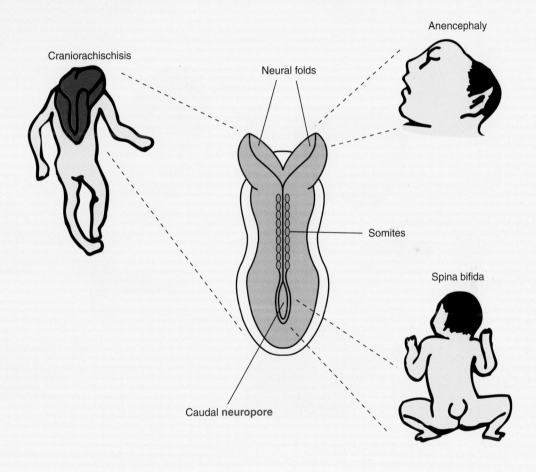

---

[3] For more information see Copp, A. J. and Greene, N. D. (2010) Genetics and development of neural tube defects. *J. Pathol.*, **220**, 217–30.

Neuropore an opening at one or other end of the neural tube that normally closes eventually

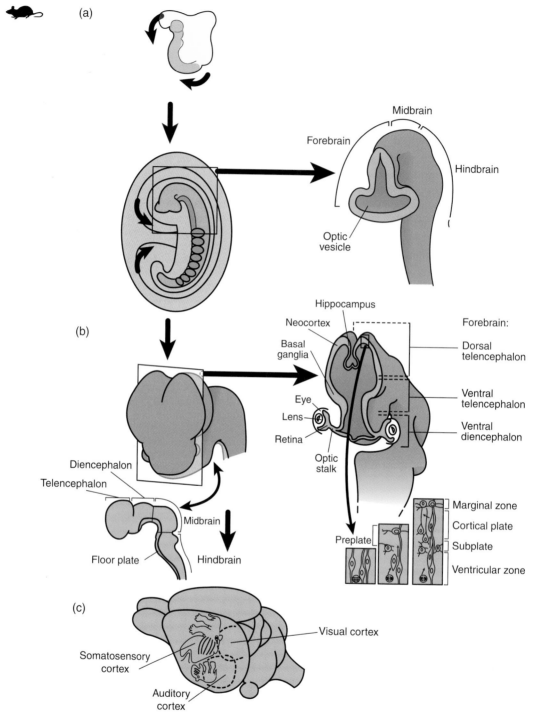

Fig. 2.8 Development of the mouse brain, continued from Figure 2.6(a) A reversal in the embryo's shape is caused by movements indicated by thick arrows. The drawing at the top is a simplified version of the drawing in Figure 2.6(d). Drawing on the right shows more detail of formation of the forebrain, midbrain, hindbrain and optic vesicles. (b) Subsequent growth and specialization increase brain complexity. Growth is achieved through continuing cell divisions in the brain's ventricular zone followed by migration of these cells towards the outer surface of the brain where they differentiate (see also Fig. 5.16 for more detail). (c) The mature brain, containing maps of sensory surfaces such as the skin (more on this in Chapter 9).

Box 2.2   Development of the mammalian eye

(a) As the cranial neural folds fuse (diagram taken from Fig. 2.6(a)), two pits appear bilaterally in the region destined to become forebrain. These pits are called the optic sulci (singular: sulcus). (b) The optic sulci continue to deepen laterally and bulge from the two sides of the forebrain to become the optic vesicles. (c) The optic vesicles remain connected to the developing forebrain by the optic stalks, which will become the optic nerves, and approach the surface ectoderm, with which they interact. (d) The neuroectoderm under the surface ectoderm changes its shape forming the optic cup. The layer on the inside of the cup becomes the retina. (e) The lens forms from a vesicle derived from the surface ectoderm (called the lens placode, see Fig. 2.11) overlying the optic cup. (f) The mature eye.

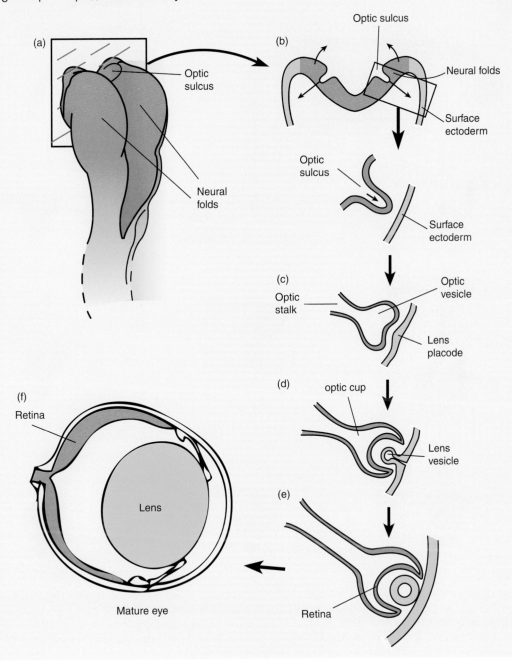

2.5 Secondary neurulation in vertebrates

While primary neurulation generates much of the neural tube of higher vertebrates (Fig. 2.9(a)), the lumen of its caudal part is formed by the hollowing out of an initially solid rod of cells rather than the rolling of the neural plate. This is called **secondary neurulation** (Fig. 2.9(b)).

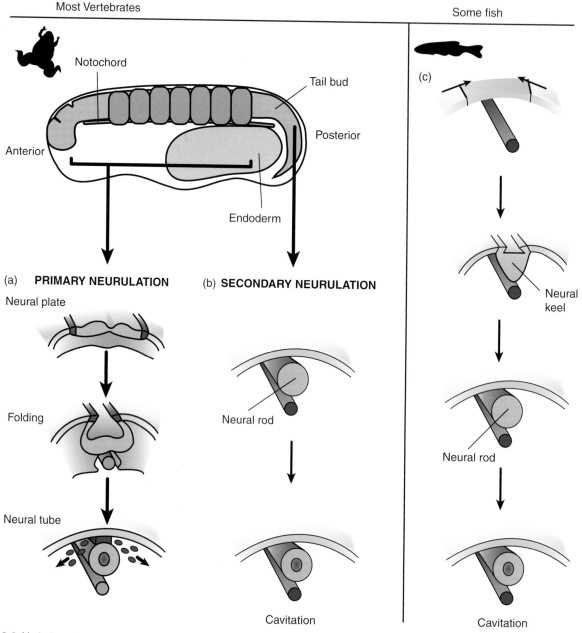

Fig. 2.9 Variations in neurulation at different positions along the neural tube and in different species. (a) Primary neurulation, involving the rolling or folding of the neuroectoderm around a central lumen, occurs along much of the length of the neural plate in most vertebrate species. (b) In posterior regions, secondary neurulation involves the initial formation of a rod of cells which then cavitates. (c) In some species of fish such as zebrafish, the neural tube forms by a thickening of the neural plate into a so-called neural keel due to movement of neuroectodermal cells towards the midline (arrows); the keel becomes a rod of cells that cavitates.

Secondary neurulation occurs as the vertebrate body elongates along its rostral to caudal axis. A structure called the tail bud forms at its caudal end (Fig. 2.9). Cells from the caudal end of the neuroectoderm generate a solid caudally located rod that cavitates to form the caudal neural tube. Interestingly, they also generate mesodermal cells that contribute to the tail bud, notochord and somites; it is possible that caudal neuroectodermal and mesodermal cells originate from caudally-located **stem cells** that have the ability to generate several different types of differentiated cell (i.e. are **multipotent**). The outcome of secondary neurulation is the generation of the caudal neural tube which is continuous with neural tube generated by primary neurulation. Secondary neurulation resembles the process that generates the entire neural tube in some species of fish. In these animals, the first step in neurulation generates a neuroectodermal structure called the neural keel, which is a thickening of the neural plate along its rostral to caudal axis Fig. 2.9(c). Subsequent steps result in the formation of a solid rod of cells that cavitates along its length.

stem cell a relatively unspecialized cell that can divide repeatedly to regenerate itself (self-renewal) and give rise to more specialized cells, such as neurons or glia.

2.6 Formation of invertebrate and vertebrate peripheral nervous systems

The descriptions above have concentrated largely on the development of central nervous systems. Peripheral nervous systems are made up from all the neurons that reside or extend axons outside the central nervous system. They are essential for extracting sensory information from the animal's internal and external environment and for controlling the actions of the body.

2.6.1 Invertebrates

The sensory nervous system of *Drosophila* provides an excellent model for the study of mechanisms regulating the development of specific cell types. It is represented largely by small sense organs called **sensilla** (singular: sensillum); a diagram of one is on the right. These comprise one or more **bipolar neurons** and a number of **support cells**. There are different types of sensillum for different sensory modalities. The most visible type is the sensory bristle, which consists of one sensory neuron and three support cells that form the bristle shaft and socket, and a sheath cell for the neuron (shown on the right, taken from Fig. 2.2 earlier in this chapter).

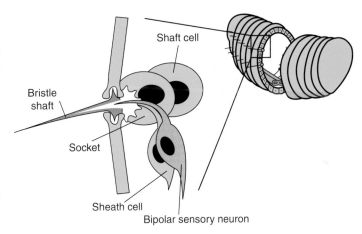

Sensilla develop from individual ectodermal cells called **sense organ precursors (SOPs)** (also known as sensory mother cells). Their locations and development were illustrated earlier, on the left-hand side of Fig. 2.2(b)–(d). SOPs appear in a segmentally repeated pattern just like neuroblasts, except that they are derived mostly

bipolar neuron a neuron with two projections emanating from the cell body or soma.

multipolar neuron a type of neuron that has a single axon and several dendrites extending from its body.

from the lateral ectoderm. Each SOP then divides in a highly stereo-typic manner to give the four cells that differentiate to give the sensillum. Depending on the location of the SOP, a fifth cell from this lineage either dies, forms a glial cell, or forms a separate **multipolar neuron**. At the end of embryogenesis, there are just 43 sensory neurons on each side of each larval body segment, although there are many more in the head.

The adult is also covered with sensilla (flies are notably bristly), but these arise much later in the pupa during metamorphosis. Within the pupa are epithelial sheets of undifferentiated ectodermal cells called imaginal discs, which give rise to the external cuticle of the fly. SOPs for adult sensilla are formed in these imaginal discs in patterns that are highly stereotypic. This feature of the larval and adult PNS has made them extremely useful in uncovering basic genetic mechanisms of neural development; this work will be discussed further in Chapters 4 and 5.

2.6.2 Vertebrates: the neural crest and the placodes

In vertebrates, most cells of the peripheral nervous system come from the **neural crest** (Figs 2.4(c), 2.6(d) and 2.10), which originates from

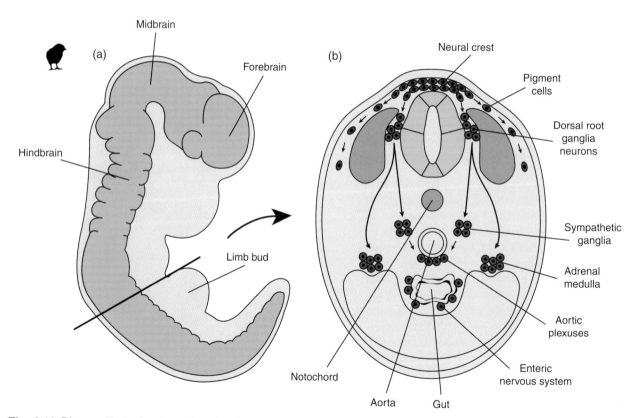

Fig. 2.10 Diagram illustrating the paths taken by neural crest cells in the trunk of a chick embryo. (a) The embryo seen from the side is cut as shown by the line to give (b) a cross section through the trunk. Some neural crest cells migrate under the skin and form melanocytes (pigment cells); others migrate in more ventral directions to regions alongside the neural tube (where they form dorsal root ganglia), near to the aorta (where they form autonomic neurons, aortic plexuses and adrenal medulla) and around the gut (where they form the enteric nervous system).

the lateral edges of the neuroectoderm. Once these edges have joined to form the neural tube, neural crest cells end up dorsally along the line of fusion (Fig. 2.4(c)). Neural crest cells migrate widely throughout the body, contributing sensory neurons, **autonomic neurons**, neurons that innervate internal organs such as the gut, **Schwann cells** and other peripheral glial cells (Fig. 2.10). The neural crest also generates non-neural cells. Some of these contribute to structures including the adrenal medulla; others are pigment cells (called melanocytes) that migrate to the skin, hair and eyes. Rostrally, neural crest cells from cranial regions contribute to non-neural head structures including bone, cartilage and connective tissue.

Throughout the body, peripheral neurons and glia gather into dense collections called **ganglia** (Fig. 2.10). Ganglia in the head of vertebrates, such as the trigeminal ganglion (which transmits sensation from the face), the vestibulo-cochlear ganglion (which transmits signals from the ear) and others, are derived not only from neural crest but also from bilateral thickenings of the ectoderm of the vertebrate head, called **cranial placodes** (Fig. 2.11). As well as contributing neurons to sensory cranial ganglia, the placodes generate sensory structures including the olfactory sensory epithelium, lens and inner ear.

autonomic neurons neurons in the peripheral nervous system that control body functions below the level of consciousness, such as respiration, heart rate, digestion, and so on.

Schwann cells glial cells of the peripheral nervous system that produce the myelin sheath around axons.

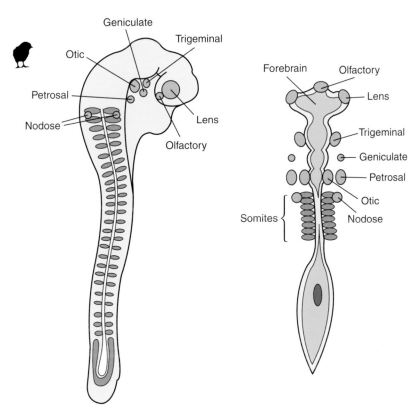

Fig. 2.11 The cranial placodes, shown on a diagram of a chick embryo. Similar to SOPs in *Drosophila* (Fig. 2.2 and Section 2.6.1), the cranial placodes arise in lateral ectoderm. Most rostral are the olfactory placodes, which generate the olfactory epithelium and its sensory neurons, and the lens placodes. Further caudally lie the trigeminal, geniculate, petrosal and nodose placodes, all of which contribute neurons to cranial sensory ganglia, and the otic placode, which generates the inner ear including its sensory epithelium and the auditory and vestibular ganglia.

2.6.3 Vertebrates: development of sense organs

The way in which the lens develops from the lens placode has already been described in Box 2.2. The development of the inner ear provides another good example of how vertebrate sense organs develop.

The vertebrate inner ear is made up of a labyrinth of fluid-filled chambers. These are derived from the **otic placode**, whose position alongside the developing hindbrain is shown in Fig. 2.11. The otic placode invaginates (a bit like the lens vesicle, Box 2.2) and pinches off from the surface ectoderm to form the **otic vesicle** (or otocyst) (Fig. 2.12). As the otic vesicle grows its shape changes dramatically, generating the complex structure of the inner ear (Fig. 2.12). Specific parts of the otic vesicle give rise to (i) the hair cells that detect the sensory stimuli and (ii) the auditory sensory neurons that

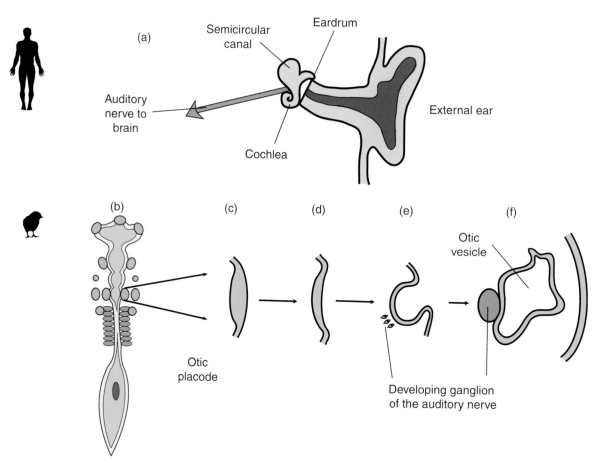

Fig. 2.12 (a) The ear in humans showing its major components, including the vestibulo-cochlear nerve (also known as the auditory or eighth **cranial nerve**) responsible for transmitting information on sound and balance to the brain. (b) to (f) Steps in the early formation of the inner ear studied in chick, from the otic placode through the formation of a cup and eventually a fluid-filled chamber with the vestibulo-cochlear ganglion of the auditory nerve developing on its medial side.

innervate them. The molecular mechanisms which control inner ear hair cell formation will be discussed in Chapter 5.[4]

2.7 Summary

- The early embryos of animals are organized into three primary tissues called the germ layers: an outer layer called the ectoderm, a middle layer called the mesoderm and an inner layer called the endoderm. Ectodermal derivatives include the epidermis (or skin) and the nervous system, which is derived from the neuroectoderm.
- There is great variation from species to species in the shapes of the three germ layers but their presence and relative positions remain conserved.
- Formation of the germ layers occurs at gastrulation. Gastrulation involves the movement of cells from the outer surface of the embryo to its inside.
- The mature central nervous system of vertebrates is hollow. In most species this reflects its origin from a hollow structure in the embryo known as the neural tube, which is formed by the folding of an earlier structure called the neural plate.
- The anterior part of the neural tube forms the forebrain, the midbrain and the hindbrain. The posterior part of the neural tube forms the spinal cord.
- Most cellular proliferation occurs on the inner side of the neural tube closest to its lumen. Cells destined to become neurons migrate away from this proliferative zone towards the outside of the tube to differentiate into mature neurons.
- Cells along the dorsal neural tube give rise to the neural crest.
- The peripheral nervous systems of flies develop from ectodermal cells called sense organ precursors (SOPs). In vertebrates, most cells of the peripheral nervous system come from the neural crest. Others are derived from bilateral thickenings of the ectoderm of the vertebrate head, called cranial placodes. The placodes generate sensory structures including the olfactory sensory epithelium, lens and inner ear.

---

[4] For more on this topic, see Ladher, R. K., O'Neill, P. and Begbie, J. (2010) From shared lineage to distinct functions: the development of the inner ear and epibranchial placodes. *Development*, **137**, 1777– 85.

Neural Induction: An Example of How Intercellular Signalling Determines Cell Fates

3

3.1 What is neural induction?

In biology, **induction** means the same as it does in other sciences or in everyday life. In physics, for example, we might induce a current in a wire by bringing a magnet close to it. In developmental biology induction refers to the process by which one tissue (the inducer) causes a change in the development of another tissue (the responder). In the case of **neural induction**, the inducing tissue tells the responding tissue to adopt a neural fate. Whether it is a person or a material or a tissue that is being induced to do something, the process of induction involves communication of some sort between the inducer and the responder.

The implication of these observations is that embryonic cells that turn into a nervous system do not carry all the information they need to make that transition. They have the potential to become neural but to realize this potential they need communication from other cells, a process known as **intercellular signalling**. This process often involves the binding of signalling molecules produced by one cell to receptor proteins on the surface of another. Other forms of intercellular communication are possible: for example lipid soluble molecules such as some hormones can diffuse across the cell membrane or in some situations cells are linked by junctions that allow small molecules to diffuse directly between them.

Although *neural* induction is the main topic of this chapter, it is important to realize that induction occurs throughout the subsequent development of the nervous system (and it also happens in non-neural tissues). Following the initial induction of neural tissue, further inductive processes generate specialized types of neural cell, giving them their morphological, molecular and functional characteristics appropriate for their age and location. Many of the concepts that apply in the case of neural induction will reappear throughout the rest of this book. Since neural induction is an excellent illustration of recurrent themes, we shall take the opportunity towards the end of this chapter

Building Brains: An Introduction to Neural Development, First Edition.
David Price, Andrew Jarman, John Mason and Peter Kind.
© 2011 John Wiley & Sons, Ltd. Published 2011 by John Wiley & Sons, Ltd.

to discuss more generally the mechanisms by which intercellular signalling works to affect what cells do next.

3.2 Specification and commitment

Before describing what is known about the mechanisms of neural induction, we should discuss two variable properties of developing cells (wherever they are and whatever their type and age): their **specification** and their **commitment**. A specified cell or tissue is one that has some level of information directing it towards its fate (e.g. neural). Commitment is a measure of how firmly a developing cell adheres to that fate. Cells might, if perturbed, alter their fates. Analogies to human behaviour are easily made: in the same way that cells can be specified to develop towards a particular fate under the influence of inducing tissues, people can be induced to follow certain paths through life, by their parents or friends for example. However, just because someone starts out on a particular path through life does not mean that they are irrevocably committed to that path. It is easy to envisage how one might test a person's commitment to the path they are following by, for example, offering them a different job. In this way we would learn something about the things that really matter to that person. In the same way, a cell that is specified by an inducing tissue is not necessarily committed under all circumstances to a particular fate. In the case of many developmental processes including neural induction, these are important principles because they provide a framework within which to design experiments to identify how the fates of cells are determined normally. In this chapter we shall see, for example, that although the dorsal ectoderm of vertebrates is normally specified to a neural fate, manipulating its cells (by isolating them in culture or by other experimental approaches) can alter their fates. Such experiments provide an insight into the mechanisms that normally keep cells developing along a correct path.

3.3 The discovery of neural induction

The earliest work that defined clearly the concept of neural induction was carried out during the first quarter of the twentieth century by Hans Spemann and Hilde Mangold. Working on amphibian embryos, these scientists discovered that if the dorsal lip of the **blastopore** is transplanted to a new location in a different embryo, it induces the formation of a second body axis, complete with a second **neural plate** which becomes a second neural tube and eventually a second mature nervous system (Fig. 3.1). The generation of two body axes creates an organism that resembles Siamese twins, each with its own nervous system. A critical point to appreciate here is that the second body axis is derived from cells of the *host* (or recipient) embryo (i.e. the one into which the graft was made) and does not come from the donor tissue itself. As a result of this work, the dorsal lip of the blastopore in amphibians became known as the **organizer** (Fig. 3.1(a)), in view of its ability

blastopore the opening formed at gastrulation by the invagination of cells to form the mesoderm and endoderm in an early embryo; it is the entry to the primitive gut and in some species it becomes the anus.

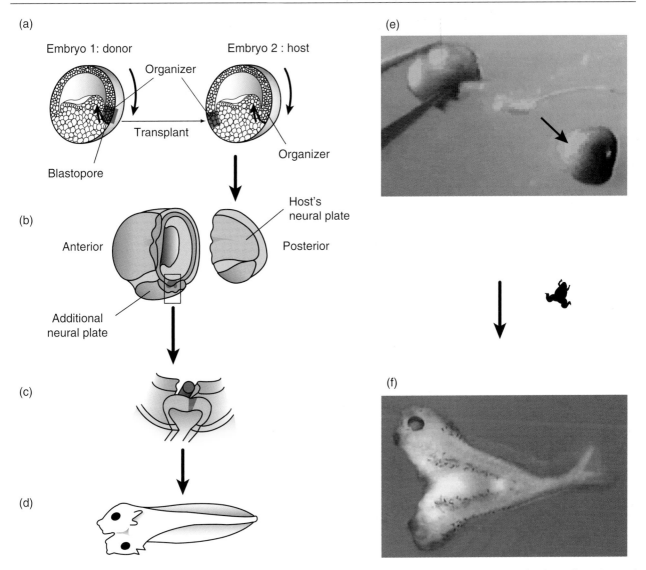

Fig. 3.1 Transplantation experiments show that the dorsal lip of the amphibian blastopore can induce the formation of neural tissue (parts (a)–(c) are adapted from Fig. 2.4 in Chapter 2). (a) The dorsal lip of the blastopore (shown in red) is taken from embryo 1 (the donor) and placed at a different location in embryo 2 (the host), which now has a new donor lip and its own lip. (b) This results in the generation of an additional neural plate in embryo 2; while some cells in this structure come from the donor (marked in red), most come from the tissues of the host embryo showing that the donor tissue has not itself generated the additional neural plate but has induced the host cells to do so. (c) The additional neural plate neurulates (Section 2.4 in Chapter2) to generate a second nervous system. (d) The second nervous system is, in fact, a component of an entire second body axis. (e) Photograph of transplantation in progress: the arrow shows where the graft (held on a fine needle) that has been cut from the donor embryo (held in fine forceps) will be placed in the host embryo (arrow). (f) Photograph of the resulting embryo. Photographs are reproduced by permission from Macmillan Publishers Ltd: De Robertis, E. M. (2006) Spemann's organizer and self-regulation in amphibian embryos. *Nat. Rev. Mol. Cell Biol.*, **7**, 296–302, copyright 2006.

to organize an appropriately patterned second axis from host tissue. Subsequent research showed that in mammals, birds and reptiles the organizer is in **Hensen's node** (see Figs 2.5 and 2.6 in Chapter 2). The discovery of the organizer provided the first example of a discrete tissue that induces surrounding tissue to adopt a particular fate. Many other examples of regions that induce neighbouring neural tissues to adopt appropriate fates have since been discovered and examples can be found in later chapters (e.g. see Chapter 4, Section 4.5.4).

Spemann and Mangold's experiments showed that cells in the early embryo that would normally form the surface ectoderm (and eventually the skin) can be induced to change their fates by an organizer transplanted into their midst. These cells must, therefore, retain the ability, or **competence**, to adopt other fates. So, successful neural induction takes place when signals from cells of the organizer are received by cells that are competent to respond to those signals. Normally, only the dorsal ectoderm cells detect the signal and respond, although cells elsewhere in the embryo have the potential to do it. Hans Spemann was awarded the Nobel Prize in Physiology or Medicine in 1935 for his work on embryonic induction.[1]

3.4 A more recent breakthrough: identifying molecules that mediate neural induction

Following the discovery of the organizer, many decades of relatively inconclusive research attempted to identify the molecules that it produces to induce neural tissue. Progress was finally made during the 1990s and led to the development of a hypothesis, known as the **default model**, to explain neural induction. As we shall see, more recent research has indicated that the default model cannot fully explain neural induction but, in many species, it still forms an important basis for our understanding.

The model came mainly from work on tissue that is induced to a neural fate in the blastula of amphibian embryos. This tissue is called the **animal cap** (it is the region above the red dotted lines at the top of Fig. 3.2(a)). When animal caps were dissected and then cultured intact as dense collections of cells, they did not develop into neural tissue (as they would in the embryo) but instead became epidermis (Fig. 3.2(a)). However, when cells of animal caps were separated from each other (a process called dissociation), then they did form neural cells (Fig. 3.2(a)). One suggestion to explain these results was that dissociation allowed molecules that *prevent* neural induction to escape from around the animal cap cells into the surrounding fluid, thereby reducing the concentration of those blocking molecules and allowing the cells to adopt a neural fate by default.

What might the molecules preventing neural induction be? A family of about 20 secreted intercellular signalling molecules called **bone morphogenetic proteins** (**BMPs**), originally identified during the 1980s through work on bone, mediate signalling between cells in many locations and at many stages of development. Members of this family, including BMP2, BMP4 and BMP7, were found in the animal cap of the blastula. The ability of dissociation to turn animal cap cells into neural cells was counteracted by adding BMPs to the cultures (Fig. 3.2(a)); under

---

[1] www.nobelprize.org/nobel_prizes/medicine/laureates/1935/spemann-lecture.html [20 November 2010]. An excellent review providing more detail of his work and the related work of others can be found in De Robertis, E. M. and Kuroda, H. (2004) Dorsal-ventral patterning and neural induction in Xenopus embryos. *Ann. Rev. Cell Dev. Biol.*, **20**, 285–308.

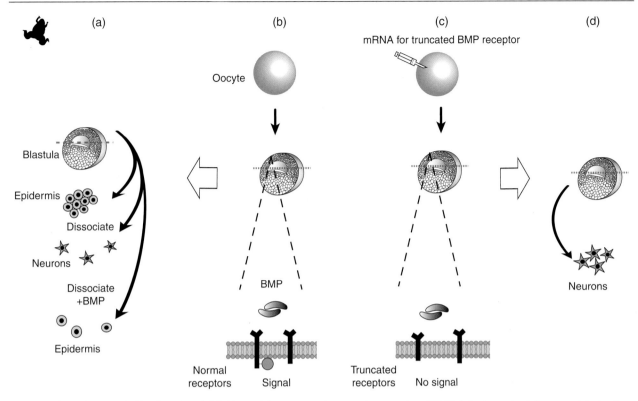

Fig. 3.2 Experiments indicating that inhibition of bone morphogenetic proteins (BMPs) is important in neural induction. (a) Cultured animal cap cells (dissected from the region above the broken red line) form epidermis if they are kept together. They form neurons if they are dissociated unless BMPs are added to them in which case they form epidermis. (b) Normal oocytes generate embryos with BMP receptors that dimerize in response to BMPs, causing them to signal. (c) If embryos are made to produce truncated non-functional receptors for BMPs in addition to normal receptors then, during dimerization, the truncated receptors interfere with the ability of cells to respond to BMPs. (d) If animal cap cells from embryos produced as in (c) (with BMP signalling inhibited) are cultured intact then they form neurons and not epidermis.

these circumstances only epidermal cells were produced, indicating that BMPs might be critical molecules preventing neural induction. Further experiments gave more support to this idea: when animal caps dissected from embryos in which BMP signalling had been blocked were cultured intact (i.e. not dissociated), their cells now adopted neural fates (Fig. 3.2(b)–(d)). These experiments showed that neural induction can be brought about by interfering with BMP signalling.

These experiments indicated that the organizer might promote neural induction because it produces molecules that inhibit BMPs in the animal cap, so preventing its cells from acquiring an epidermal fate; but what are the active molecules produced by the organizer to induce neural tissue?

During the early 1990s, Richard Harland's laboratory at the University of California at Berkeley was studying frog embryos exposed to ultraviolet light. These frogs lacked neural tissue and Harland's laboratory was trying to find ways of reversing this defect. They found that treatment of these embryos with a pool of **cDNA** molecules that made proteins normally generated by the organizer reversed the defects. By dividing the starting pool into ever smaller pools they homed in on the active protein and called it noggin. The name came from the finding

cDNA DNA molecules able to generate proteins since they are copies of mRNAs.

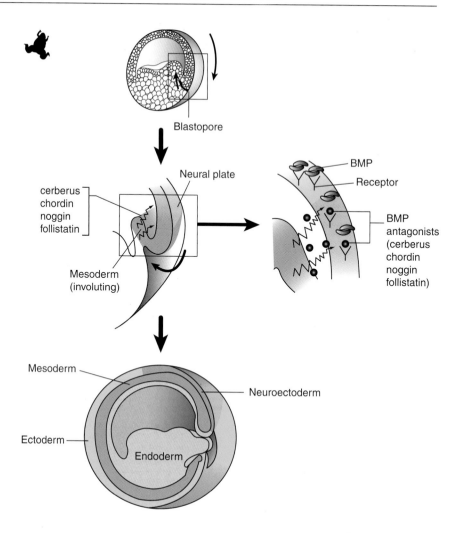

Fig. 3.3 The default model of neural induction based largely on work in amphibians: mesoderm dorsal to the blastopore secretes molecules that antagonize BMPs present in the part of the overlying ectoderm dorsal to the blastopore, converting it to neuroectoderm.

that high concentrations of this protein produce embryos with abnormally big heads (noggin is slang for head).

At the same time, other laboratories were finding other potentially important proteins present specifically in the organizer, including chordin (named because of its presence not only in the organizer but later in the notochord), follistatin (which was already known in a different context, as a component of ovarian fluid) and cerberus (named after the three-headed dog guarding the entrance to the underworld in Greek mythology). Experiments showed that (i) noggin, chordin, follistatin and cerberus can all bind to and inhibit the activity of BMPs, (ii) if these proteins are depleted in *Xenopus* embryos using morpholino oligonucleotides (see Fig. 1.4 in Chapter 1) there is a severe loss of neural plate tissue. Based mainly on this research in amphibians, a default model of neural induction summarized in Fig. 3.3 was proposed.[2]

---

[2] For more details of the experimental work done in the 1990s to support the default model, we suggest a review by Hemmati-Brivanlou, A. and Melton, D. (1997) Vertebrate neural induction. *Annual Reviews of Neuroscience*, **20**, 43–60.

3.5 Conservation of neural induction mechanisms in *Drosophila*

Work in invertebrates added strength to the default model by indicating that its major component (neural induction achieved through inhibition of BMP signalling) is conserved even in highly divergent species. Molecules involved in the vertebrate neural induction model described above have homologues in invertebrates. The *Drosophila* gene *decapentaplegic* (*dpp*) encodes a **homologue** of vertebrate BMP2 and BMP4. The gene encoding vertebrate chordin is homologous to the *Drosophila* gene *short gastrulation* (*sog*). These genes are critical for inducing *Drosophila* neuroectoderm.

Drosophila oocytes and early embryos contain a concentration gradient of a protein called Dorsal (Fig. 3.4). Dorsal concentrations are highest ventrally (somewhat confusingly!). Dorsal activates the production of other molecules – which molecules depends on the concentration of Dorsal relative to two thresholds (Fig. 3.4). At high levels, Dorsal activates the production of mesoderm-inducing molecules such as Snail. Intermediate levels of Dorsal activate the production of SOG protein in the bilateral neuroectodermal regions. DPP protein is produced dorsally, where Dorsal is at very low levels or absent. In Chapter 4 we shall return to the actions of these and related molecules in setting up the dorsoventral axis of the *Drosophila* CNS.

DPP and SOG antagonize each other, as do their vertebrate counterparts BMP and chordin. In mutant *Drosophila* embryos in which *sog* gene function is lost, the epidermis expands and the extent of the neuroectodermal regions is reduced, due to the absence of *sog*'s check on *dpp*. In *Drosophila* mutants that have lost the activity of *dpp*, the neuroectoderm expands while the epidermis is reduced in extent. Experimental findings such as these have led to the conclusion that, even though the ventrally located neurogenic region in flies is on the opposite side of the embryo to the dorsally located neuroepithelium in vertebrates, the molecular mechanisms that induce neural fates are highly conserved.

3.6 Beyond the default model – other signalling pathways involved in neural induction

Results from more recent experimental work have indicated that, in most species tested, the straightforward version of the default model outlined above is insufficient to explain neural induction. For example, in chicks the times and places at which BMPs and their antagonists are found suggest that things are more complicated. (i) The BMP antagonists noggin and follistatin are not in the organizer at appropriate stages suggesting that they are not required for neural induction. (ii) The BMP antagonist chordin is in the organizer, but is still there even after this tissue has lost its neural inducing activity, suggesting that it is insufficient to induce neural tissue and additional factors are important. (iii) BMPs themselves are only present at very low levels in ectoderm before neural induction begins, indicating

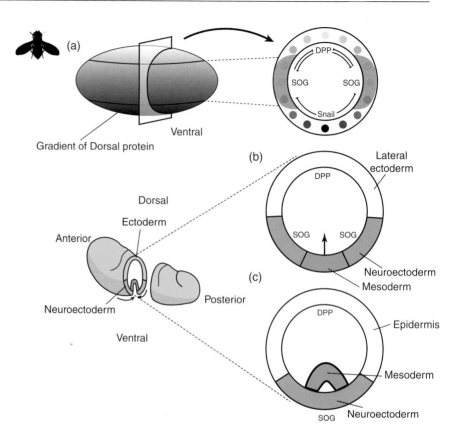

Fig. 3.4 Neural induction in *Drosophila*: (a) the oocyte and early embryo have a concentration gradient of Dorsal protein along the dorsoventral axis (grey shading). High, intermediate and low levels of Dorsal relative to two thresholds activate different sets of genes in ventral, intermediate and dorsal regions respectively. High levels of Dorsal result in the specification of mesoderm ventrally. Intermediate levels of Dorsal result in the specification of neural tissue (orange) ventrolaterally on each side of the embryo. This lateral neural tissue contains SOG protein, a homologue of vertebrate chordin, which antagonizes DPP protein, a homologue of vertebrate BMPs. (b) and (c) As the embryo develops, mesoderm moves into the embryo's interior, lateral neural tissues move ventrally and fuse, and dorsal tissue forms epidermis (see also Fig. 2.2 in Chapter 2).

Box 3.1 Chordates

The chordates are a large and diverse animal group comprising vertebrates (animals with backbones) and protochordates. Protochordates lack backbones but resemble vertebrates in some important respects: of particular relevance here is that at some stage of their life history they have a dorsal neural tube and notochord. For example, sea-squirts (ascidians) go through a larval stage with a neural tube and notochord although these structures are lost at metamorphosis when the mature sea-squirt forms as a barrel-shaped blob. These diagrams show the organization of **ascidian** embryos: the section on the left shows the antero-posterior axis, the section on the right shows a cross section.

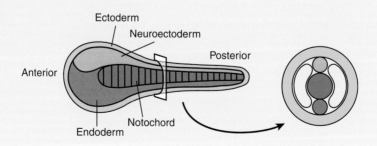

that there is not much to antagonize. Furthermore, in experimental work in which BMP antagonists were added to chick **epiblast**, neural tissue was not always induced, again suggesting that additional factors are important.

There is evidence from many species of chordate (including members of the protochordates – Box 3.1) for the involvement of other signalling molecules in neural induction. Prominent among these are **fibroblast growth factors** (**FGFs**) and **Wnts**, families of molecules that were initially discovered in other contexts. FGFs were discovered during the 1970s and early work showed that they induced the proliferation of fibroblasts; there are over 20 FGF family members in mammals. Wnts were discovered during the 1970s and 1980s through a convergence of work on homologous genes in *Drosophila* and mammals; there are about 20 Wnt family members in mammals. These signalling molecules are implicated in the regulation of many different events throughout development, as will become apparent in the coming chapters.

In some species the default model does not seem to explain neural induction at all. In protochordates such as the ascidians (Box 3.1), FGFs rather than antagonists of BMPs are responsible for neural induction, suggesting that the default model has little if any relevance in these species. In vertebrates, some experiments have provided evidence that inhibition of Wnt signalling or activation of FGF signalling can lead to neural induction in animal cap tissue. The inducing molecule cerberus antagonizes not only BMPs but also Wnts. The following paragraph outlines some current ideas on how FGF signalling and Wnt antagonism combine with BMP antagonism to induce neuroectodermal development. More research is needed to gain a clear understanding; a detailed account of current work is outside the scope of this book, but excellent reviews can be found in the literature.[3]

The balance of evidence suggests that in vertebrates FGFs are not direct neural inducers but that FGF signalling is required for neural induction by BMP antagonists. One hypothesis comes from knowledge of the processes that occur within cells when they are stimulated by BMPs and FGFs, which will be discussed in the next section. Looking ahead to Fig. 3.5, it can be seen that FGFs cause changes within cells that antagonize the changes caused by BMPs, thereby contributing to the same overall outcome as antagonists of BMPs themselves. Another hypothesis proposes that FGFs act through two separate pathways, one that represses the production of BMPs and the other that does not involve BMPs or their signalling pathways. Regarding Wnt signalling, there is evidence that neural induction requires activation of the canonical Wnt signalling pathway resulting in the translocation of β-catenin to the nucleus (shown below in Fig. 3.6) where it blocks the activation of the BMP gene.

FGFs and Wnts have also been implicated in bringing the elongation of the vertebrate body axis to an end. Neural induction continues while the embryo is gastrulating, but must be stopped in a

epiblast the layer of cells in the early embryos of birds, reptiles and mammals that gives rise to the three germ layers at gastrulation.

---

[3] For example, Stern, C.D. (2005) Neural induction: old problem, new findings, yet more questions. *Development*, **132**, 2007–2021.

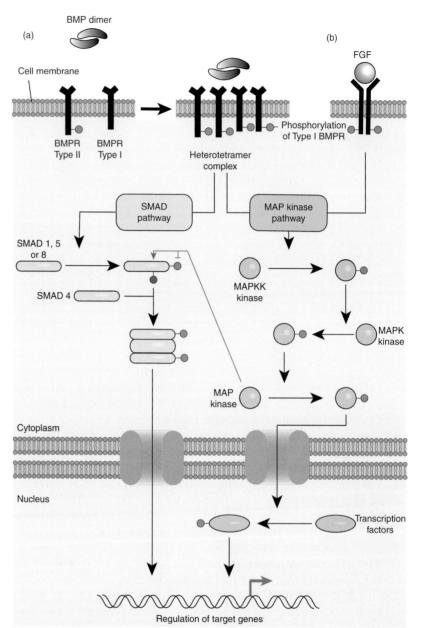

kinase an enzyme that transfers phosphate groups onto specific molecules, a process called phosphorylation.

autophosphorylation the phosphorylation of a kinase protein by its own enzymatic activity.

Fig. 3.5 (a) **BMP signalling**: there are two types of BMP receptor (BMPR), Types I and II. BMP molecules bind together forming dimers and then bind to Type II receptors, causing the formation of complexes comprising four receptor proteins, two Type I and two Type II (complexes of this type are called heterotetramers). This causes phosphorylation of the Type 1 receptors and the activation of two pathways: (i) the SMAD pathway and (ii) the mitogen-activated protein **kinase** (MAPK) pathway (phosphorylation causing activation is indicated by small green circles). BMPR Type I phosphorylation leads to the phosphorylation of SMADs 1, 5 or 8 which then combine to form complexes with SMAD4 and enter the nucleus to regulate the transcription of specific target genes. It also causes the sequential phosphorylation of three molecules each of which is a type of kinase: first, a MAPKK kinase (MAPKKK), second a MAPK kinase (MAPKK) and finally a MAP kinase (MAPK) itself. Phosphorylated MAPK proteins can enter the nucleus to phosphorylate and hence activate transcription factors controlling the transcription of specific target genes. There are many different MAPKKKs, MAPKKs and MAPKs. (b) **FGF signalling**: there are several FGF receptors (FGFRs), which are receptor tyrosine kinases. Binding of FGFs causes FGFRs to dimerize, **autophosphorylate** on their tyrosines and activate the MAPK pathway. As well as regulating gene transcription, MAPKs can also have cytoplasmic functions, one of which is to phosphorylate SMAD1 in a central rather than a terminal position (small red circle), thereby inhibiting this pathway (this inhibitory pathway is in the figure's centre and is in red). During neural induction, the net effect of BMP antagonism and FGF signalling is inhibition of SMAD1 activity.

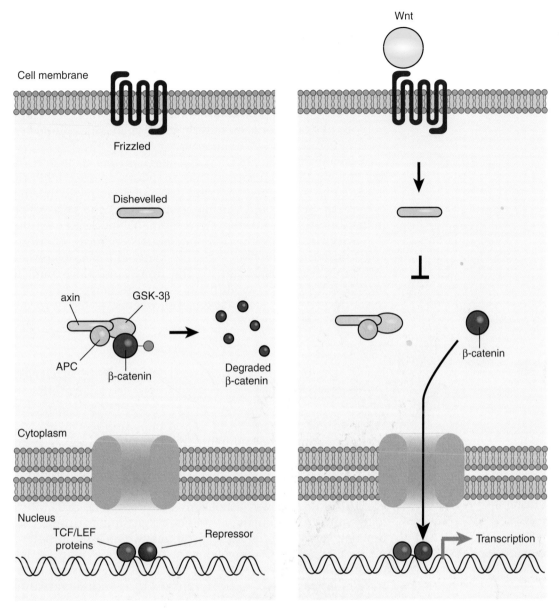

Fig. 3.6 **Wnt signalling**: Wnts can signal through several pathways and only the best-known is illustrated here. This is the canonical Wnt pathway (now often referred to as the Wnt/β-catenin pathway) and its major components are conserved from *C. elegans* to mammals. Wnt proteins bind to cell-surface receptors of the Frizzled family causing them to activate intracellular Dishevelled family proteins. When Dishevelled is activated it inhibits a complex of proteins including axin, glycogen synthase kinase 3 (GSK-3) and adenomatous polyposis coli (APC). In the absence of Wnt signalling, this complex causes phosphorylation (small green circle) of β-catenin which is then **degraded proteolytically**; inhibition of the complex prevents phosphorylation and degradation of β-catenin, which enters the nucleus where it displaces a repressor protein and, in combination with proteins of the TCF/LEF (T-cell factor/lymphoid enhancer-binding factor) family, affects the transcription of specific target genes.

proteolytic degradation the breakdown of proteins into peptides and amino acids.

somites segmental masses of mesoderm lying on either side of the notochord and neural tube during the development of vertebrate embryos.

controlled way to give vertebrates their characteristic body lengths and numbers of **somites** (somites are illustrated in Figs 2.4–2.7 in Chapter 2). It is thought that ectodermal cells lose their competence to respond to neural induction around the end of gastrulation, at which time differentiation at the tail end of the nervous system is associated with loss of FGF and Wnt signalling.[4] The process of axis elongation is intimately tied up with patterning of the nervous system along its anteroposterior axis (anteroposterior patterning is discussed in Chapter 4).

In conclusion, research on the mechanisms of neural induction has led to the realization that in many species BMP signalling needs to be modulated *at several stages* throughout early embryogenesis, both before and during gastrulation, for successful neural induction and neural plate development. Molecules implicated in these events include the BMP antagonists cerberus, chordin, noggin and follistatin as well as FGFs and Wnts and possibly other signalling molecules. Regulation of the times and places and levels of production of these modulators from the early stages of embryo formation, before gastrulation even begins, is likely to be critical and to vary between species.

3.7 Signal transduction: how cells respond to intercellular signals

Work on the mechanisms of neural induction has demonstrated the critical importance of signalling between developing cells in specifying their fates. It provides an excellent example of the principle that the modulation of intercellular signalling can have profound effects on cell specification. We shall see in later chapters that, throughout the rest of development, not only does this same principle hold but many of the very same molecules and signalling pathways continue to function often in different developmental processes at different ages. Intercellular signalling involving the binding of a **ligand** to its specific receptor activates cascades of biochemical reactions within a cell (intracellular reactions), a process referred to as **signal transduction**.

ligand a molecule or ion that binds to a receptor molecule, for example on the cell surface, to generate a biological response.

phosphorylation the addition of a phosphate group to a molecule often causing its activation or deactivation.

Signal transduction is achieved through the sequential catalytic activation of intracellular enzymes. Enzymes can be activated in various ways, for example some are activated by **phosphorylation** causing reversible conformational changes in the enzyme. The whole process is a domino effect in which activation of one enzyme leads to activation of the next, and so on. Small amounts of ligand can have large effects on the cell, because activated enzymes can modify large numbers of substrate molecules. Thus, an important property of these signal transduction cascades is that they amplify the original signal, thereby increasing its magnitude relative the background activity of the biochemical pathways within the cell (i.e. the signal-to-noise ratio is increased).

---

[4] For further details, see a review by Wilson, V., Olivera-Martinez, I. and Storey, K. (2009) Stem cells, signals and vertebrate body axis extension. *Development*, **136**, 1591–1604.

Another important property of signal transduction pathways is the crosstalk that occurs between them. This can be appreciated by studying the BMP and FGF transduction pathways shown in Fig. 3.5. Prominent in these pathways is a family of molecules called SMADs. These are homologues of the proteins encoded by a *C. elegans* gene called *sma* and a *Drosophila* gene called *mothers against decapentaplegic*, or *mad* (*decapentaplegic* is discussed above in Section 3.5). Whereas BMP signalling activates SMAD1 by phosphorylating a region at its end, FGF signalling phosphorylates a region in the middle of SMAD1, which inhibits it (marked in red in the middle of Fig. 3.5). This means that FGFs and antagonists of BMPs can generate the same outcomes, helping to explain why both sets of molecules can induce neural tissue.

Fig. 3.6 shows the canonical Wnt signalling pathway. The BMP, FGF and Wnt pathways, in common with many other signal transduction pathways, result eventually in changes in the transcription of specific genes. These changes have profound effects on the molecular constitution and hence the fate of the cell. They are discussed in the next section.

3.8 Intercellular signalling regulates gene expression

Intercellular signalling influences profoundly the specification of cell fates through its effects on gene transcription. In some cases, proteins of a signal transduction pathway (e.g. MAPKs, Fig. 3.5) activate regulatory DNA-binding molecules; in others, they themselves bind to DNA and regulate gene transcription (e.g. SMADs, Fig. 3.5).

3.8.1 General mechanisms of transcriptional regulation

In all embryos, it takes some time after fertilization before genes start to be transcribed (the exact time varies from species to species). During this very early phase, it is the products of maternal genes that were loaded into the egg during its formation that control development. Eventually, developmental control is transferred to the young embryo's genome. In some species this occurs very early, for example in mouse it happens around the two-cell stage, whereas in others it occurs later, for example in *Xenopus* and *Drosophila* it happens before and around gastrulation. The mechanisms that regulate the transition are not well understood. Once the embryonic genome has been activated, normal development relies on its being controlled correctly by the embryo itself.

Proteins that bind to DNA to regulate gene transcription are called **transcription factors**; there are about 2500 different transcription factors in humans. Transcription factors bind to particular regions of the DNA called **regulatory elements**, which include **promoters** and **enhancers**. Transcription factors regulate the transcription of DNA to mRNA, which is then available for translation to protein, a process known as **gene expression**. Transcription factors determine which genes are switched on (activation) and which are switched off (repression) in cells at different places and times in development.

Box 3.2   How transcription factors work

Enzymes that generate RNA (i.e. RNA polymerases) bind to specific regions in the genome. They bind at sites called promoters. In order for them to bind, other proteins must also be present: all these proteins are called transcription factors. Many transcription factors bind non-specifically to promoters throughout the genome. Others bind only at specific sites by recognizing specific sequences. These site-specific transcription factors are particularly interesting because they exert control over the expression of specific target genes. Their level can determine whether or at what level the genes that they control are expressed within a cell and hence the developmental path taken by that cell. In this book the transcription factors we focus on are site-specific. As shown in the diagram, the complexes created by transcription factors and other so-called co-activator proteins can stimulate gene transcription by (i) recruiting **histone** modifying enzymes (HMEs) that alter the **chromatin** (chromatin is the name given to DNA combined with its associated proteins) locally and render conditions more favourable for transcription, or (ii) by recruiting kinases that phosphorylate RNA polymerase in the complex, thereby activating it to synthesize RNA (green circles indicate phosphorylation). In the former case, modification of histones involves their acetylation (i.e. introduction of an acetyl group). Histones are proteins around which DNA wraps itself tightly in living cells and **nucleosomes** are the structures formed by this packing. Efficient packing of DNA is essential because uncoiled DNA contained by a chromosome is up to about 10 cm long! It would be wrong, however, to think that chromatin is organized in this way simply to pack a great length of DNA into a small space. Compaction physically restricts access by transcription factors to the genome and there is good evidence that chromatin structure alters dynamically in a highly regulated way through development. Chromatin modifications are likely to be important determinants of whether particular parts of the genome are expressed and, as a consequence, are likely to be important in the regulation of development.[5]

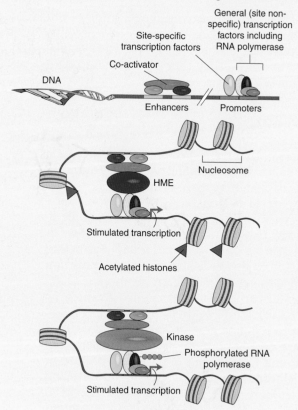

[5] For further reading on this topic, see: (i) Ho, L. and Crabtree, G. R. (2010) Chromatin remodelling during development. *Nature*, **463**, 474–84; (ii) Kwon, C. S. and Wagner, D. (2007) Unwinding chromatin for development and growth: a few genes at a time. *Trends Genet.*, **23**, 403–12.

Of most interest for understanding how cells are specified during development are those transcription factors that are expressed only in specific cells at particular times during development. Such transcription factors have the potential to establish the specific properties of developing cells. Other transcription factors are produced ubiquitously by most or all cells; while they are needed for the transcriptional machinery to work, they do not explain how differences between cells are acquired. Box 3.2 gives further information on how specific and general transcription factors are thought to combine to regulate gene transcription.

Many different transcription factors combine to specify cells from the earliest stages of development onwards. Transcription factor proteins have specialized regions called **motifs** that allow them to interact with DNA. Box 3.3 shows some examples of the three-dimensional structures of well-known classes of DNA-binding motifs found in transcription factors that are known to specify many aspects of neural development.

Box 3.3 Examples of DNA-binding motifs found in three classes of transcription factor

(a) The **homeodomain** comprises about 60 amino acids that are folded into three helices, one of which interacts directly with DNA, connected by short loops. (b) **Basic helix–loop–helix (bHLH)** domains are characterized by two helices connected by a loop and usually form dimers (shown in blue and green). (c) **Zinc finger** domains comprise a helix that interacts with the DNA and a sheet of amino acids stabilized and held in position relative to each other by a zinc atom; some transcription factors contain multiple zinc fingers arranged in tandem. The individual members of each class of transcription factor have different amino acid sequences but share structural motifs. For any given transcription factor it is still largely unknown which genes are targeted and whether the set of targeted genes varies with location and developmental time; much research is now focused in this area.

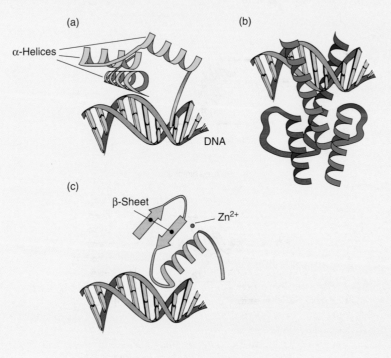

Box 3.4   Methods for detecting gene expression

Two commonly used methods for detecting gene expression, using the chick embryo shown in Fig. 3.7 as an example: the top line shows that, in both cases, the tissue is placed in solution containing either a nucleic acid probe that is **complementary** to the mRNA of interest or an antibody that binds specifically to the protein made from that mRNA. The aim is to stain the cells that express the mRNA or protein of interest. (a) *In situ* **hybridization**: two cells side-by-side straddling a boundary of gene expression are enlarged, one expresses the mRNA of interest, the other does not. The nucleic acid probe (red) binds specifically to complementary mRNA of interest. The probe is labelled. The label is used in a second reaction that marks the expressing cells by, for example, generating a coloured product in them. (b) **Immunocytochemistry**: a primary antibody (orange) binds specifically to the protein of interest. Another antibody, called a secondary antibody, is often used to recognize the primary antibody and so indicate where the primary antibody has bound. The secondary antibody carries a label that can be used to mark the cells that contain the protein of interest.

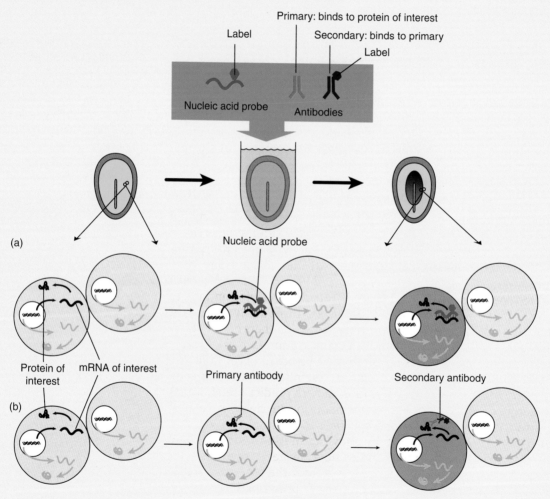

complementary describes a strand of DNA or RNA that can bind to a second strand because each base on one strand can pair, in order, with the base on the opposite strand (A and T pair, C and G pair).

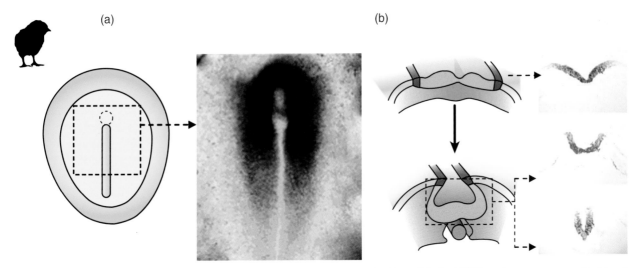

Fig. 3.7 (a) In this experiment, mRNA from a *Sox* gene has been detected using a labelled RNA probe, a process called *in situ* hybridization (see Box 3.4 for a description of the method), revealing transcription of this gene in the intact epiblast of the chick embryo (purple stain), which is competent to develop as neural tissue (for a description of the anatomy of epiblast development, see Fig. 2.4 in Chapter 2). (b) In this experiment, the same method has been used on sections cut through the neural plate to show transcription of a *Sox* gene restricted to the developing neural plate. (Photographs are from Rex, M. *et al.* (1997) Dynamic expression of chicken Sox2 and Sox3 genes in ectoderm induced to form neural tissue. *Dev. Dyn.*, **209**, 323–32, and Wakamatsu, Y. *et al.* (2004) Multiple roles of Sox2, an HMG-box transcription factor in avian neural crest development. *Dev. Dyn.*, **229**, 74–86.)

3.8.2 Transcription factors involved in neural induction

Returning to the specific case of neural induction, we have discussed how intercellular signalling through BMPs, FGFs and Wnts affects development by affecting the expression and activity of transcription factors, but what transcription factors are affected (aside from those already mentioned, i.e. SMADs and β-catenin)? We now know that cells induced to a neural fate express specific sets of transcription factors which distinguish them from other cell types; particularly important in both vertebrate and invertebrate embryos are members of the evolutionarily highly conserved SOX family of transcription factors.

There are about 30 *Sox* genes in vertebrates. Ectodermal cells that are competent to become nerve cells express members of the *Sox* gene family, indicating that SOX transcription factors predict the ability of cells to adopt a neural fate. Following neural induction, expression becomes restricted to cells that are specified to a neural fate (Fig. 3.7; Box 3.4 complements this figure by showing methods for detecting gene expression). Our understanding of how *Sox* genes operate is far from complete. One unresolved issue stems from the observation that numerous SOX factors are expressed in overlapping patterns in the developing CNS and PNS. Why are there so many? Answers to this question will come from continuing research on the detailed functions of each factor individually and in combination with others.

Churchill is another example of a transcription factor expressed by the developing neural plate and required for neural plate specification. It was discovered in chick and is expressed by neural tissue in response to FGF. It is required (i) for the expression of molecules that then

primitive streak a structure formed when epiblast cells move anteriorly along the midline of a vertebrate embryo.

repress the expression of a mesodermal gene and (ii) to stop epiblast cells migrating too far through the **primitive streak** to form mesoderm.

3.8.3 What genes do transcription factors control?

Transcription factors control the expression of genes often referred to as downstream targets. Cells develop differently because they vary in the sets of transcription factors and downstream targets that they express; but what downstream target genes are controlled by each transcription factor and how do they cause the cell to adopt its fate? For example, how do SOX transcription factors specify the development of neural tissue? Here our knowledge becomes hazy.

Some of the downstream targets of a transcription factor are direct targets activated or repressed by the binding of the transcription factor to their regulatory elements. Many, however, are indirect targets activated or repressed via the actions of directly regulated genes. Working out whether the downstream targets of a transcription factor are directly or indirectly regulated is a complex process whose description is outside the scope of this book.[6] When we consider that just the *direct* targets of a single transcription factor might number in the tens or hundreds and that they might change with age and with cell type, depending on what other transcription factors are also expressed, it is hardly surprising that we still know relatively little about the molecular pathways through which transcription factors work. They regulate networks of interacting genes that are likely to be extensive and complex; an example of a relatively simple network is shown in Fig. 3.8. Increasing understanding in this area is a major challenge for future research. It will require not only experimental biological methods but, increasingly, the ability to analyse computationally the very large amounts of data generated by examining the activities of potentially many thousands of genes simultaneously. This area is known as **bioinformatics**.[7]

3.8.4 Gene function can also be controlled by other mechanisms

In Chapter 1, we described how small RNA molecules generated by an experimenter and injected into cells can be used to block, and so assess the functions of, specific mRNAs (see Fig. 1.4). It has been realized only in the last couple of decades that cells also produce their own very small RNA molecules that regulate the functions of the genes they express; in 2006 Andrew Fire and Craig Mello were awarded a Nobel Prize for their groundbreaking work on mechanisms of **RNA interference**.[8] Naturally-occurring small regulatory RNAs are called **microRNAs** (Fig. 3.9). They were first discovered in 1993 in *C. elegans*

---

[6] For further information, try Holstege, F. C. and Clevers, H. (2006) Transcription factor target practice. *Cell,* **124**, 21–23 and references cited therein.

[7] For further reading, see Rister, J. and Desplan, C. (2010) Deciphering the genome's regulatory code: the many languages of DNA. *Bioessays*, **32**, 381–384.

[8] http://nobelprize.org/nobel_prizes/medicine/laureates/2006/mello-lecture.html [20 November 2010].

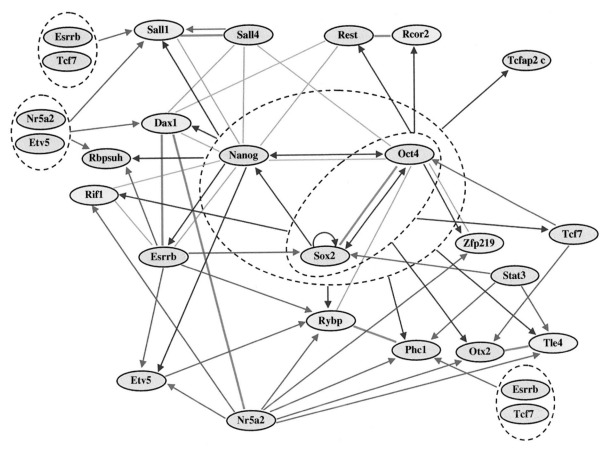

Fig. 3.8 An example of a gene regulatory network in mouse stem cells: this network appears complicated but is a relatively simple example. It includes a *Sox* gene that regulates itself as well as other genes, some directly and others indirectly. *Sox* genes are discussed in this chapter; the other genes are not discussed and are only named here to illustrate the nature of the network. Those genes in yellow encode proteins that interact with proteins encoded by genes in pink; orange and green lines represent protein interactions. Blue and pink arrows indicate regulatory interactions; arrows from a dashed ellipse indicate that the targets are regulated by all of the regulators inside the ellipse. Some regulators appear multiple times in the network to reduce the number of intersecting arrows. Reproduced from Zhou, Q, Chipperfield, H, Melton, D. A. and Wong, W. H. (2007) A gene regulatory network in mouse embryonic stem cells. *Proc. Natl Acad. Sci. USA*, **104**,16438–43. Copyright 2007 National Academy of Sciences, USA.

by Victor Ambros, Rosalind Lee and Rhonda Feinbaum working in Dartmouth Medical School in the USA.

MicroRNAs are about 22 nucleotides long and they bind to complementary sequences in multiple target mRNAs, usually limiting or preventing their translation. Exactly how they do this is not well understood, although it is known that they act on mRNAs in collaboration with a protein complex called the RNA-induced silencing complex (or RISC). We now know about many hundreds of different microRNAs in many organisms across all kingdoms; humans probably have well over 1000. MicroRNAs have come to be seen as an ancient and vital component of genetic regulation.

MicroRNAs are encoded by sequences found in the regions between protein coding genes (intergenic) as well as in introns of protein coding regions (intragenic). These regions are transcribed to generate

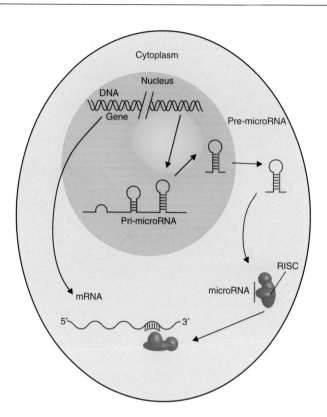

Fig. 3.9 Control of gene function by microRNAs: some sequences in the genome are transcribed to give mRNAs, which are exported to the cytoplasm for translation; other sequences can be transcribed to give pri-microRNAs which form hairpin structures from which pre-micro-RNAs and eventually microRNAs are cut following export from the nucleus. Mature microRNAs combine with the RNA-induced silencing complex (RISC) to bind to and inhibit or block translation from specific mRNAs. Typically, microRNAs bind in the 3′ untranslated regions of target mRNAs (i.e. the regions of mature mRNAs that do not code for proteins).

primary transcripts called pri-microRNAs. We still know very little about how the transcription of microRNA-encoding sequences in the genome is regulated; clearly, this is a very important question. Once produced, pri-microRNAs fold back on themselves to form multiple distinct hairpin structures. These molecules are processed in the nucleus by RNAase enzymes including Drosha, which recognize and cut out the hairpin structures to make pre-microRNAs. Pre-microRNAs are exported from the nucleus where the active micro-RNA is finally generated by processes that involve another RNAase enzyme called Dicer.

Identifying the mRNAs that microRNAs target has proved a major challenge since most microRNAs do not bind to mRNAs with full complementarity. Much more work is needed before we understand what RNAs are regulated by this mechanism and when during development.[9]

3.9 The essence of development: a complex interplay of intercellular and intracellular signalling

In this chapter we have described how intercellular signalling molecules such as BMPs, FGFs and Wnts act on cell-surface receptors to

[9] For more information on this topic from one of its discoverers, see Ambros, V. (2004) The functions of animal microRNAs. *Nature*, **431**, 350–5.

activate intracellular signal transduction pathways leading to alterations in gene expression. We have seen that the binding of signalling molecules to their receptors can be modulated by other molecules such as the BMP antagonists. We have discussed how transcription factors act as mediators between the signalling processes and the morphological and functional development of neural cells by regulating which genes are active in each cell; in fact, it is likely that they act not just in a binary fashion, switching genes on or off, but more subtly to control levels of activity.

Transcription factors are effectively the molecular switches and rheostats set by signals from outside each cell and dictating the next step in its development. As is the case with intercellular signalling molecules, the same transcription factors play numerous different roles throughout development. Their functions at any particular place and time are determined by the intracellular and extracellular environment in which they operate, for example which other transcription factors are co-expressed with them.

The fates of cells depend on the combinations of transcription factors they express. These combinations are influenced by intercellular signalling. Signalling itself is regulated by transcription factors, which control the production of signalling, receptor and signal transduction molecules. This complex interplay between intercellular signalling and intracellular regulation of gene expression lies at the heart of the regulation of development of all tissues.

3.10 Summary

- Induction refers to the process by which one tissue causes a change in the development of another tissue. In neural induction, the inducing tissue, called the organizer, instructs the responding tissue to adopt a neural fate.
- Research in vertebrates showed that neural induction takes place when signals from the organizer are received by ectodermal cells, which are competent to respond to those signals.
- The default model of neural induction proposed that ectodermal cells adopt a neural fate if the BMP signalling between them is inhibited by molecules produced by the organizer. The default model has since been extended and modified and may not apply in all species.
- A major component of the default model- that neural induction is achieved through inhibition of BMP signalling- is conserved between vertebrates and invertebrates.
- Signalling between cells (intercellular signalling) specifies cell fates via intracellular transduction pathways that regulate gene expression and hence a cell's molecular constitution. Many signalling pathways are used over and over again for different purposes throughout development.
- The control of gene expression is mediated by the actions of networks of transcription factors. Other molecules such as microRNAs are also likely to influence this process.

Patterning the Neuroectoderm

4

4.1 Regional patterning of the nervous system

Once the **neuroectoderm** has been specified, the next step is to divide it up into areas that will lay the basis for regional specializations in the structure of the mature nervous system. This process is known as regional patterning or **regionalization** of the neuroectoderm. Regional patterning happens progressively, starting (in vertebrates) at the neural plate stage, and continuing during and after neurulation (Chapter 2, Section 2.4). As an example, the chick anterior neural tube is initially simple, but becomes progressively divided up to form the different regions of the brain (Fig. 4.1). In fact the process of regionalization begins even before any morphological differences are visible: in the early neuroectoderm, future brain regions are laid out as discrete gene expression domains, particularly of genes encoding **transcription factors** (in *Drosophila* this stage is sometimes called **prepatterning**). These transcription factors influence the behaviour and properties of the neuroectodermal cells within these domains, most notably in influencing the patterns of neural cell production that subsequently occur in different regions. The formation of neural cells within the neuroectoderm – **neurogenesis** – is the subject in the next chapter. In this chapter, we concentrate on the mechanisms that subdivide the neuroectoderm into distinct regions.

neuroectoderm the neurogenic region of the ectoderm which develops into the nervous system.

transcription factors proteins that bind to DNA to regulate gene transcription.

4.1.1 Patterns of gene expression are set up by morphogens

To a large extent, regionalization involves long-range signalling that provides cells with information about their location within the neural epithelium. Such information is known as **positional information**, and it involves signalling molecules with very particular properties. We have seen already that cells can influence the fate or behaviour of other cells through the production of diffusible signals (e.g. as occurs in neural induction, Chapter 3). A cornerstone of patterning in developmental biology is the idea that some diffusible signals can induce more than one type of response in recipient cells, depending on the *amount* of the signal the cells receive. If such a signalling molecule diffuses from a source to form a concentration gradient, then a recipient

Building Brains: An Introduction to Neural Development, First Edition.
David Price, Andrew Jarman, John Mason and Peter Kind.
© 2011 John Wiley & Sons, Ltd. Published 2011 by John Wiley & Sons, Ltd.

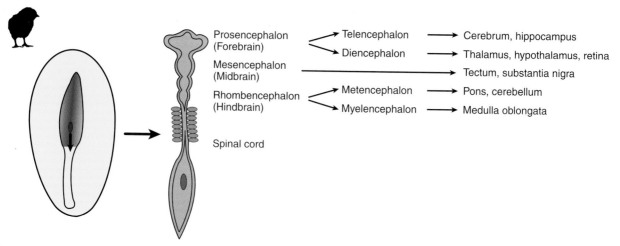

Fig. 4.1 Regional specializations emerge in the anteroposterior (AP) axis of the chick neural tube (often known as the rostrocaudal axis; see Chapter 2, Section 2.2). After neurulation, the anterior or rostral end of the neural tube becomes progressively subdivided early on into the regions that will form the brain. More posteriorly, the neural tube is rather uniform and gives rise to the spinal cord.

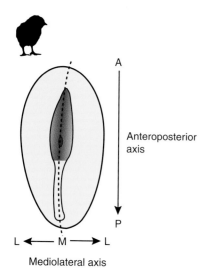

Fig. 4.2 The neuroectoderm has two axes. Here, the chick neural plate is being formed by the anterior-to-posterior retreat of Hensen's node. Its long axis is the anteroposterior axis, as featured in Figure 4.1. At right angles to this is the mediolateral axis. Because chick is a bilaterally symmetrical animal, this axis comprises left and right halves separated by a midline (the dashed line). A = anterior; P = posterior; M = medial; L = lateral.

cell's response will reflect its distance from the source. Hence, the cell has received positional information. By this mechanism, signals may organize and pattern cell behaviour over long ranges. For this reason, the signalling source is often called an **organizer** (this term can apply to any inducing tissue, as seen in neural induction, Chapter 3). A signal that provokes more than one cellular response in a concentration-dependent manner is called a **morphogen** (Box 4.1).

4.1.2 Patterning occurs within a monolayer epithelium

How does the simple concept of positional information allow the construction of a complex three-dimensional nervous system? As will be apparent from Chapter 2, complex tissue folding and cell movements generate the three-dimensional structure of the nervous system. The neural tissue is much simpler, however, at the stage at which patterning begins. Although the morphology of the embryo differs markedly between different organisms, the neuroectoderm essentially begins as a simple two-dimensional sheet of cells. Therefore, one can imagine that two morphogen systems working at right angles to each other could be enough to instruct cells with all the positional information they need about their location within the neuroectoderm (Fig. 4.2). We shall see that this is essentially what happens. In one direction, patterning occurs in the axis running from anterior to posterior (the **anteroposterior** (AP) axis). The second axis is at right angles to the AP axis, and is termed either the **dorsoventral** (DV) axis or the **mediolateral** (ML) axis, as will be explained later in this chapter (Section 4.5). Ultimately the cells of the neuroectoderm integrate the information in both axes and respond accordingly.

4.1.3 Patterning happens progressively

Another principle that helps to explain how complexity is built is that patterning occurs progressively. We shall see that broad domains are

Box 4.1 The French Flag model of morphogens and positional information

The concept of the morphogen was famously encapsulated in the 1960s by Lewis Wolpert in his French Flag analogy. In a hypothetical epithelium, a signal is produced by a group of cells (an **organizer**) on one side of the cell field. This signal diffuses to form a concentration gradient. Cells respond to the level of this signal to become 'blue, white or red' cell types. Close to the source, cells receive a signal above the highest threshold (blue line) and respond to become 'blue' cells. Beyond this, cells respond to a lower dose to become 'white' cells. Further still, cells do not receive enough signal to respond, and become 'red' cells by default. In the absence of any signal (e.g. in a mutant), all cells would become default red cells.

The cellular response to a morphogen is usually not the acquisition of a specific cell fate directly. Instead, the immediate response is the expression of specific transcription factors in domains within the epithelium. Expression of these transcription factors acts as a read-out of the morphogen gradient, and subsequently they influence cell behaviour or fates through affecting the expression of other genes.

Recipient cells have an intrinsic ability to respond appropriately to the morphogen gradient, which depends on their previous developmental history. This is known as **competence**. Thus, in another part of the developing embryo, cells may respond to a gradient of the above morphogen by activating green, white and orange genes (the Irish flag). The **context-dependence** of cellular response to signalling is key to explaining how a small toolkit of signalling pathways is used over and again in neural development with a huge variety of outcomes.

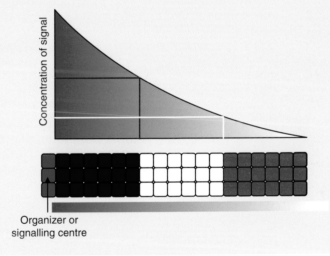

Organizer or
signalling centre

defined initially, and then these are subdivided further to build more and more complexity. In addition, in some organisms the body is divided into **segments** along the AP axis. This is particularly clear in the external body plan of insects where, for instance, the thorax is divided into three segments, each bearing a pair of legs. The insect nervous system is also divided into 15 segmental units called **ganglia**, each containing some 800 neurons by the end of embryogenesis (Chapter 2, Fig. 2.2). Segmentation has clear developmental benefits in terms of simplifying the patterning process. The task of determining the arrangement of large numbers of neurons in the embryonic CNS is divided up into two more manageable tasks: first, the neuroectoderm is divided into a reiterated series of domains (segments); then a common local blueprint of neural cell arrangements is patterned within each segment. Segmentation is a strategy

segments many animals are divided up into reiterated units called segments. In some cases this is clearly visible (e.g. the segments of an earthworm) but in many cases segments are only apparent during development. Also known as metameres.

that is also used in patterning vertebrate hindbrain, but it is not a feature of the rest of the CNS. In the next section, we examine how AP patterning is achieved in *Drosophila*.

4.2 Patterning the anteroposterior (AP) axis of the *Drosophila* CNS

Historically, studying the AP patterning of the *Drosophila* embryo has provided us with dramatic insights into the genetic mechanisms by which complex patterns can emerge from simple beginnings. It was the first developmental process to be subjected to a systematic genetic screen to identify mutations in genes that caused pattern disruptions (e.g. see Box 1 in Chapter 1). This work was so influential that it led to two of the scientists involved, Christiane Nüsslein-Volhard and Eric Wieschaus, receiving the Nobel Prize for Medicine in 1995.[1] Although their screen was based on **epidermis** pattern features, the genes uncovered are also relevant to the nervous system because both tissues rely on patterning within the embryonic ectoderm, which later becomes segregated into epidermis and neuroectoderm (Chapter 3, Section 3.5).

4.2.1 Creating domains of transcription factor expression

Patterning in the *Drosophila* AP axis involves a cascade of regulatory events which divides the early embryo into broad domains and then into a greater number of smaller domains, corresponding to the segments. The starting point is the production of morphogen gradients along the entire AP axis of the embryo (Fig. 4.3). A major morphogen is encoded by the *bicoid* gene. *bicoid* mRNA is synthesized in the mother's **nurse cells** and then deposited in the maturing egg, where it becomes anchored in the cytoplasm at the anterior end. After fertilization, Bicoid protein is synthesized and diffuses posteriorly to form a concentration gradient. Unusually for a signalling molecule, Bicoid is a transcription factor. At this early stage, the *Drosophila* embryo is a **syncytium**: it consists of many nuclei in a common cytoplasm. Since there are no cell membranes separating the nuclei until later in development, Bicoid is free to diffuse and enter nuclei throughout the embryo. The first task of Bicoid is to induce the synthesis of another transcription factor, Hunchback, which also forms an AP concentration gradient.

Nuclei at different locations along the AP axis are exposed to different levels of Bicoid and Hunchback. These different levels induce the expression of proteins encoded by the **gap genes** in broad AP domains (Fig. 4.3). Gap genes are so named because when mutated, whole regions of the embryo are missing corresponding to the domain of their expression. The regulation of the gap genes nicely illustrates the concentration-dependent effects of morphogens at the molecular level.

epidermis the outermost layers of cells covering the exterior body surface.

nurse cells cells that contribute material to a growing egg cell within the ovary.

---

[1] http://nobelprize.org/nobel_prizes/medicine/laureates/1995/index.html [20 November 2010].

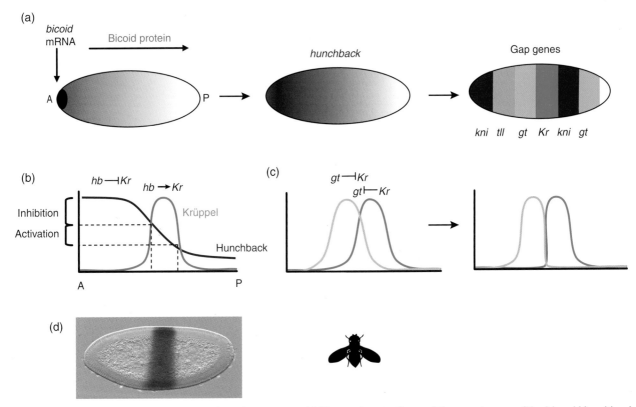

Fig. 4.3 Establishing the regional expression of gap genes. (a) Expression gradients of the morphogens, Bicoid and Hunchback (HB), are formed in the syncytial blastoderm embryo. These switch on the gap genes in different regions along the AP axis, including *knirps* (*kni*), *tailless* (*tll*), *giant* (*gt*) and *Krüppel* (*Kr*).(b) Regulation of the *Krüppel* (*Kr*) gene by HB protein is shown as a graph representing protein levels along the AP axis of the embryo. HB inhibits *Kr* expression at high concentrations (near the anterior) but activates at moderate concentrations (in the middle). (c) Initially, the gap genes (e.g. *gt* and *Kr*) are expressed in broad overlapping domains. Cross-repressive interactions sharpen the boundaries between these domains. (d) Image of an embryo in which *Kr* mRNA has been detected by *in situ* hybridization (see Box 4 in Chapter 3 for an explanation of this method). (Image from Haecker, A., Qi, D., Lilja, T., Moussian, B., Andrioli, L. P., Luschnig, S. and Mannervik, M. (2007) *Drosophila* brakeless interacts with atrophin and is required for tailless-mediated transcriptional repression in early embryos. *PLoS Biology*, **5**, e145. (Creative Commons Attribution Licence).)

For instance, the expression domain of the gap gene, *Krüppel*, is positioned due to its regulation at different threshold levels of Hunchback protein. At high levels in the anterior, Hunchback is a transcriptional repressor of the *Krüppel* gene. At lower levels, it becomes an activator of *Krüppel*, but at lower levels still (in the posterior), Hunchback is unable to affect *Krüppel* expression (Fig. 4.3). The upshot is that Krüppel protein is expressed in a discrete domain in the middle of the embryo. The gap gene products themselves are transcriptional repressors. They are initially expressed in rather fuzzy overlapping domains, but mutual repression between the gap genes acts to sharpen the boundaries of their expression to give discrete domains (Fig. 4.3).

With these broad bands of gap gene expression, the nuclei of the early embryo have received their first dose of patterning along the AP axis. In order to refine this crude initial subdivision, the gap gene products regulate two further sets of genes – the pair-rule genes and the homeotic genes.

Fig. 4.4 (a) Pair-rule and Hox genes are activated by Hunchback and the gap genes. Pair-rule genes such as *eve* and *ftz* are activated in seven stripes, marking the segments. The gap genes and pair-rule genes combine to activate Hox genes in different groups of segments. Note that by the stage of Hox gene activation, the embryo has reached the 'germ-band extended' stage where the posterior end of the embryo loops over the rest of the body (see Chapter 2, Section 2.2). (b) Image of *ftz* mRNA expression as detected by *in situ* hybridization in a fixed embryo. The nuclei of the embryo glow brightly due to a fluorescent stain while *ftz* mRNA is seen as seven dark stripes corresponding to odd-numbered segments (image courtesy of Ilan Davis, University of Oxford). (c) In this embryo, seven different Hox gene mRNAs have been detected using multiple fluorescent probes (image from Lemons, D. and McGinnis, W. (2006) Genomic evolution of Hox gene clusters. *Science*, **313**, 1918–1922.)

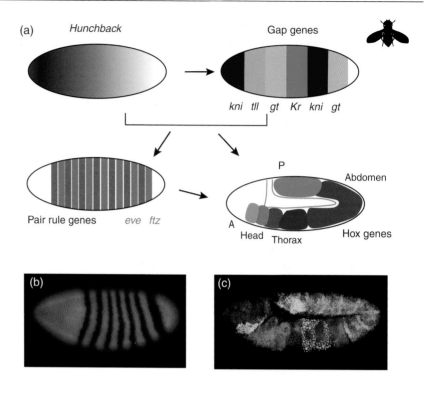

4.2.2 Dividing the ectoderm into segmental units

Gap gene products activate the **pair-rule genes** in a reiterated pattern of smaller domains. Their expression establishes the number and position of segments. The pair-rule gene *even-skipped* (*eve*) is activated in seven stripes marking domains that will become the even-numbered segments (hence, when mutated, even-numbered segments are lost or 'skipped' – Fig. 4.4). *fushi tarazu* (Japanese for 'not enough segments') is expressed in a complementary pattern of stripes, thereby marking the odd-numbered segments. There are many other pair-rule genes with complex regulatory interactions between them that refine the extent and boundaries of the segments.

4.2.3 Assigning segmental identity – the Hox code

The basic pattern of neurogenesis is largely the same in each segment, each giving rise to an individual segmental ganglion (look ahead to Fig. 4.20). However, this pattern must be modified according to the segment's location along the AP axis. For instance, thoracic segments have different musculature compared with abdominal segments, and so require a somewhat different pattern of motor neurons within their segmental ganglia. This is particularly apparent in the adult fly in which thoracic segments have legs and wings, which require sophisticated musculature that is not present in abdominal segments. A mechanism is therefore required to give segments individual identity.

homeotic typically referring to a mutation that causes the change of one body part or region to resemble another, such as leg to wing, or thoracic segment to abdominal segment.

In the 1940s, Ed Lewis began studying a distinctive class of genes. Instead of causing loss or malformation of body parts, mutations of these genes (now known generally as **Hox genes**) caused **homeotic** transformations in segment identity. That is, a segment would be transformed perfectly to resemble another segment. For instance, mutation of *Ultrabithorax* (*Ubx*) causes the third thoracic segment to develop as though it had the identity of the second thoracic segment: the resulting mutant fly has a pair of wings on its normal second segment and an extra pair on its now transformed third segment. The normal function of Hox genes, therefore, is to assign identity to a segment, and they are also known as **selector genes**. Lewis's work eventually led to his sharing the Nobel Prize with Nüsslein-Volhard and Wieschaus.

With the advent of molecular cloning, the homeotic genes were discovered to encode a family of related transcription factors. Each of the genes shares a related sequence called the **homeobox**, which encodes the DNA-binding domain (the **homeodomain**) of the transcription factor proteins (Chapter 3, Box 3). We now know that during evolution all of the Hox genes arose by a series of **tandem duplications** of a single primordial Hox gene. The duplicated genes remain clustered together on the chromosome (although this has become split into two separate clusters relatively recently in *Drosophila* evolution – Fig. 4.5).

The different Hox genes are expressed in an overlapping series of domains in the AP axis. Strikingly, the order of these domains reflects the order of the genes on the chromosome (Fig. 4.5). As a result of the overlapping expression domains, each segment expresses a unique combination of Hox genes and it is thought that these combinations give different AP regions their identity. This is known as the **Hox code**.[2]

With the expression of gap genes, pair-rule genes and Hox genes, the ectoderm is divided into segments, and each segment is supplied with information about its location on the AP axis. The next step entails local patterning within each segment. In this step, **segmentation genes** are activated in narrow stripes within each segment. However, we shall consider this process after first addressing early AP patterning in vertebrates.

selector gene a gene that regulates an entire developmental programme (e.g. thoracic segment vs abdominal segment) rather than specifying particular cell types. Examples are Hox genes. Mutation of a selector gene tends to be homeotic.

tandem duplication the evolutionary process by which a section of DNA (e.g. containing one or more genes) becomes duplicated so that the chromosome now has two copies of the section in tandem. A common way in which gene families are initially formed.

4.3 Patterning the AP axis of the vertebrate CNS

4.3.1 Hox genes are highly conserved

One of the most significant milestones in developmental biology was the discovery that Hox gene complexes are highly conserved in both structure and function in a whole host of animals, from *C. elegans* to humans. It is astonishing to think that the common ancestor of insects and vertebrates already had a sophisticated Hox gene system for nervous system patterning. Early in vertebrate evolution the entire cluster of genes became duplicated several times, giving rise to four separate Hox gene clusters (Fig. 4.5). Just as in *Drosophila*, these genes are expressed in an overlapping series of domains along the AP axis of the neural tube, with the order of expression corresponding to the

---

[2] For further reading on the Hox code, see Myers, P. Z. (2008) Hox genes in development: the Hox code. *Nature Education*, **1**(1).(http://www.nature.com/scitable/topicpage/hox-genes-in-development-the-hox-code-41402 [20 November 2010]).

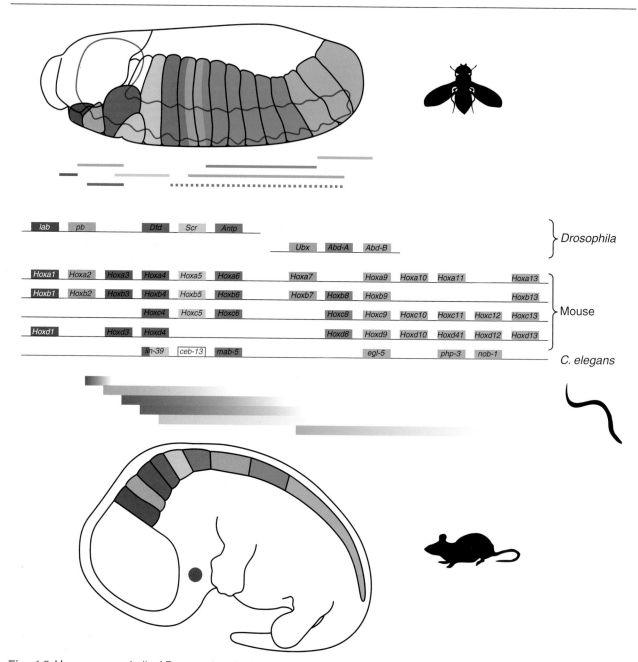

Fig. 4.5 Hox genes underlie AP patterning. In the centre are represented the chromosomal arrangement of Hox genes (in 'gene clusters') in *Drosophila*, mouse and *C. elegans*. The genes are colour-coded to show their sequence homology across species. In *Drosophila*, the cluster has been split into two. In mouse, the cluster has been duplicated twice, and there have been subsequent losses or duplications of certain genes in each cluster. The cluster is also conserved in a simplified form in *C. elegans* even though this organism is not segmented. The embryos are coloured to represent the regions that are most affected by each gene – note that the order is the same as the order of genes on the chromosome. Next to each embryo is depicted the approximate expression domains of the genes. Note how in mouse the area affected by each gene is coincident with the anterior limit of its expression domain. (Redrawn with permission from Macmillan Publishers Ltd: Pearson, J. C., Lemons, D. and McGinnis, W. (2005) Modulating Hox gene functions during animal body patterning. *Nature Reviews Genetics*, **6**, 893–904, copyright 2005.)

gene order in the clusters. Hox genes are important for patterning the vertebrate hindbrain and spinal cord, as will be addressed later.

4.3.2 Initial AP information is imparted by the mesoderm

Given the dramatic conservation of Hox gene function in all animals, one might think that other aspects of *Drosophila* AP patterning are also conserved in vertebrates. However, this is not generally the case (with some important exceptions). The mechanism involving Bicoid, the gap genes and pair-rule genes does not function in vertebrates. Instead, initial AP patterning is triggered by signals from the mesoderm, and is closely connected with the process of neural induction itself, the topic of Chapter 3. This process has been well investigated in *Xenopus*. Recall that neural induction results from the secretion of **bone morphogenetic protein** (BMP) antagonists by the mesoderm as it slides underneath the dorsal ectoderm during gastrulation (Section 3.4). These BMP antagonists counteract the anti-neural effects of BMP in the overlying dorsal ectoderm, leading to formation of the **neural plate**. In his initial transplant experiments that demonstrated the inductive properties of mesoderm, Spemann discovered that transplanting the dorsal lip of the blastopore from *late*-stage gastrulating embryos induced neural tissue with posterior fates only, showing that it behaved as an inducer differently from *early*-stage dorsal lip. Hence, initial AP information is imparted by the mesoderm at the same time as neural induction. This led to a two-signal model for the mesoderm's role in neural induction and patterning: first an **activation signal** (inducing signal) generally induces neuroectoderm formation but this has an anterior character by default. In the posterior of the embryo, the mesoderm secretes an additional **transformation signal** which confers posterior identity information (Fig. 4.6).

As was discussed in Chapter 3, the activation signal involves antagonists of BMPs. The nature of the transformation signal is problematic. Fibroblast growth factors (FGFs), Nodal, retinoic acid (RA) and Wnts have all been implicated. Particularly strong candidates are RA (Box 4.2) and, more recently, Wnt (Fig. 3.6 in Chapter 3). In the case of

bone morphogenetic proteins a family of about 20 secreted intercellular signalling molecules with functions throughout development, but particularly important in the establishment of neuroectoderm and its patterning.

neural plate a sheet of neuroectoderm that rolls up to form the neural tube.

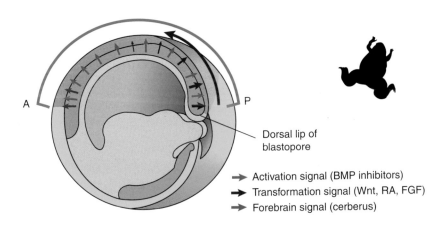

A

P

Dorsal lip of blastopore

→ Activation signal (BMP inhibitors)
→ Transformation signal (Wnt, RA, FGF)
→ Forebrain signal (cerberus)

Fig. 4.6 In *Xenopus*, AP patterning of the neural plate is induced by the mesoderm. The bracket denotes the AP axis of the neuroectoderm overlying the mesoderm. Activation signals (red) promote neural induction, while graded transformation signals (blue) are required to confer posterior neural identity. In the absence of transformation signals (in the anterior), the neural tissue adopts an anterior character. This transformation signal may be produced either by the posterior mesoderm (short blue arrows) or by the late-stage dorsal lip of the blastopore itself (curved blue arrow), or both. More recently, it has been found that a separate anterior signal is required for forebrain induction (green).

Box 4.2 The retinoic acid (RA) signalling pathway

Unlike most of the signals involved in neural development, RA is not a protein, but a small organic molecule related to vitamin A. Its signal transduction pathway is relatively simple. RA diffuses across the membrane of recipient cells into the cytoplasm where it complexes with a receptor protein (RA receptor or RAR). The RA-RAR complex translocates into the nucleus, where it activates target genes by binding to a DNA sequence called the retinoic acid response element (RARE). Such sequences regulate the expression of some of the Hox genes.

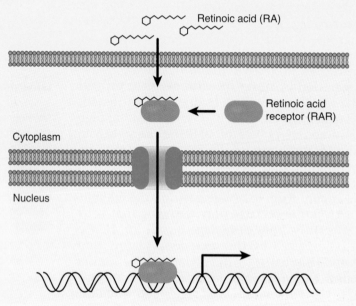

chick, the expression gradients of these signals are likely to be laid down during the anterior-to-posterior retreat of Hensen's node during axis extension (see Chapter 3, Section 3.6).[3]

Recently, it was discovered that the activation–transformation model is not enough to pattern the whole AP axis. In addition to the posteriorizing signals, specific signals are required for the extreme anterior of the nervous system. These signals emanate from the early-stage dorsal lip of the blastopore during gastrulation and from the anterior-most mesoderm that is formed at this stage (known as the **prechordal plate**). One of these signals is cerberus, the head inducer that we met in Chapter 3 (Section 3.4). This signal is secreted by the prechordal plate and has very strong forebrain inducing activity (Fig. 4.7). It seems that cerberus is a multifunctional inhibitor of BMP, nodal and Wnts, which may explain its powerful effect in promoting head development.

---

[3] For more information of this aspect, see Wilson, V., Olivera-Martinez, I. and Storey, K. G. (2009) Stem cells, signals and vertebrate body axis extension. *Development*, **136**, 1591–1604.

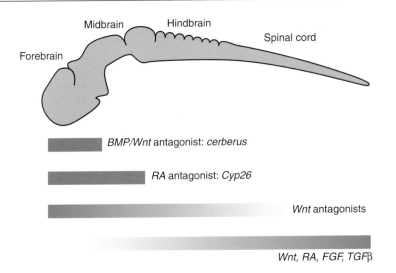

Fig. 4.7 Expression domains of some of the signals and other molecules implicated in long-range AP axis patterning in vertebrates. Some of these are morphogens with graded effects along the AP axis. Wnt signalling directly regulates regionally expressed genes which encode transcription factors; for example, it represses the anterior patterning gene, *Otx2*. The initial effect of RA, however, might be to establish AP patterning within the mesoderm, which subsequently affects the overlying neuroectoderm. In zebrafish, an RA degrading enzyme (Cyp26) is produced at the anterior end, and this restricts RA action to more posterior regions. Similarly, Wnt antagonists are also produced anteriorly.

4.3.3 Mesoderm signals set up domains of transcription factor expression

As with the *Drosophila* gap genes, the initial response to these patterning signals is the activation of transcription factors in different AP expression domains within the neural plate. In the anterior, a set of genes encoding transcription factors respond to head signals and the absence of transformation signals to define the regions of the anterior brain (Fig. 4.8). For instance, the **midbrain–hindbrain boundary** is defined by abutting expression domains of the genes *Otx2* and *Gbx2* which encode homeodomain transcription factors. *Otx2* is critical to anterior brain formation: in mouse *Otx2* mutants, the entire forebrain and midbrain are missing. The **forebrain–midbrain boundary** arises between the expression domains of the transcription factor genes *Pax6* and *En1*. Within the forebrain, a boundary is formed at the junction of *Six3* and *Irx3* expression domains. This is called the **zona limitans intrathalamica** (ZLI), and is important for patterning within the **diencephalon**.

Within the forebrain, the telencephalon is itself further subdivided by the regional expression of further transcription factor genes. For example, *Emx1* and *Emx2* divide the telencephalon into regions that

diencephalon a component of the early forebrain of vertebrates, situated caudal to the telencephalic vesicle, giving rise to adult structures including the thalamus.

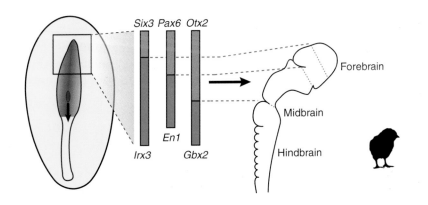

Fig. 4.8 Regions in the anterior brain are defined by domains of transcription factor expression in the neural plate. The bars represent the AP extent of expression for pairs of genes, such as *Six3* and *Irx3*. Each pair of genes defines a border between two future brain regions, as becomes apparent later in development (on the right). Thus, the interface of *Otx2* and *Gbx2* expression defines the midbrain–hindbrain boundary. In a manner reminiscent of *Drosophila* gap genes, the genes of each pair are initially activated in broad, somewhat overlapping domains, and then their borders are sharpened by mutual repression.

Box 4.3 Human congenital diseases due to mutations in anterior regionalization genes

A number of disorders of the nervous system are caused by mutations in patterning genes. In most cases, the disorders are apparent in individuals who are heterozygous for the gene mutation (and therefore also have one normal copy of the gene). Homozygous mutation is very rare, but can be expected to lead to catastrophic failure in brain development, resulting in lethality before or just after birth.

SIX3: Mutations in the human *SIX3* gene can result in a disorder called holoprosencephaly. In a severe form of this disease the left and right forebrain hemispheres fail to separate during the development of the prosencephalon. This is consistent with *SIX3*'s role in regionalization of the anterior neural tube.

PAX6: Heterozygous mutations in *PAX6* result in a spectrum of eye abnormalities and more subtle defects in the olfactory system and the brain. Many such mutations are known. Very rare cases have both *PAX6* genes affected, resulting in lethality with a catastrophic loss of head and forebrain structures (as shown in (a) and (b) below).

EMX2: Individuals who have one defective *EMX2* gene show severe schizencephaly in which large portions of the cerebral hemispheres may be completely absent (as observed in computerised tomography (CT) scans in (c) and (d) below).

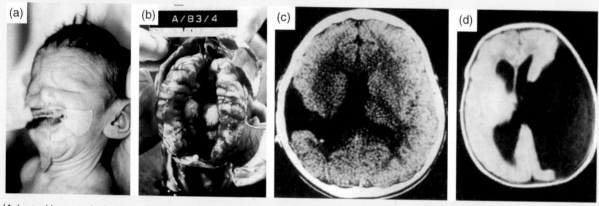

(Adapted by permission from Macmillan Publishers Ltd. Brunelli, S. *et al.* (1994) Glaser, T. *et al.* (1996) *PAX6* gene dosage effect in a family with congenital cataracts, aniridia, anophthalmia and central nervous system defects. *Nature Genetics*, **12**, 94–96, copyright 1996 (left) and Brunelli, S. et al. (1994) Germline mutations in the homeobox gene EMX2 in patients with severe schizencephaly. Nature Genetics, 7, 463–471, copyright 1994 (right).)

homologue a gene or structure that is similar in different species since it was derived from their common ancestor during evolution.

will form the anterior (mainly motor) and posterior (mainly sensory) halves of the cerebral hemispheres. Mutation of *Emx2* can cause severe congenital defects in humans (Box 4.3). The function of *Emx2* in subdividing the cerebral hemispheres will be discussed again in Chapter 9. Intriguingly, *Otx2* and *Emx1/2* are **homologues** of two genes which similarly play a role in *Drosophila* anterior brain regionalization: *orthodenticle* (*otd*) and *empty spiracles* (*ems*). Although there is probably little in common structurally between the insect and vertebrate brain, this homology implies a very ancient mechanism for patterning the anterior end of the CNS.

4.3.4 The hindbrain is organized into segments called rhombomeres

The patterning of the anterior brain does not involve true segmentation (in the sense of reiterated segmental units). However, patterning

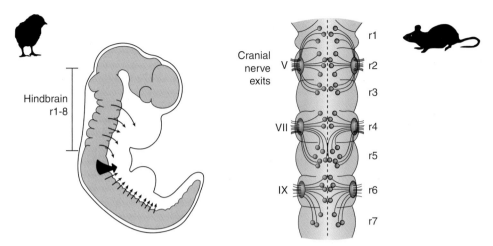

Fig. 4.9 As the neural tube develops, the hindbrain is characterized by swellings called rhombomeres; in chick (left) there are eight rhombomeres, but only seven are visible in mouse (right). Rhombomeres are segmental units, each of which exhibits a similar pattern of neurons later in development. In addition, there are differences between odd- and even-numbered rhombomeres, as illustrated by the arrangement of cranial nerve exits (right) and also the formation of neural crest cells (not illustrated here).

of the hindbrain **primordium** (the **rhombencephalon**) is achieved via a process of segmentation. The first visible sign of segmentation is the transient appearance of eight swellings in the neural tube soon after closure. These are termed **rhombomeres** and are designated r1–r8 (Fig. 4.9). These segments are a crucial developmental stage in the later anatomical and functional organization of the hindbrain. For instance, the initial formation of neurons within the hindbrain shows a clear segmentally repeated pattern, although this later becomes obscured by the shear scale of neurogenesis. The arrangement of **cranial nerve** exits shows an underlying two-segment repeating pattern: odd- and even-numbered segments have different patterns of neurons, and motor axon exit points derive only from even-numbered rhombomeres. The molecular pathway of rhombomere formation is quite distinct from that of *Drosophila* segmentation.

primordium an embryological term for a region that will subsequently give rise to a particular organ or tissue.

cranial nerves the nerves emerging from the vertebrate hindbrain.

4.3.5 How rhombomeres are specified

Our knowledge of how rhombomeres are specified is surprisingly patchy. Much of what we know originally came from studies in chick, and more recently from genetic studies in zebrafish. The first stage of rhombomere specification is the activation of transcription factors in odd- or even-segment patterns in response to initial AP signalling (similar to the pair-rule genes in *Drosophila*). One of the first such genes discovered was *Krox20*, which encodes a zinc-finger transcription factor (Figure 4.10). This gene is expressed in regions that become r3 and r5. In *Krox20* knock-out mice r3 and r5 are missing, and r2, r4 and r6 become fused together. Conversely, enforcing *Krox20* expression in even-numbered rhombomeres makes them take on odd-numbered characteristics. Thus, *Krox20* is required for their odd-segment identity.

As with *Drosophila* segments, rhombomeres have distinct identities. For instance, r1 will form the **cerebellum**. These identities are

cerebellum meaning 'little brain' it is a discrete structure at the base of the brain that lies above the brainstem. It regulates a range of functions including motor control, attention and cognition.

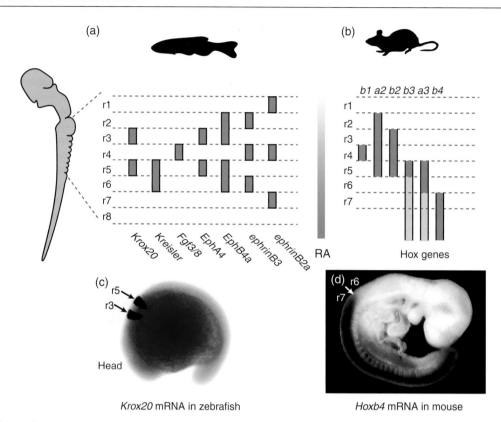

Fig. 4.10 Expression patterns of genes involved in rhombomere specification. (a) Summary of genes expressed in rhombomere-specific patterns. These are primarily based on chick and zebrafish studies. *kreisler* encodes a transcription factor that probably helps to regulate *Krox20*. Ephs and ephrins are involved in keeping the rhombomeres separate (see next figure). We have little idea at present how these domains of expression are set up in response to the graded AP signals such as RA. One important event is the setting up of a new signalling centre in the future r4, from which FGF signals emanate. These act locally in cooperation with RA to set up gene expression domains in r5 and 6. (b) The Hox gene expression patterns are from mouse – there are some differences in other vertebrates. (c) Expression of *Krox20* mRNA in prospective rhombomeres 3 and 5 of a zebrafish embryo. *Krox20* is a homologue of *Drosophila Krüppel* (image courtesy of Qiliang Lin and David Wilkinson). (d) Expression of *Hoxb4* mRNA in the mouse neural tube posterior to r6. (Image from. Brend, T., Gilthorpe, J., Summerbell, D. and Rigby, P. W. J. (2003) Multiple levels of transcriptional and post-transcriptional regulation are required to define the domain of Hoxb4 expression. *Development*, **130**, 2717–2728.)

likely to be conferred by the Hox genes (Fig. 4.5). Hox gene activation precedes segmentation, but subsequently there is extensive cross-regulation by rhombomere specification genes such as *Krox20*, which establishes sharp borders of Hox gene expression that coincide with rhombomere boundaries (Fig. 4.10). The function of Hox genes in rhombomere identity is not yet entirely established, but there are some striking experimental observations. In chick, ectopic expression of *Hoxb1* (a gene normally expressed exclusively in r4) causes a transformation of r2 to resemble r4. Conversely, r4 is transformed to resemble r2 when *Hoxb1* is mutated in mouse. Thus, *Hoxb1* is a **homeotic selector gene** for r4 identity. However, mutations of other Hox genes often have more complex phenotypes that include loss of rhombomeres. Consequently, it has been suggested that Hox genes play a role in the process of segmentation as well as segment identity, unlike their *Drosophila* counterparts.

As might be expected, Hox genes are regulated by the early posteriorizing signals, thereby converting graded posterior-to-anterior information into the sequence of Hox gene expression domains. Indeed, some Hox genes are directly regulated by RA (Box 4.2). In addition, in posterior regions RA and FGF regulate Hox genes via intermediate transcription factors encoded by the *Cdx* gene family. These are related to the *Drosophila* gene *caudal*, which regulates gap and Hox genes in the posterior *Drosophila* embryo.

In addition to the hindbrain, more posteriorly expressed Hox genes create regional differences along the spinal cord. In chick, the cervical (neck) region of the spinal cord is defined by the expression of *Hoxc6*, whereas more caudal parts (such as the thoracic spinal cord) express genes such as *Hoxc9* (Fig. 4.5). Forcing the expression of *Hoxc6* in the thoracic neural tube induces it to produce motor neurons of a type normally found only in the cervical region (namely, those that innervate the forelimbs).

Although the spinal cord exhibits an obvious repeating pattern in terms of nerve roots, this does not appear to represent true segmentation (in the sense of reiterated developmental modules). Instead, this periodicity is induced in the neural tube at a relatively late stage by signals emanating from the adjacent mesodermal **somites**.

somites segmental masses of mesoderm lying on either side of the notochord and neural tube during the development of vertebrate embryos.

4.4 Refining AP axis patterning within regions and segments

In both *Drosophila* and vertebrates, the mechanisms that we have covered so far divide the AP axis rather coarsely into regions and segments. Subsequently, fine-tuned patterning occurs within these regions to define subregions and local patterns of neurogenesis. A common theme that emerges in different organisms is that short-range signalling occurs between the cells at the boundaries of adjacent regions to keep the regions distinct. In addition, these interactions often lead to the appearance of distinct populations of boundary cells between domains, which then act as signalling centres to organize local patterning within the domains.

4.4.1 Rhombomere cell populations are kept separate by Eph–ephrin signalling

The sharp boundaries that are formed between rhombomeres result from differences in proteins on the membranes of cells in odd and even segments, which cause them to avoid contact with each other. The repulsion between cells of adjacent rhombomeres sharpens their boundaries and maintains them as independent developmental units. The molecules mediating this repulsion appear to be members of the **Eph-ephrin** families of cell surface molecules, which are expressed in different combinations of rhombomeres (Figs 4.10 and 4.11). Expression of the genes encoding these proteins is under the control of the segmentation and segment identity transcription factors. For

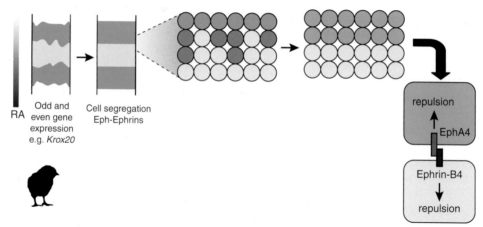

Fig. 4.11 At the boundary between two rhombomeres, ephrins on the cell surface bind to their Eph receptor partners on adjacent cells. Unusually, the Eph–ephrin interaction appears to cause a response in both cells (signalling is bidirectional). The response is mutual repulsion between cells. The upshot is that cells in adjacent rhombomeres attempt to minimize their contact by rearranging, which sharpens the boundaries.

Fig. 4.12 In *Drosophila*, expression of genes encoding two signalling molecules, *wg* and *hh*, initiates fine-tuned patterning within each segment. Their mRNAs are expressed in narrow abutting stripes and the secreted protein products diffuse, leading ultimately to activation of other segmentation genes in 1–2 cell-wide stripes, represented schematically here. The image shows expression of one of the segmentation genes, *engrailed*. This is expressed in the anterior of each segmental compartment. *engrailed* encodes a transcription factor that is important for *hh* activation.

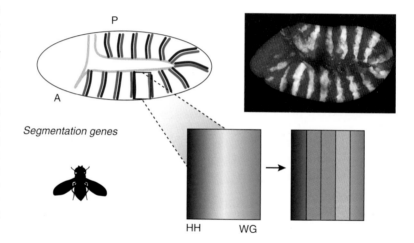

example, the *EphA4* gene is directly activated by *Krox20* in rhombomeres 3 and 5. Ephs and ephrins play well-known roles in other aspects of neural development (Chapters 6, 8, 9).

4.4.2 Boundaries organize local patterning in Drosophila segments

Revisiting *Drosophila* segmentation, the pair-rule genes define segments and they cooperate to regulate a further series of genes within each segment – the **segmentation** genes. An important initial step is the activation of segmentation genes *wingless* (*wg*) and *hedgehog* (*hh*) in adjacent stripes in each segment (Fig. 4.12). *wg* encodes a Wnt signal protein (Chapter 3, Section 3.6); *hh* encodes a highly conserved signal protein whose homologues feature prominently later in this chapter (Box 4.4). The juxtaposition of *wg* and *hh* expression stripes defines the boundaries of discrete developmental units similar to rhombomeres.

Box 4.4   The hedgehog (HH) signalling pathway

The signal transduction pathway for HH is rather convoluted. The cell's receptor for HH is the transmembrane protein, Patched. In the absence of HH, Patched prevents another transmembrane protein, Smoothened, from reaching the cell surface. Upon HH binding, the Patched receptor is down-regulated, thereby allowing Smoothened to move to the surface. Here it inhibits a protease complex that normally cleaves a GLI family transcription factor (encoded by the *cubitus interruptus* gene in *Drosophila*). The cleaved form of the GLI protein is a transcriptional repressor whereas the uncleaved form is an activator. Thus the upshot of HH binding to a cell is the conversion of GLI from a repressor to an activator, with consequent changes in the expression of target genes.

HH was discovered because when mutated, the embryos are covered with spiny denticles (resembling a hedgehog's spines), indicating a disruption of epidermal patterning in the segments. Subsequently, several vertebrate homologues were found. One of these plays an important role in vertebrate neural patterning and is known as Sonic hedgehog (SHH) (unfortunately named after a video game character). The signalling pathway is highly conserved, with a major difference in vertebrates being that when Smoothened protein reaches the cell surface in response to SHH signalling, it moves into a cellular outgrowth called the primary **cilium**, where it carries out its function.

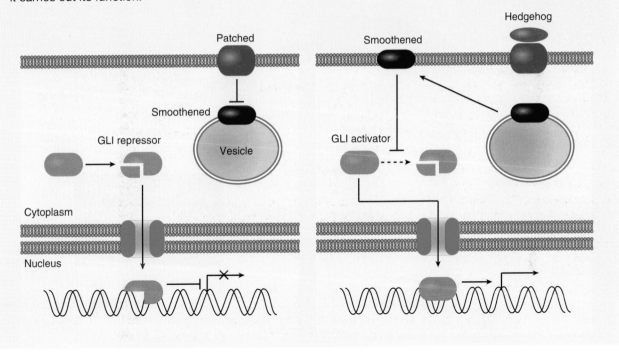

Each boundary now acts as a local organizer with *wg* and *hh* diffusing into each segment and acting as local morphogens. Their action eventually leads to the expression of a series of other segmentation genes in abutting 1–2 cell wide stripes across the segment (Fig. 4.12). As a result of this local patterning, ectodermal cells have very precise information about their location within a segment.[4]

---

[4] More information on Hedgehog's role in *Drosophila* segmentation is included in Ingham, P. W. and Placzek, M. (2006) Orchestrating ontogenesis: variations on a theme by sonic hedgehog. *Nature Reviews Genetics*, **7**, 841–850.

4.4.3 In the vertebrate brain, boundaries organize local patterning

In the vertebrate CNS, the boundaries between anterior brain regions also become key local signalling centres (Fig. 4.13). The best-studied example of this is the **isthmic organizer**, a group of cells formed close to the future midbrain–hindbrain border. This expresses FGF8 and WNT1, which diffuse locally to activate a number of genes. In particular, the transcription factors encoded by *En1* and *En2* (homologues of *engrailed*) are expressed on both sides of the organizer, where they are required to specify the **tectum** anteriorly and the **cerebellum** posteriorly (Fig. 4.13). Interestingly, *En1/En2* are activated in a graded manner. Later in development, these gradients may be directly involved in

tectum in non-mammalian vertebrates, the site in the brain that receives innervation from retinal ganglion cells. Known as the superior colliculus in mammals.

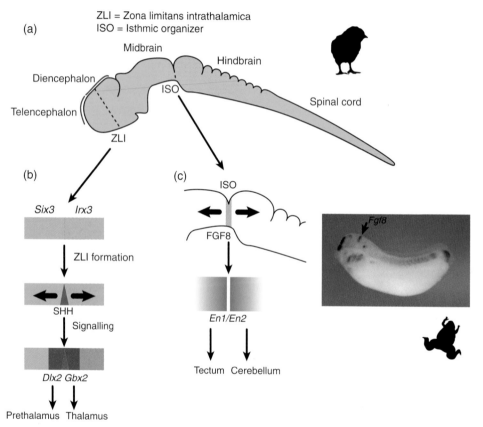

Fig. 4.13 The boundaries between brain regions become new signalling centres for local patterning. (a) Two signalling centres are illustrated here: the zona limitans intrathalamica (ZLI) forms in the diencephalon, and the isthmic organizer (ISO) forms at the midbrain–hindbrain boundary. (b) The ZLI forms at the boundary between *Six3* and *Irx3* expression domains. SHH signalling from the ZLI locally induces the expression of the *Dlx2* anteriorly and *Gbx2* posteriorly, leading to the specification of the prethalamus and thalamus respectively. This difference in cellular response to SHH arises because of the expression of different transcription factor genes on each side of the ZLI (*Six3* and *Irx3*), which cause the SHH signal to be interpreted differently. (c) At the ISO, FGF8 diffuses into the midbrain and first rhombomere, where it activates the *En1* and *En2* genes. This results in the formation of the tectum and cerebellum. The image shows *Fgf8* mRNA expression in a *Xenopus tropicalis* embryo. The stripe of expression at the ISO is indicated by the arrow. (Image from Lea, R., Papalopulu, N., Amaya, E. and Dorey, K. (2009) Temporal and spatial expression of FGF ligands and receptors during *Xenopus* development. *Developmental Dynamics*, **238**, 1467–1479.)

forming expression gradients of Ephs and ephrins in the tectum, which guide neuronal interactions during retinotectal map formation (Chapter 9).

The same signal diffusing both anteriorly and posteriorly from a signalling centre often elicits different transcriptional responses on either side. The ZLI patterns the diencephalon locally by producing Sonic hedgehog (SHH). SHH is one of three vertebrate homologues of *Drosophila* Hedgehog (Box. 4.4). In chick studies, SHH signalling from the ZLI activates the transcription factor genes *Dlx2* on the anterior side and *Gbx2* on the posterior side. This differential response to SHH leads to the formation of the **prethalamus** and **thalamus,** respectively. The basis of this difference depends on the pre-existing expression of the gene *Irx3* posterior to the ZLI. Recall that *Irx3* is one of the two genes implicated in defining the border in the first place (Section 4.3.3). If *Irx3* is ectopically expressed anteriorly to the ZLI, the anterior cells now activate *Gbx2* in response to SHH rather than *Dlx2*. Thus, in general, early subdivisions in the neural plate not only create boundaries that form local secondary organizers, but also define they way in which cells respond to the signals from these organizers (i.e. they define cellular **competence**).[5]

In summary, the boundaries between the initial transcription factor expression domains take on roles as secondary signalling centres for fine-tuned local patterning. Signalling from these boundary cells promotes local patterning of gene expression within domains that directly influence fine-tuned patterns of neurogenesis at a local level. The concept of repeated rounds of patterning, from long-range to local, is a key factor for building complexity in the nervous system.

prethalamus a subdivision of the diencephalon of the vertebrate brain.

thalamus a structure in the centre of the vertebrate brain that transmits sensory input to the cerebral cortex, and receives reciprocal output from the cortex.

4.5 Patterning the dorsoventral (DV) axis of the nervous system

4.5.1 Patterns of neurons in the DV axis of the spinal cord

The **dorsoventral** (DV) axis of the nervous system is at right angles to the AP axis and has a somewhat simpler organization. The result of patterning in this axis can be seen in a cross section of the vertebrate spinal cord (Fig. 4.14). Here, the nervous system has a **bilaterally symmetrical** structure (the left-hand side is a mirror image of the right). On each side, distinct classes of neurons arise at different positions along the DV axis of the neural tube, as classified by morphology, function and gene expression patterns (Fig. 4.14). In fact, at least 11 distinct neuronal domains can be identified. The vertebrate neural tube that forms the spinal cord has provided a good model for exploring mechanisms of patterning.

bilaterally symmetrical most animals have bodies divided into roughly mirror-image halves (left and right).

---

[5] For more detail on boundaries in neural development, see Kiecker, C. and Lumsden, A. (2005) Compartments and their boundaries in vertebrate brain development. *Nature Reviews Neuroscience*, **6**, 553–564.

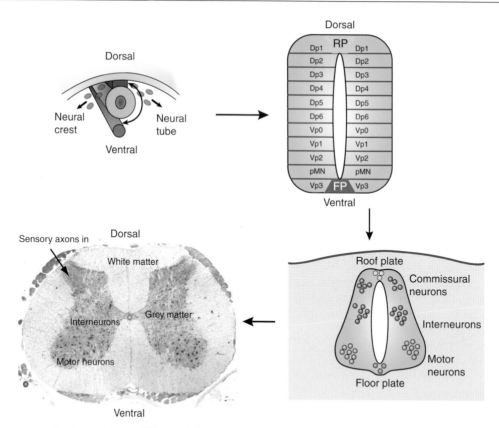

Fig. 4.14 Neural organization within the DV axis of the spinal cord. The photograph (lower left) shows a cross section through the mature cat spinal cord revealing its bilateral symmetry and dorsoventral structure. Motor axons exit ventrally while sensory axons from the dorsal root ganglia enter dorsally. Patterning occurs in the DV axis of the neural tube. Neurons are produced from a series of progenitor domains arranged along the DV axis. For example, pMN contains progenitors of the motor neurons whereas Vp2 gives rise to the V2 interneurons. Neurons involved in sensory input are generated dorsally (including commissural neurons). In addition, specialized glia form the floor plate (FP) and roof plate (RP) at the ventral and dorsal points of the neural tube, respectively. These will later be seen to be crucial for DV patterning.

4.5.2 Embryonic origin of the DV axis

mediolateral the axis of a bilaterally symmetrical organism from its midline to its sides.

The DV axis of the neural tube can be traced back to a **mediolateral** axis in the neural plate. The left and right halves of this axis are separated by a midline. Upon neurulation the midline becomes the ventral apex of the neural tube while the lateral edges of the neural plate join to form the dorsal apex (Fig. 4.15).

As with the AP axis, the molecular mechanisms of patterning in the DV axis involve graded signalling from organizers which are interpreted to give domains of transcription factor expression; these eventually lead to different patterns of neurogenesis. However, a notable difference from the AP axis is that no process of segmentation is involved. Before considering the molecular mechanisms of vertebrate neural tube patterning, we examine what is known about DV patterning in *Drosophila*.

4.5.3 DV neural patterning in Drosophila

Like the neural plate of vertebrates, the *Drosophila* neuroectoderm has a midline in a central position along a mediolateral axis. However, as it

(a)

(b)

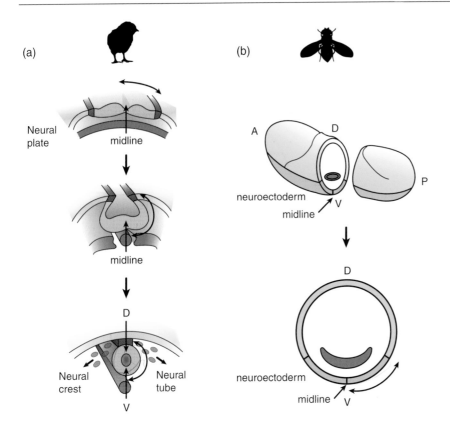

Neural plate
midline
midline
D
Neural crest
Neural tube
V

A
D
P
neuroectoderm
midline
V
D
neuroectoderm
midline
V

Fig. 4.15 Origins of the neural DV axis. (a) In the vertebrate neural plate, the midline defines a central position along the bilaterally symmetrical mediolateral (ML) axis (double-headed arrow) (refer back to Fig. 4.2). However, after neurulation, the midline becomes the *ventral* apex of the neural tube, defining its DV axis. Thus, the ML axis becomes the DV axis. (b) In *Drosophila*, the neural midline also defines a central position along the mediolateral axis in the neuroectoderm. However, this is usually referred to as the DV axis because it is part of the entire DV axis that extends around the circumference of the ectoderm.

also corresponds to the ventral pole of the DV axis of the whole embryonic ectoderm, the mediolateral axis is usually simply called the DV axis (Fig. 4.15). In the previous chapter (Section 3.5), we learnt that neural induction divides the *Drosophila* ectoderm into two large domains marked by high expression of *dpp* dorsally and *sog* (a *dpp* antagonist) ventrally. This also represents the first step in neural patterning along the DV axis, since the *sog* domain (the neuroectoderm) gives rise to the CNS **neuroblasts** and the *dpp* domain (the lateral ectoderm) will later produce the PNS precursors (**sense organ precursors**). How these precursors are produced will be described in Chapter 5.

Subsequently, *dpp* acts as a morphogen in the neuroectoderm. Complex interactions occur between *dpp* and *sog* that result in the diffusion of DPP protein laterally into the neuroectoderm to form a dorsal-to-ventral gradient of activity. Additionally, the transcription factor Dorsal (DL) continues to be expressed in an opposing ventral-to-dorsal gradient. These gradients regulate three genes encoding homeodomain transcription factors so that they are expressed in non-overlapping DV columns (Fig. 4.16). These **columnar genes** are *ventral nervous system defective* (*vnd*), *intermediate defective neuroblasts* (*ind*) and *muscle segment homeobox* (*msh*). The three genes respond to different threshold levels of DL and DPP. For instance, *vnd* expression requires high DL activity and is the most sensitive to inhibition by DPP; together this confines *vnd* expression to cells closest to the future CNS midline.

We now know that the columnar gene system is a very ancient mechanism for dividing up the DV axis of the nervous system. Homologues of the columnar genes are expressed in similar spatial

neuroblasts dividing cells that will develop into neural cells; the term can be used in mammalian and non-mammalian species but is more commonly used in describing insect development.

sense organ precursors (SOPs) (or sensory mother cells) individual ectodermal cells from which sense organs or sensilla develop in insects.

Fig. 4.16 Activation of the *Drosophila* columnar genes. Morphogen gradients of DL and DPP expression combine to activate the expression of *vnd*, *ind* and *msh* in different domains ('columns') along the DV axis in the neuroectoderm. Lower left shows a schematic cross section through the columns, whereas on the right is a lateral view of a fixed embryo showing expression columns of mRNAs of *dpp*, *msh*, *ind* and *vnd* running from top to bottom. Below right shows some of the interactions that regulate the columnar genes. *vnd* is activated by high levels of DL but is very sensitive to inhibition by DPP. This confines its expression close to the ventral midline. *ind* is activated by DL, but is inhibited near the midline by *vnd*, ensuring that its expression is restricted to the middle column abutting *vnd*. In turn *ind* inhibits *msh*, but is itself more susceptible to DPP inhibition than is *msh*. As a result *msh* is expressed in the most dorsal (lateral) part of the neuroectoderm. (Image from Kosman, D., Mizutani, C. M., Lemons, D., Cox, W. G., McGinnis, W. and Bier, E. (2004) Multiplex detection of RNA expression in *Drosophila* embryos. *Science*, **305**, 846).

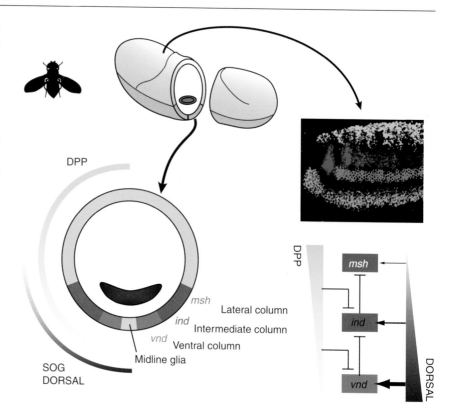

neural crest part of the ectoderm located between the neural tube and the epidermis that contributes neurons and other cells throughout the body of vertebrates.

arrangements at the earliest stages of DV neural patterning in a wide range of organisms, including vertebrates, segmented worms and primitive chordates.[6]

4.5.4 DV patterning in vertebrates

Although homologues of the columnar genes are expressed in the vertebrate neural tube, their expression is only a small component of a more extensive system of DV patterning. If the columnar genes represent an ancient patterning system, vertebrates seem to have subsequently acquired further sophistication in DV patterning. We saw earlier that there are at least 11 progenitor domains in the neural tube. How are these set up? This involves two opposing signals, BMP and Sonic hedgehog (SHH; Box 4.4). The role of BMP is remarkably reminiscent of the role of its *Drosophila* homologue, DPP, whereas Hedgehog does not play a role in DV patterning in *Drosophila*. These signals first act in the neural plate following on from neural induction itself. After neural induction, BMP diffuses from lateral ectoderm to promote cellular responses in adjacent lateral regions of the neural plate (Fig. 4.17). Cells on the lateral edge of the neural plate are induced to become **neural crest** cells via activation of the gene *snail*. More significantly for neural tube patterning, signalling also induces the formation of a specialized glial population called the **roof plate**. After neural tube

---

[6] For more detail on BMPs in DV patterning, see Mizutani, C.M. and Bier, E. (2008) EvoD/Vo: the origins of BMP signalling in the neuroectoderm. *Nature Reviews Genetics*, **9**, 663–677.

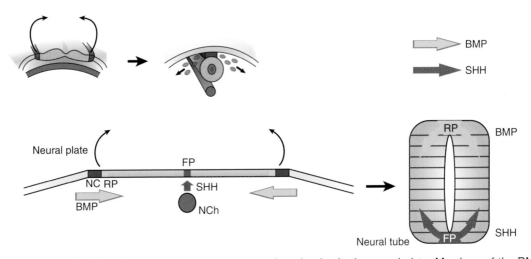

Fig. 4.17 Patterning of the DV axis of the vertebrate neuroectoderm begins in the neural plate. Members of the BMP family (mainly BMP4 and 7) diffuse in from the lateral ectoderm to induce the formation of neural crest precursors (NC) and roof plate cells (RP). SHH signalling from the notochord (NCh) induces the formation of floor plate cells (FP) at the midline. After neural tube closure, the floor plate and roof plate become new signalling centres for SHH and BMP respectively.

formation, the roof plate forms a secondary source of BMP at the dorsal apex of the neural tube.

In the early 1990s, transplantation experiments in chick revealed that mediolateral patterning in the neural plate, and consequently DV patterning in the neural tube, is organized by a signal emanating from the **notochord**, a mesodermal structure that underlies the neural plate's midline. For instance, transplanting a second notochord under the lateral neural plate would induce the formation of an ectopic ventral apex, with the floor plate flanked by motor neurons in the lateral region (Fig. 4.18). Subsequently, it was found that the inductive signal produced by the notochord is SHH. At this early stage of development,

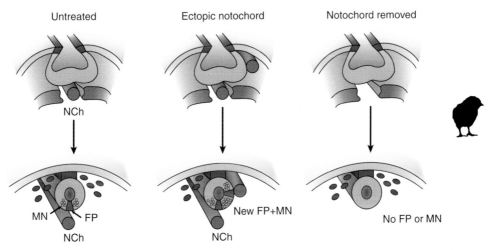

Fig. 4.18 The notochord induces ventral neural tube patterning. In chick, transplantation of an ectopic notochord next to the lateral neural plate leads to the appearance in the neural tube of a second floor plate flanked by motor neurons. Conversely, when the notochord is surgically removed, these ventral cell types fail to appear in the neural tube. The conclusion is that the notochord is both *necessary* and *sufficient* for the induction of ventral types in the chick neural tube. The direct effect of notochord signalling is to induce the floor plate. The induction of other ventral fates (e.g. motor neurons) occurs secondarily via signalling from the floor plate.

floor plate the most ventral region of the neural tube.

the effect of SHH is primarily to induce the **floor plate** via the induction of expression of the winged-helix transcription factor FOXA2 (Fig. 4.17). Like the roof plate, the floor plate is another specialized glial cell population, and it becomes an important SHH-producing signalling centre after neural tube closure. Thus, the primary role of early BMP and SHH signalling is to set the locations of new BMP and SHH signalling centres within the neural tube itself.

(a)

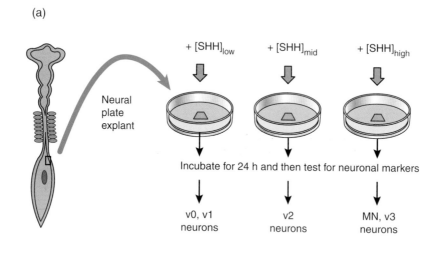

(b)

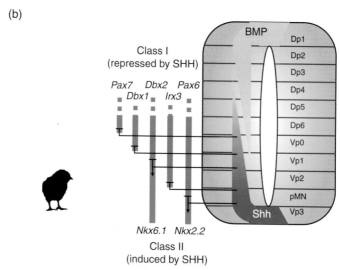

Fig. 4.19 SHH signalling from the floorplate patterns the neural tube as a morphogen. (a) The concentration-dependent effect of SHH on neural tube differentiation was demonstrated in chick explant experiments. Pieces of naïve neural plate were cultured *in vitro* in media containing different concentrations of SHH. Some 24 hours later, the types of neurons produced in each explant varied in a manner that correlated *in vivo* with the proximity of the neurons to the floor plate. In other words, explants treated with high concentrations of SHH produced neuronal subtypes that are normally found close to the floor plate, while explants exposed to lower SHH concentrations made neurons of a type normally found in more dorsal domains, further from the floor plate. (b) SHH defines neuronal progenitor domains via the activation and inhibition of homeodomain transcription factors. One group of factors (Class II) is activated at different threshold concentrations of SHH, leading to their expression in ventral regions of differing dorsal extent. Conversely, Class I genes are repressed at different SHH concentrations, leading to their expression in dorsal regions of differing ventral extent. Unique combinations of these factors thereby determine the identity of each progenitor domain. BMP probably has a similar role in the dorsal neural tube.

4.5.5 Morphogens set up DV progenitor domains

After neural tube closure, the floor plate and roof plate take on the role as new sources of SHH and BMP respectively. The molecules diffuse into the lateral neural tube to set up opposing concentration gradients. They act as classical morphogens (Box 4.1) to induce different neural fates at different levels of the neural tube in a concentration-dependent manner. In the case of SHH, there is much experimental evidence to support this, particularly from chick studies (Fig. 4.19). Thus, high concentrations of SHH close to the floor plate induce the formation of the progenitor domain Vp3, whereas steadily decreasing concentrations further from the floor plate induce pMN, Vp2, Vp1 and Vp0 respectively (Fig. 4.19). As might be anticipated, SHH acts by regulating the expression domains of transcription factors, particularly of the homeodomain family. It is believed that each progenitor domain is thus defined by the expression of a unique combination of these transcription factors – a so-called **homeodomain code** (Fig. 4.19).

The precise role of BMP in inducing dorsal progenitor fates is less well established. Recent evidence from chick explant studies, however, suggests that it too induces dorsal fates in a concentration-dependent manner, and it therefore has an equivalent morphogen function to *Drosophila* DPP. Extending the similarity with *Drosophila* even further, it has been suggested that BMP inhibitors from the notochord (such as chordin, the homologue of *sog*) help to set up the DV concentration gradient of BMP.

4.6 Bringing it all together

At the beginning of this chapter, it was stated that patterning in two axes could provide neuroectodermal cells with the positional information they require. The *Drosophila* CNS has provided a clear illustration of how AP and DV patterning are integrated to determine patterns of neurogenesis. Within each segment, the 800 neurons derive from a fixed array of 60 **neuroblasts** with unique identities that depend on the location at which they arise from the neuroectoderm (Fig. 4.20) (see Chapter 2, Fig. 2.2 for a recap). Each neuroblast is unique and divides stereotypically to generate a specific group of neurons according to its location. Unique neuroblast identities are conferred by AP (segmentation) and DV (columnar) genes, which together subdivide the neuroectoderm in a grid-like structure. The intersection of expression of these genes provides each nascent neuroblast with a unique combination of patterning factors, and thus a distinct identity. In one example, neuroblast 5–2 arises from the neuroectodermal location that expresses *gooseberry* (*gsb*) and *vnd* (Fig. 4.19). This neuroblast identity information subsequently influences the types of neurons produced when the neuroblast divides.

A similar principle applies to the integration of AP and DV axis information in vertebrates, although neural progenitor identities are defined on a regional basis rather than the precise cell-by-cell manner of *Drosophila*. For example, we saw that SHH induces motor neurons in a ventral domain of the neural tube (pMN) via the activation of *Nkx2.2*. The particular *type* of motor neuron produced from pMN, however, depends on the position along the AP axis (e.g. the cervical or thoracic

Fig. 4.20 Patterning of neuroblast identities in *Drosophila*. This diagram brings together the functions of the AP and DV patterning genes shown in Figs 4.12 and 4.16. In the image is shown a ventral view of *Drosophila* embryo in which a marker has been used to stain the neuroblasts. The dotted lines represent the ventral midline and the segmental boundaries. Neuroblasts arise from the neuroectodermal cells in stereotyped locations; they appear in several waves, and only the neuroblasts of the first waves are shown. The cartoons show a single segment, with the neuroblasts as larger pale cells on the neuroectoderm (therefore this is a view *from inside* the embryo). Each neuroblast has a unique identity. These identities are assigned according to location by combined information from the AP and DV systems of patterning in the neuroectoderm. For example, the 5–2 neuroblasts express the unique combination of *vnd* and *gsb*. Similarly, the intersection of *wg* and *ind* defines neuroblast 4–2.

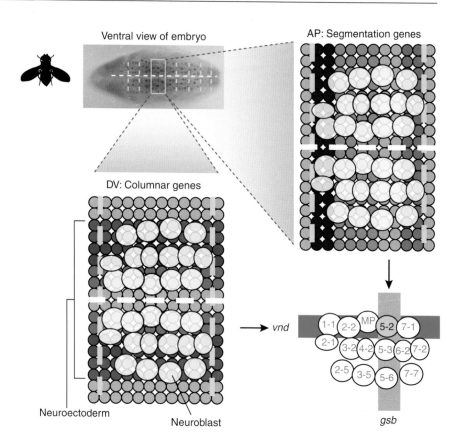

spinal cord). This corresponds to the intersection of *Nkx2.2* and various AP expression domains of Hox genes.

4.7 Summary

- The nervous system is differentiated into specialized areas, such as the brain at the anterior end. Patterning mechanisms provide the information by which this is achieved.
- Patterning entails graded signals (morphogens) that are interpreted to give discrete domains of gene expression along an axis.
- Patterning begins in the neuroectoderm. Patterning therefore occurs in two axes: the AP and DV axes.
- In the case of insects and the vertebrate hindbrain, regionalization involves segmentation.
- Finer-scaled patterning occurs within the initial broad domains. This often entails the setting up of new signalling centres at domain borders.

Generally, the output of patterning mechanisms affects subsequent neuron and glial cell formation (neurogenesis and gliogenesis) in a number of ways, including influencing the timing and rate of neuron production, as well as determining the types of neuron that are generated. How these processes are regulated is the subject of the next chapter.

Neurogenesis: Generating Neural Cells 5

5.1 Generating neural cells

As the nervous system develops, a vast number of neurons and glia (together termed **neural cells**) must be generated from relatively few initial **neural progenitor** cells in the neural epithelium. The process of generating neurons is called **neurogenesis**. Depending on the system and the species, this process can extend over a considerable period of time, from after the initial formation and patterning of the neuroectoderm until birth or even beyond. In general, progenitor cells undergo repeated cell divisions (proliferation). Some of the daughter cells remain as dividing progenitors whereas others are **committed** to become neurons or glia. These cells are termed **neural precursor** cells – they no longer divide (they are post-mitotic) and eventually undergo **differentiation** to attain their mature form as neurons or glial cells.

Neurogenesis is therefore a balance between proliferation and commitment to differentiation. This balance must be carefully regulated to ensure that the correct numbers of neurons of the right kinds are made in the appropriate locations. Only a fraction of cells must undergo commitment at any one time to ensure that the proliferating population is not exhausted.

Neurogenesis must be coordinated with mechanisms that generate differences between neural cell types in terms of structure (e.g. **pyramidal neurons**), function (e.g. motor neurons), and neurotransmitter type (e.g. **glutamatergic** neurons). This is termed **neural subtype specification**. Different types of neuron are produced in different regions of the nervous system, such as motor neurons and commissural interneurons in the ventral and dorsal spinal cord respectively. It follows that a major consequence of the patterning processes described in the previous chapter is to ensure that newly generated neural precursor cells differentiate appropriately according to their location.

In addition to spatial differences in neural subtypes, in many locations different neural cells are generated at different times. For instance, in the spinal cord, cells that are generated early become neurons whereas later born cells become glial cells. We shall see in this

neural progenitor defined in this book as a cell that divides to give daughter cells, some of which will differentiate as neural cells. Progenitor cells are often multipotent. Cf **neural precursor**.

pyramidal neuron a major type of neuron in the vertebrate brain, characterized by a triangular-shaped cell body.

glutamatergic a neuron or synapse that uses the neurotransmitter glutamate.

Building Brains: An Introduction to Neural Development, First Edition.
David Price, Andrew Jarman, John Mason and Peter Kind.
© 2011 John Wiley & Sons, Ltd. Published 2011 by John Wiley & Sons, Ltd.

chapter that the mechanisms of controlling commitment to differentiation, maintenance of cell proliferation and neuronal subtype specification are intimately connected.

5.2 Neurogenesis in *Drosophila*

Progenitor cells have the potential to differentiate as neurons: they are said to have neural **competence**. At any one time, only a fraction of such cells go on to differentiate as neurons – a process termed neuronal **commitment**. A central question of neurogenesis is: what mechanism triggers progenitor cells to commit to neural differentiation? Insight into the mechanisms of competence and commitment initially came from genetic studies in *Drosophila*.

5.2.1 Proneural genes promote neural commitment

As outlined in Chapter 2, the *Drosophila* CNS is formed by progenitors called neuroblasts (Section 2.3.2) while the PNS is formed by **sense organ precursors** (SOPs) (Section 2.6.1). These cells come from the neuroectoderm and lateral ectoderm respectively (Fig. 5.1). In this system, the ectodermal cells have neural competence, but only a proportion become committed as neuroblasts or SOPs. Forward genetic analysis (see Box 1.1 in Chapter 1) led to the identification of two groups of genes that are crucial for this process.

The first group of genes was identified because their mutation results in loss of neuroblasts and SOPs. These are called **proneural genes** because their activity is absolutely required for both competence and commitment. Proneural genes include *achaete*, *scute* and *atonal*, and they encode transcription factors characterized by a protein motif called the basic helix–loop–helix (**bHLH**) domain (Chapter 3, Box 3.3). As might be expected, proneural genes are initially expressed

sense organ precursor (SOP) individual ectodermal cells from which sense organs or sensilla develop in insects. Although called precursors, they are in many respects like progenitors since they undergo cell division.

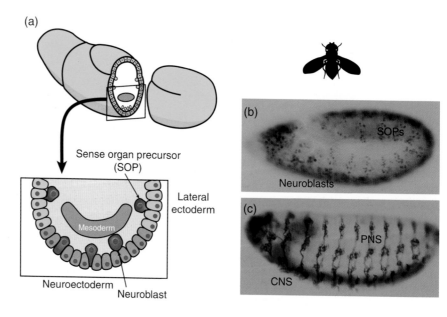

Fig. 5.1 In *Drosophila*, neuroblasts and sense organ precursors (SOPs) generate the CNS and PNS respectively. (a) Neuroblasts and SOPs are ectodermal cells that leave the epithelial layer. (b) These cells can be detected in the developing embryo (seen here in side view) using antibodies against cell-specific proteins that are often described as being 'markers'. Note the segmentally repeated pattern of SOPs. (c) In an older embryo, these cells have divided and some of their progeny have differentiated into the neurons of the CNS and PNS. The CNS forms a ventral nerve cord (see Fig. 2.2 in Chapter 2).

in the ectoderm, where the proteins are present in discrete groups of cells called **proneural clusters** (Fig. 5.2). Only cells in these clusters have neural competence. Subsequently, expression becomes restricted to a single cell in each cluster, which corresponds to the committed neural cell – either SOP or neuroblast depending on the location.

bHLH a DNA-binding structure found in many developmentally important transcription factor proteins, characterized by two helices connected by a loop and usually forming dimers.

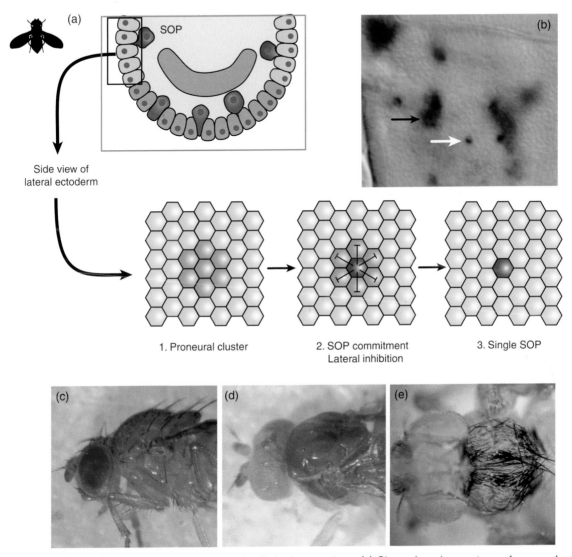

Fig. 5.2 Proneural genes are expressed in clusters of cells in the ectoderm. (a) Shown here is a cartoon of one such cluster (light green) in the lateral ectoderm. The cells of each cluster have the potential (competence) to become SOPs. A single cell attains this fate (dark green) and it then inhibits the remainder of the cells (lateral inhibition). The same process produces neuroblasts in the neuroectoderm. (b) Expression pattern of a proneural gene (*scute* mRNA) in the developing wing of the fly. A number of proneural clusters are visible (e.g. black arrow). Expression is also observed in individual cells (white arrow), which represent already committed SOPs (stage 3 of panel (a)). *scute* mRNA was detected by *in situ* hybridization (Chapter 3, Box 3.4). (c) Each SOP will form a sensory bristle. These bristles can be seen projecting from the back of the fly. (d) A *scute* mutant fly, showing lack of bristles due to failure in SOP commitment. This mutation was first described in the 1930s. (e) When the *scute* gene is ectopically expressed throughout the ectoderm (using the GAL4/UAS system, Chapter 1, Box 1.2), many more ectodermal cells become SOPs, and the fly becomes very bristly.

lateral inhibition a process in which one cell inhibits neighbouring like-minded cells from acquiring the same fate.

epidermis the outermost layers of cells covering the exterior body surface.

5.2.2 Lateral inhibition: Notch signalling inhibits commitment

Within a proneural cluster, only one cell makes the step from neuronal competence to commitment. This cell prevents its neighbours from following suit via an inhibitory intercellular signalling pathway. The receptor of this pathway is called Notch (Box 5.1). The committed cell expresses a Notch **ligand**, known as Delta, on its surface where it can contact Notch receptors on the surrounding cells of the proneural cluster. This results in production of HES proteins – transcriptional repressors that inhibit proneural gene expression. This mechanism of fate determination is very widespread in developmental biology and is known as **lateral inhibition**. The upshot of lateral inhibition is that cells surrounding the committed neural cell shut down their proneural gene expression, lose their neural competence and eventually take on a default alternative fate as **epidermal** cells. As might be expected,

---

Box 5.1   The Notch signalling pathway

This highly conserved pathway is named after the receptor, Notch, which is expressed on all cells. The Notch receptor is itself named after one of the phenotypes observed when the gene is mutated: notched wings. Unlike most of the other signalling pathways we have come across, Notch ligands are not diffusible signals, but are transmembrane proteins on the surface of the signalling cell. This is therefore a contact signalling pathway. In the committed neural cell (the signalling cell, shown on the left), the proneural factor triggers expression of the Notch ligand, Delta. Delta protein on the surface then binds to the Notch receptor of adjacent cells, triggering the **proteolytic cleavage** of Notch protein by presenilin. The intracellular domain of Notch (NotchICD) then moves to the nucleus where it complexes with a transcription factor called Suppressor of Hairless (SU(H)). The complex activates transcription of *Enhancer of split* (*E(spl)*) genes (members of the *HES* family), which encode bHLH transcriptional repressors that inhibit proneural gene expression in the recipient cell, blocking its neural competence.

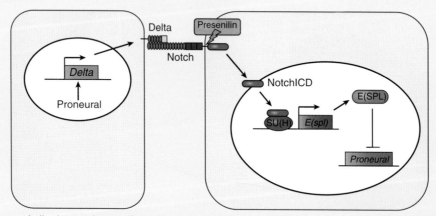

The pathway is very similar in vertebrates. There are four *Notch* genes in mouse and several *HES* genes, which stands for *Hairy/Enhancer of split*. This alludes to the fact that *E(spl)* genes are also related to the **pair-rule gene**, *hairy*.

---

proteolytic cleavage the breakdown of proteins into simpler peptides and amino acids.

mutations in genes of the Notch pathway have the opposite effect to proneural gene mutations: they result in the commitment of too many ectodermal cells in each proneural cluster, leading to the formation of too many neural cells.

What leads to the initial decision by just one cell to commit? Before commitment, it is thought that all cells of a proneural cluster compete for the prize of becoming an SOP because each cell initially expresses Delta ligand. Each cell therefore inhibits its neighbouring cells, but since all cells are receiving inhibition, none are able to commit. The stand-off thus created is called **mutual inhibition** (Fig. 5.3). Subsequently, one cell appears to escape inhibition, enabling it to inhibit its neighbours more efficiently thereby shutting down their proneural gene expression. Thus, mutual inhibition transitions into lateral inhibition. Currently, it is not entirely clear what triggers this transition, but one possibility is that one cell initially expresses slightly more proneural factor than the rest (perhaps by chance), giving it an advantage in inhibiting the other cells.

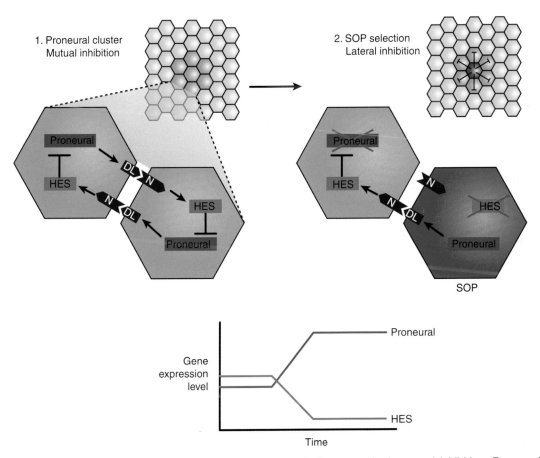

Fig. 5.3 Initially, Notch signalling between all cells in the proneural cluster results in mutual inhibition. Proneural factors and their HES antagonists are co-expressed at this stage, and all cells maintain their neural competence. Subsequently this shifts to lateral inhibition in which just one cell signals to the rest of the cluster. This cell (the SOP) expresses only proneural factor and the surrounding cells express only HES. The graph represents the transition in gene expression that occurs in the SOP.

5.3 Neurogenesis in vertebrates

5.3.1 Proneural genes are conserved

Following on from the *Drosophila* research, several vertebrate homologues of proneural bHLH genes have been discovered, many of which play fundamental roles in generating neurons in the PNS and CNS. For instance, *Ascl1* (*achaete-scute-like 1*) is expressed in **neural crest**, some sensory **placodes** (Chapter 2, Section 2.6), and some parts of the neural tube; mouse knock-out studies have shown that it is required for a variety of central and sensory neurons. Neurogenin genes (*Ngn1* and *Ngn2*) are related to the *Drosophila* proneural gene, *atonal*, and are required for much of the neurogenesis in the spinal cord and brain.

As in *Drosophila*, vertebrate proneural bHLH genes are opposed by the function of Notch signalling. A good example of this is seen in sensory cell development within the otic sensory placode, which forms the **inner ear** (Chapter 2, Section 2.6) (Fig. 5.4). In the developing sensory epithelium of the inner ear, cells are made competent to become sensory hair cells by the expression of *Atoh1* (*Atonal homologue 1*), another gene related to *Drosophila atonal* (which, interestingly, is itself required for *Drosophila* auditory sensory neurons). Lateral inhibition ensures that only a proportion of placode epithelial cells become hair cells, whereas the remainder differentiate as support cells.

5.3.2 In the vertebrate CNS, neurogenesis involves radial glial cells

When it comes to the vertebrate CNS, there are important differences in neurogenesis compared with *Drosophila*, mostly because much larger numbers of neurons must be generated. In the vertebrate neural tube, neurons are generated from progenitor cells called **radial glia**, so named because historically they were thought to be glia – their

neural crest part of the ectoderm located between the neural tube and the epidermis that contributes neurons and other cells throughout the body of vertebrates.

placodes bilateral thickenings of the ectoderm of the vertebrate head that generate sensory structures.

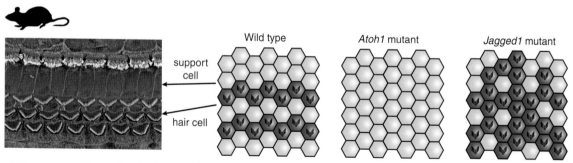

Fig. 5.4 Sensory cell formation in the mouse inner ear. Cells in the otic epithelium differentiate as sensory 'hair cells', which mediate auditory sensory transduction, and non-sensory support cells. A proneural gene, *Atoh1*, is expressed in the otic epithelium and promotes commitment to hair cell fate. In mouse knock-out mutants of *Atoh1*, no hair cells are formed and all cells become support cells by default. *Jagged1* encodes a *Notch* ligand. In *Jagged1* mutants, some support cells differentiate as extra hair cells. This is due to a reduction of lateral inhibition. Loss of inner ear hair cells is a major cause of hearing loss – through trauma or age. There is much interest in attempting to reactivate *Atoh1* expression in the inner ear to provoke the formation of new hair cells in order to restore hearing. (Image provided by Elizabeth Orton and Karen Steel, Sanger Institute, Cambridge, UK.)

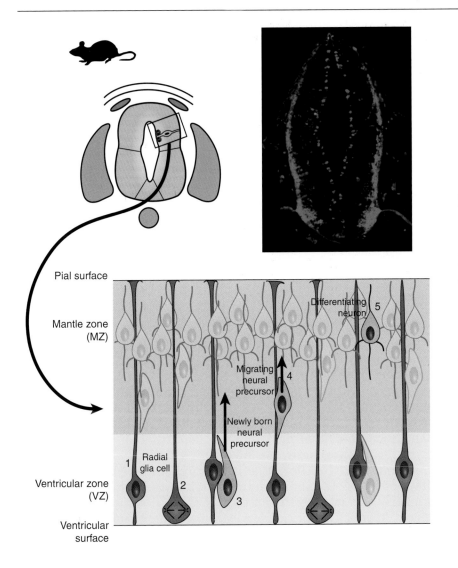

Fig. 5.5 A generalized view of neurogenesis in the vertebrate neural tube. The neuroepithelium consists of neural stem cells called radial glia (brown), which stretch across the epithelium (1 in the lower cartoon). These undergo repeated divisions in the ventricular zone (2). Some of the daughter cells leave the cell cycle to become post-mitotic neural precursors (3). These migrate along the remaining radial glia (4) into the mantle zone, where they differentiate (5). The image (upper right) is from a slice through a mouse neural tube. The nuclei of radial glia (blue) are in the ventricular zone on each side, while maturing neurons (green) have moved out into the mantle zone (image adapted by permission from Macmillan Publishers Ltd: Petersen, P. H. *et al.* (2002) Progenitor cell maintenance requires *numb* and *numblike* during mouse neurogenesis. *Nature.* **419**, 929–934, copyright 2002).

progenitor role was discovered only relatively recently. These cells reside at the luminal (inner) surface of the neural tube epithelium. This region is often described as the **ventricular zone** (refer back to Fig. 2.6 in Chapter 2). Radial glia extend long processes that span the neural epithelium (Fig. 5.5). They are **neural stem cells**, which are defined by two properties: (i) multipotency – they are capable of producing progeny cells that can differentiate into a range of both neuronal and glial cell types; (ii) self-renewal – whilst some of their progeny exit the cell cycle to differentiate, a proportion of the progeny retain their neural stem cell characteristics, thus maintaining the pool of progenitor cells that divide repeatedly over an extended period of development.

The progeny that exit the cell cycle migrate along the processes of the remaining radial glia until they reach the outer surface of the neural tube where they accumulate and differentiate to form the future grey matter of the central nervous system. Prior to differentiation, these post-mitotic cells are termed neural precursors and the layer that they form is called the **mantle zone** or, in the particular case of those precursors that form the cerebral cortex, the **cortical plate**. The migration of these precursors is discussed in Chapter 6.

5.3.3 Proneural factors and Notch signalling in the vertebrate CNS

Although neurogenesis in the vertebrate CNS appears rather different from *Drosophila*, proneural genes are still central to the process. In the neural tube, proneural genes such as *Ngn2* are expressed in progenitor cells of the ventricular zone. The proneural factors become upregulated in committed neural precursors where they are thought to activate a variety of genes required for cell cycle arrest, neuronal cell migration and eventually neuronal differentiation. They also inhibit the function of transcription factors such as those encoded by the *Sox* genes, which are known to be important for maintaining the stem cell character of neural progenitors (*Sox* genes were discussed in Chapter 3, Section 3.8.2).

The antagonistic bHLH/Notch interaction is also maintained in the CNS: neural tube progenitors are characterized by co-expression of proneural proteins and their HES antagonists, just like *Drosophila* cells at the mutual inhibition stage (Fig. 5.6). An important difference in the neural tube, however, is that Notch inhibition does not become permanent, with inhibited cells taking on a different, non-neural fate. Instead, they are only temporarily inhibited and retain their competence as neural progenitors. Therefore, by preventing commitment Notch inhibition maintains the population of progenitor cells for further neurogenesis. An interesting consequence of this difference compared with *Drosophila* is that mutation of *Notch* (in mouse knock-outs) has the counterintuitive effect of *reducing* total neuron numbers. This happens because there is brief, early flush of neurogenesis in which all progenitors become committed to neuronal differentiation. Although the earliest neurons are formed, no pool of proliferating progenitors remains to form the vast majority of neurons needed to form a mature brain.

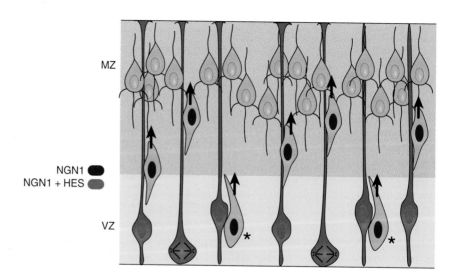

Fig. 5.6 The progenitor cells (radial glia) in the ventricular zone of the neural tube are characterized by co-expression of proneural factors (including NGN1) and their HES antagonists. This gives them neural competence but also maintains their stem cell nature. Maintenance of this state is likely to entail Notch signalling between the cells. Over time, some of the cells lose HES expression (as shown by the asterisks). Proneural factor function is then able to commit them to exit the cell cycle, migrate and differentiate. Compare this to SOP commitment in Fig. 5.3.

MZ

NGN1
NGN1 + HES

VZ

Thus, in vertebrate neurogenesis, proneural factors trigger neural commitment, while Notch signalling maintains the neural progenitor state (Fig. 5.6). We shall see later that cell division patterns also have an important impact in regulating commitment and progenitor maintenance.

Besides the bHLH genes that have proneural functions, other genes of the bHLH family are activated in neural cells only after they have been committed to differentiation. These include *NeuroD*, which is expressed generally in post-mitotic neural precursor cells. *NeuroD* is a powerful regulator of terminal differentiation itself. This was shown in overexpression experiments in which *NeuroD* mRNA was injected into fertilized *Xenopus* eggs. The resulting embryo developed with many extra neurons formed throughout the whole ectoderm.

5.4 The regulation of neuronal subtype identity

5.4.1 Neural precursors already have intrinsic identity

Newly generated neural precursor cells will eventually differentiate to form the wide variety of different subtypes of neuron in the nervous system. In general, a variety of transcription factors are expressed in different neuronal populations during differentiation, where they regulate genes involved in various aspects of neuronal phenotype, such as neurotransmitter type.

How do newly generated neural precursors acquire their neuronal subtype identity? There are at least two ways in which this might happen. It could be that progenitor cells generate unspecialized neural precursors, which subsequently differentiate as specialized subtypes according to their regional environment (an extrinsic mechanism). Alternatively, progenitor cells may utilize intrinsic information they have about their location to produce neural precursors destined to differentiate as specific neuronal subtypes. We shall see later that environment has an important influence on cell differentiation (Section 5.6.5, but also see Chapter 11 for the role of neuronal activity). In general, however, a neuron's subtype fate is heavily influenced at its birth by transcription factors already expressed in the progenitor cell as a consequence of regional patterning mechanisms (Chapter 4). Thus, progenitor cells generally have restricted potential to produce certain subtypes of neuron. Regional patterning factors activate a regulatory cascade of transcription factors within the progenitors, that continues in the newly generated neuronal precursor cells, and finally into the differentiating neurons to regulate aspects such as different dendritic morphologies, neurotransmitter expression patterns and migration behaviours.

This cascade of gene regulatory interactions is complex and the details are poorly known in many cases, but some examples are given in the following sections. One particularly clear paradigm in *Drosophila* has already been described in the previous chapter: the acquisition of unique neuroblast identities as a consequence of regulation by anteroposterior (AP) and dorsoventral (DV) patterning factors (Section 4.6).

These unique identities are defined by the activation of different 'neuroblast identity' transcription factors in the neuroblasts, which influence subsequent neuron differentiation.

5.4.2 Different proneural genes – different programmes of neurogenesis

One influence of regional patterning on neuronal subtype identity is that different proneural genes are activated in different regions of the nervous system. These genes not only trigger neurogenesis but also regulate distinct neural differentiation programmes to generate different neuronal subtypes. This was first demonstrated in the *Drosophila* PNS, where different proneural genes (including *scute* and *atonal*) drive the formation of characteristic subtypes of sensory neuron. Misexpression of each proneural gene using the GAL4/UAS system (Chapter 1, Box 1.2) results in the overproduction of distinct types of sensory neuron. In the vertebrate neural tube, different proneural genes are activated in specific progenitor domains, where they generate neurons with different subtype identities (Fig. 5.7).

5.4.3 Combinatorial control by transcription factors creates neuronal diversity

There are too few proneural genes to explain the range of neuronal identities in the nervous system. Instead, the genes function in

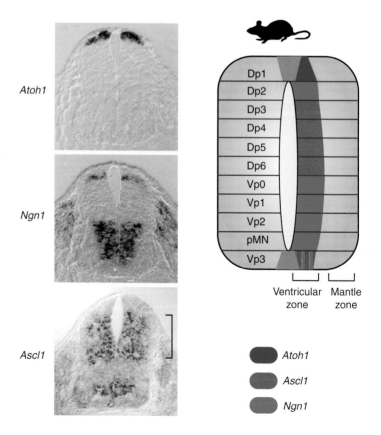

Fig. 5.7 One consequence of regional patterning is that neurogenesis is triggered by different proneural factors in different regions of the nervous system. This contributes to regional differences in the production of neuronal subtypes. This example shows the expression of mRNAs for different proneural genes in distinct progenitor domains along the DV axis of the mouse neural tube. Refer back to Fig. 4.14 in Chapter 4 for an explanation of the neural tube schematic. (Images reproduced from Muroyama, Y., Fujihara, M., Ikeya, M., Kondoh, H. and Takada, S. (2002) Wnt signalling plays an essential role in neuronal specification of the dorsal spinal cord. *Genes Dev.*, **16**, 548–553.)

combination with many other transcription factors of different families. We saw in Chapter 4 how dorsoventral domains in the neural tube are defined by the expression of unique combinations of transcription factors (Section 4.5.5). This carries over into subsequent neurogenesis: neural cell types are specified by the expression of unique combinations of transcription factors in the progenitors of each domain. For instance, the progenitors of the ventral neural tube express a number of transcription factors (including those encoded by *Pax6*, *Nkx2.2*, *Irx3*), which combine to specify distinct neuronal identities in the domains.[1]

In many different systems it has been noted that combinations of **homeodomain** and proneural bHLH factors are important for different neural cell fates. This is well illustrated in the vertebrate retina, where a 'bHLH + homeodomain' code has been proposed to direct the differentiation of the various cell types (Fig. 5.8). Whilst much is known about the specification of the major retinal cell types, it should be noted that each type exists as many distinguishable subtypes, and we know much less about how the subtypes are specified. For instance, over 20 subtypes of amacrine cell have been defined, but the factors specifying their phenotypes have not yet been established.[2] A similar subdivision of cell types occurs throughout the nervous system. In the ventral spinal cord, motor neurons form distinct 'pools' that innervate distinct muscle sets. These pools may be distinguished by the activity of different members of the LIM family of homeodomain proteins.

A principle abundantly illustrated here is one that we have come across several times already. In general, only rarely does a particular transcription factor uniquely identify a neural cell type. Such a one-to-one correspondence would require a huge number of different factors devoted to neural subtype specification. Instead, through **combinatorial** action, relatively few transcription factors can potentially encode a vast number of different neural identities.

An important corollary of combinatorial control is that a single transcription factor will have multiple functions in different locations or even at different times (i.e. depending on what other factors are co-expressed with it). This explains how a proneural gene such as *Ngn1* can generate several different neuronal types. In another example, in the early neural plate *Otx2* is a patterning gene required for anterior brain regionalization, setting up the midbrain–hindbrain boundary and defining the **thalamus** (Chapter 4, Section 4.3.3). Later it continues to be expressed in thalamic progenitors during neurogenesis, where it promotes their differentiation as excitatory glutamatergic neurons as opposed to inhibitory **GABAergic** neurons. Patterning and proneural factors all have complex and shifting roles to play in several stages of neurogenesis.

homeodomain a region in many developmentally important transcription factor proteins comprising about 60 amino acids folded into three helices, one of which interacts directly with DNA, connected by short loops.

combinatorial referring to the fact that molecules (e.g. signals or transcription factors) usually act in combinations, either to affect cell behaviour or gene expression. This means that a relatively small number of such molecules can encode a large number of different outcomes.

thalamus a structure in the centre of the vertebrate brain that transmits sensory input to the cerebral cortex, and receives reciprocal output from the cortex.

GABAergic a neuron or synapse that contains GABA.

---

[1] For more detail on transcription factor codes and neural fates, see Guillemot, F. (2007) Spatial and temporal specification of neural fates by transcription factor codes. *Development*, **134**, 3771–3780.
[2] Retinal development is an excellent system for exploring neurogenesis: for more detail see Livesey, F.J. and Cepko, C.L. (2001) Vertebrate neural cell-fate determination: lessons from the retina. *Nature Reviews Neuroscience*, **2**, 109–118.

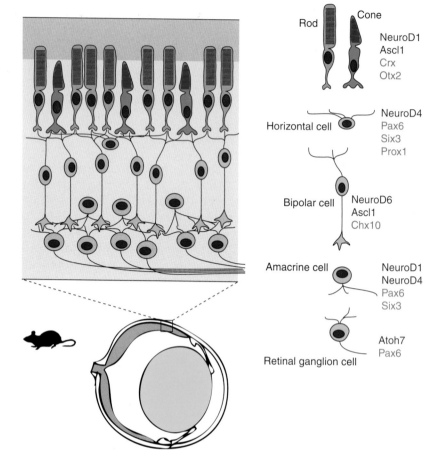

Fig. 5.8 Different combinations of bHLH (blue) and homeodomain (red) transcription factors define different classes of neuron and glial cell in the vertebrate retina. Evidence that these factors are important for subtype identity comes from analysis of mouse mutants and experimentally induced co-expression of different bHLH and homeodomain protein combinations in retinal **explant** tissues grown in culture.

explant part of an organism that has been excised and cultured in isolation.

fibroblast growth factors a family of growth factors involved in embryonic development as well as other processes such as wound healing.

cerebellum meaning 'little brain' it is a discrete structure at the base of the brain that lies above the brain-stem. It regulates a range of functions including motor control, attention and cognition.

5.5 The regulation of cell proliferation during neurogenesis

5.5.1 Signals that promote proliferation

Control of cell division is a key aspect of neurogenesis. We saw that the proneural–Notch interaction is important for maintaining the balance between proliferating progenitors and committed neural precursors. Environmental factors are also important in promoting progenitor proliferation. Such factors take the form of exogenous signals that promote or inhibit mitosis (the former are called **mitogens**). For example, in the cortex **fibroblast growth factor** 2 (FGF2) promotes proliferation of cortical progenitor cells, and this factor needs to be added to isolated cortical cells in order to keep them proliferating in culture. In the human **cerebellum**, SHH (Chapter 4, Box 4.4) acts as a mitogen for *ATOH1*-expressing progenitors of **granule neurons**, strongly stimulating their proliferation during early childhood. As might be predicted, dysregulation of proliferation signals can be harmful (Box 5.2). For instance, medulloblastomas are childhood tumours of the cerebellum. One form of medulloblastoma is associated with mutations that result in uncontrolled SHH signalling.

Box 5.2   The study of normal neurogenesis sheds light on brain cancer

Neurogenesis is a delicate balance between proliferation of progenitor cells and their differentiation into neurons and glial cells. Much evidence now shows that cancer represents the dysregulation of normal developmental processes. In many cases, cancer cells proliferate out of control and show a relatively un-differentiated morphology (i.e. they resemble progenitor cells that fail to differentiate). Factors that are asso-ciated with progenitor cells are often found to be upregulated in cancer cells. For instance, the HLH genes *OLIG1* and *ID* are required for maintenance and proliferation of **astrocyte** progenitors, and are also abnor-mally expressed in tumours derived from astrocytes (astrocytomas). *ID* is also highly expressed in neuro-blastomas, rare childhood tumours typically derived from neural progenitors in the **autonomic nervous system** or **adrenal medulla**. Conversely, factors that drive neural differentiation, such as the proneural gene *ATOH1*, inhibit tumour formation. Inactivation of such differentiation genes may be one of the causa-tive events in tumour progression.

astrocyte a type of glial cell; they are star-shaped with many processes that enwrap neuronal synapses.

5.5.2 Cell division patterns during neurogenesis

In order to generate vast numbers of neurons, such as those found in the mammalian cortex, the balance between cell cycle promotion and exit must be tightly regulated. One key aspect of this regulation is the nature of cell division itself. During cell proliferation, we commonly think of a cell dividing **symmetrically** to yield two identical daughter cells. However, the division can also be **asymmetric**, whereby the daughter cells acquire distinct developmental potentials. There are two types of asymmetric cell division, both of which are important in neurogenesis. In the first type, a cell divides to yield two daughters that differentiate differently. Such divisions can generate cellular di-versity. An example of this is seen in the generation of sense organs of *Drosophila*. Each SOP (Section 5.2.1) undergoes a limited series of asym-metric cell divisions to produce the sensory neuron and three different support cells that make up a sense organ (Fig. 5.9).

The second type of asymmetric cell division is the self-renewing division exhibited by progenitor cells: in this case, one daughter re-tains the mother's progenitor character of multipotency and high proliferative potential while the other cell is committed to differen-tiation. This mode of division is typical of **stem cells**. Such asym-metric cell divisions are important in the CNS of both invertebrates and vertebrates (Fig. 5.9).

stem cell a relatively unspecialized cell that can divide repeatedly to re-generate itself (self-renewal) and give rise to more specialized cells, such as neurons or glia.

5.5.3 Asymmetric cell division in Drosophila requires Numb

Genetic analyses in *Drosophila* have led to the discovery of several mechanisms for the control of asymmetric cell division.[3] In one

---

[3] Mechanisms not discussed here can be found in Wu, P. S., Egger, B. and Brand, A. H. (2008) Asymmetric stem cell division: lessons from *Drosophila*. *Semin. Cell Dev. Biol.*, **19**, 283–293.

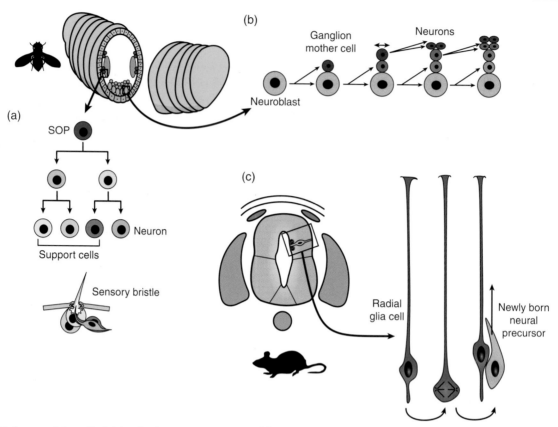

Fig. 5.9 Asymmetric cell division in the nervous system. (a) Such divisions can generate cellular diversity, as seen in the *Drosophila* PNS. Each SOP divides asymmetrically to give the sensory neuron and three support cells which form a sensory bristle on the surface of the fly. The three support cells comprise: a glial cell that ensheathes the neuron, a cell that secretes the bristle shaft and a cell that makes the socket in which the shaft sits. (b) and (c) Asymmetric cell division can also be a self-renewal or stem cell type, and this is characteristic of progenitor cells in the CNS of both *Drosophila* and vertebrates. In the *Drosophila* CNS (b), neuroblasts undergo repeated asymmetric divisions. At each division one daughter retains the neuroblast's characteristics while the second becomes a ganglion mother cell, which has very limited further division potential. It divides only once more to yield two neurons. (c) In the vertebrate neural tube, radial glial cells undergo repeated cell divisions to generate neural precursors. Progenitors are theoretically able to carry on dividing indefinitely – they have high proliferative potential. If different types of neural precursor are produced at different divisions, then the progenitor is also multipotent. These are both key characteristics of stem cells.

ground-breaking case, forward genetic screening (Box 1.1 in Chapter 1) revealed a mutation with a striking PNS phenotype: all four cells of each sense organ differentiated as one type of support cell – the socket cell (Fig. 5.10). Because the sensory neuron was absent, this mutant was named *numb*. In the SOPs of the mutant fly each division becomes symmetrical. Instead of generating two cell types (say, 'A' and 'B'), both daughter cells take the fate of the 'A' cell. Note, however, how the two cell fates vary with each different division in Fig. 5.10, and yet *numb* is required for generating diversity of cell type at each division. Thus, *numb* does not act by specifying any particular cell type, but is generally required at each division to make one cell different from the other (enabling one to become the 'B' cell).

The *numb* gene encodes a cytoplasmic protein that is made in the dividing cell and is asymmetrically distributed during division such that it is

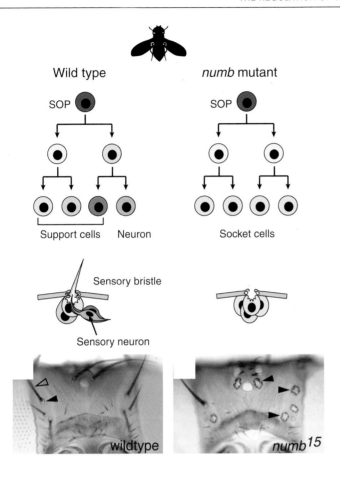

Fig. 5.10 *numb* is required for asymmetric cell division in *Drosophila* sense organs. The four cells of each sensory bristle arise from asymmetric division. Outwardly, only the shaft and socket are visible (unfilled and filled arrowheads, respectively, indicate one example on this close-up of a fly's head). Mutations that affect the cell divisions are readily visible in genetic screens by virtue of changes in external appearance of the bristles. In the *numb* mutant fly (*numb[15]*), groups of four socket cells are observed because the divisions have become symmetric. Several examples of socket clusters are indicated on the image but note that not all bristles are affected in this particular fly. (Images adapted from Berdnik, D., Török, T., González-Gaitán, M. and Knoblich, J. A. (2002) The endocytic protein α-adaptin is required for numb-mediated asymmetric cell division in *Drosophila*. *Dev. Cell*, **3**, 221–231, with permission from Elsevier).

inherited by only one daughter, where it ensures the 'B' fate (Fig. 5.11). To show that asymmetric segregation of Numb protein is important, experiments were carried out in which Numb protein was artificially boosted in the dividing cell so that both daughter cells received it (using the GAL4/UAS system described in Chapter 1, Box 1.2). In this case, both daughters now take on the 'B' cell fate at each division, and the four cells all differentiate as sensory neurons with the concomitant loss of support cells.

The role of Numb appears to be to prevent Notch receptor activity within the cell. The two daughter cells undertake a form of

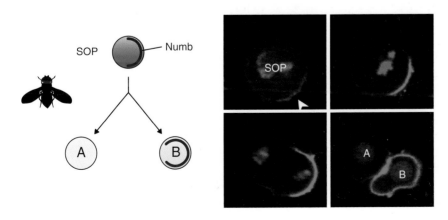

Fig. 5.11 In asymmetrically dividing cells, Numb protein (blue in the cartoon) becomes localized under the cell membrane in a crescent. This ensures that it is inherited by only one daughter cell (the 'B' cell). The images show a series of fluorescence microscopy snapshots of a dividing SOP within a living fly. Here Numb protein is visualized by being tagged with green fluorescent protein (GFP; Chapter 1, Box 1.4), and chromosomes are red. (Images adapted from Mayer, B., Emery, G., Berdnik, D., Wirtz-Peitz, F. and Knoblich, J. A. (2005) Quantitative analysis of protein dynamics during asymmetric cell division. *Current Biology*, **15**, 1847–1854 copyright (2005), with permission from Elsevier.)

Notch-dependent lateral inhibition whereby each tries to take on the 'B' fate and inhibit its sister from doing likewise. The cell that inherits Numb is immune from the inhibitory effect of Notch signalling and so is able to assume the preferred 'B' cell fate while its sister is forced to take on the alternative 'A' cell fate. Hence, Notch signalling is not only required for SOP specification in the ectoderm, but also for asymmetric cell division.

5.5.4 Control of asymmetric cell division in vertebrate neurogenesis

As we saw earlier, radial glial cells undergo repeated self-renewing asymmetric cell divisions (Fig. 5.9). Originally, indirect evidence for this came from examining cells in fixed tissues, but in recent years advances in microscopy have allowed such divisions to be observed directly in living tissues by time-lapse microscopy (Box 5.3). In chick, zebrafish and mouse, neurogenesis can be followed in cultured slices of living neural tube in which some cells express a fluorescent protein, such as **green fluorescent protein** (GFP – see Chapter 1, Box 1.4) (Fig. 5.12).

In many ways, production of neurons by asymmetric cell division of radial glial cells closely resembles neuroblast divisions in the *Drosophila* CNS. There are two homologues of *numb* that function during vertebrate neurogenesis (called *Numb* and *Numblike* in mouse). Several studies show that Numb protein is asymmetrically localized in radial glial cells and that it can be inherited by one of the resulting daughter cells. It is tempting to think therefore that Numb promotes neural precursor formation by inhibiting Notch, just as in *Drosophila*. However, determining the function of vertebrate *Numb* has proved to be complicated. Recent studies suggest that vertebrate *Numb* plays a different role from its *Drosophila* counterpart and is required to maintain attachment of progenitors at the ventricular surface. Consistent with this, mouse *Numb* mutants

Fig. 5.12 Visualization of asymmetric division in a living tissue slice taken from the chick neural tube. The images represent a series of snapshots taken over 24 hours during the division of a single radial glial cell that has been marked with GFP. Note how there are dramatic movements of the nucleus of the radial glial cell (RG) before and after division (this is called **interkinetic nuclear migration**). The newly generated neural precursor cell (NP) moves to the marginal zone while the radial glial cell re-establishes its morphology and starts to divide again. (Image adapted from Wilcock, A. C., Swedlow, J. R. and Storey, K. G. (2007) Mitotic spindle orientation distinguishes stem cell and terminal modes of neuron production in the early spinal cord. *Development*, **134**, 1943–1954.)

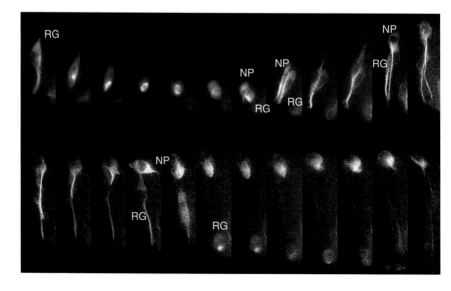

Box 5.3 Fluorescence microscopy techniques

A microscope is an essential part of the developmental neurobiologist's toolkit. Many of the images shown in this book rely on the detection of **fluorescent** molecules in embryos and tissues by fluorescence microscopy. These may be neuronal proteins detected by fluorescently labelled antibodies, fluorescent proteins introduced into a neuron (e.g. GFP), or fluorescent dyes that have been injected to trace a neuron's morphology (e.g. DiI). In this technique, light of a particular wavelength is shone on the specimen, it emits light of a different wavelength, which is extracted by optical filters in the microscope for viewing. What is seen is a bright image (the light emitted by the fluorescent molecule) on a black background. Several different fluorescent dyes can be detected simultaneously, enabling the detection of two or more different gene products (see Fig. 4.4(c) for a dramatic example of such 'multiple labelling').

However, for thick tissues like an embryo or a brain slice, much of the light being detected is scattered from out-of-focus parts of the specimen. This makes the image very blurred. A number of methods have been developed to overcome this. The most widespread is laser scanning confocal microscopy (LSCM). This technique was invented by Marvin Minsky in the 1960s, but only became generally available to developmental neurobiologists from the 1990s. In LSCM, a laser produces an intense spot of illuminating light that is scanned across the specimen. The fluorescence emitted by the specimen cannot be viewed directly; it requires an electronic detector and a computer to reconstruct the scanned image for viewing. The advantage of this form of illumination is that the light coming just from the point of focus can be filtered out while any background out-of-focus light is discarded. The image is therefore a crisp 'optical section' of just the plane of focus. Many sections can be recorded from different levels of the tissue and the computer can reconstruct these into a three-dimensional image of the whole tissue. Confocal microscopy revolutionized developmental biology and it is routinely used in labs throughout the world. Most of the fluorescence images in this book were produced using this technique.

One problem with LSCM is that because most light (the out-of-focus light) is discarded it requires extremely intense laser illumination. This is acceptable for fixed specimens, but it severely damages living embryos and cells. More recently, new methods have been used to study living cells. One is based on confocal microscopy and uses laser light of lower energy (infrared) to avoid photodamage. This is called two-photon excitation microscopy (see Box 10.4 for an example). Another technique – deconvolution microscopy – uses an entirely different method of dealing with out-of-focus light. The specimen is illuminated with a normal light source rather than a powerful laser, but the out-of-focus light is collected and 'brought back into focus' by sophisticated computational analysis based on the optical properties of the microscope. As this method does not discard the out-of-focus light, it is more sensitive and does not require such intense illumination. With these techniques, live cells can be followed as they divide, migrate, change shape, form synapses, die and so on.

show a loss of progenitors and concomitant overproduction of neurons.[4] Another unresolved question is how asymmetric cell division is coordinated with proneural gene activity during neuronal commitment.

5.5.5 In vertebrates, division patterns are regulated to generate vast numbers of neurons

There is an important difference between *Drosophila* and vertebrate neurogenesis. In *Drosophila*, the division pattern of neuroblasts is

---

[4] For further reading about possible mechanisms involving Numb, see Zhong, W. and Chia, W. (2008) Neurogenesis and asymmetric cell division. *Curr. Op. Neurobiol.*, **18**, 4–11.

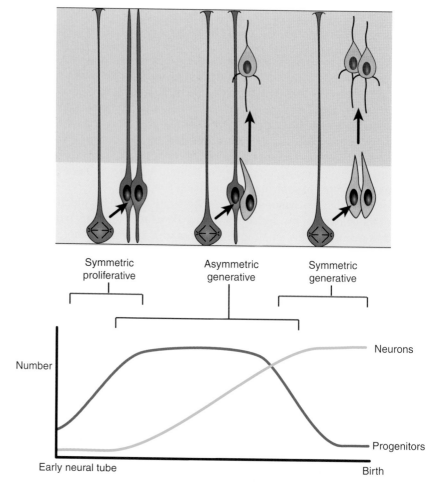

Fig. 5.13 In the neural tube, the rate of neuron production is related to the changes in division pattern over time. The first phase is expansion of the neural progenitor population by symmetric proliferative divisions. Then progenitors switch to asymmetric generative divisions, giving a steady production of neural cells. Finally, symmetric generative divisions cause all progeny to become neurons or glia, thereby exhausting the progenitor population. Changing the time of switching may be a particularly labile process in evolution. For instance, it may be the mechanism by which higher primates evolved a larger brain.

hardwired – each neuroblast divides strictly asymmetrically to produce an **invariant** sequence of offspring. In vertebrates, radial glia are more flexible in their mode of division. Cell divisions are not invariably asymmetric and regulation of division mode is an important mechanism of controlling neuron generation. In the case of the cerebral cortex, after formation of the neural tube, progenitor cells initially divide symmetrically to expand the progenitor population (Fig. 5.13). Subsequently, more and more progenitors switch to repeated rounds of asymmetric division to produce neural precursors. Towards the end of neurogenesis, there is thought to be a further switch to symmetric divisions that generate two post-mitotic neural precursors, thereby depleting the progenitor pool.[5]

Our understanding of how these switches in mode of division are regulated is at present sketchy. In *Drosophila*, the invariant asymmetric mode of division arises because neuroblasts have a network of proteins (so-called 'polarity complexes') that ensure the asymmetric localization of determinants like Numb is coordinated with the orientation of

[5] To read more about division patterns and their possible regulation, see Götz, M. and Huttner, W.B. (2005) The cell biology of neurogenesis. *Nature Reviews Molecular Cell Biology*, **6**, 777–788.

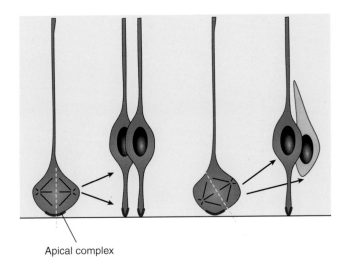

Apical complex

Fig. 5.14 Orientation of the cell division plane may determine whether a radial glial cell divides symmetrically or asymmetrically. Proteins such as PAR complex localize to an apical membrane complex. If this is bisected, both daughters inherit radial glial characteristics; if the division is off-centre, only one cell retains this fate and the other cell becomes a committed neural precursor.

the **mitotic spindle**. Consequently when the cell divides, one cell (always the one on the inner side of the neuroblast) accurately inherits the determinants. These proteins include the **PAR complex**, which was first discovered as being necessary for asymmetric cell division in the early *C. elegans* embryo. The PAR complex localizes to the opposite side of the neuroblast from Numb, and so is retained in the neuroblast during division where it maintains the cell's stem-cell-like characteristics.

In vertebrates, current research is aimed at understanding how localized proteins and the orientation of the mitotic spindle may relate to changes in the mode of cell division. In dividing radial glia, protein complexes including PAR localize to a small apical membrane patch at the ventricular side of the cell (Fig. 5.14). One attractive idea is that the orientation of cell division relative to this patch may be critical. Most symmetric proliferative divisions (those that result in the production of two radial glial cells) have been observed to result from a division plane orientated vertically relative to the plane of the epithelium so that the apical patch is bisected and inherited by both daughters. Conversely, asymmetric generative divisions tend to be associated with an off-centre division plane so that only one daughter inherits the patch. These observations suggest that inheritance of the apical membrane patch is critical for a daughter cell to retain neural progenitor characteristics (Fig. 5.14).

mitotic spindle an array of microtubules that forms during cell division and serves to pull the chromosomes into each daughter cell.

5.6 Temporal regulation of neural identity

5.6.1 A neural cell's time of birth is important for neural identity

A consequence of the stem cell division pattern is that a progenitor generates neural precursors over an extended period of time. We saw how progenitors generate neural cell types according to their location (owing to their expression of different progenitor factors). In many parts of the CNS, the type of neural cells generated also changes over

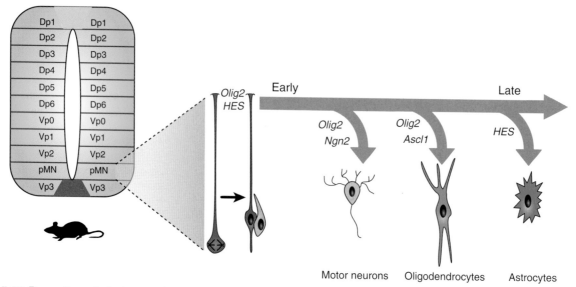

Fig. 5.15 Progenitor cells in the neural tube of the spinal cord generate different neural cells over time. For instance, those in the pMN progenitor domain (which express the genes *Olig* and *HES*) divide initially to generate precursor cells that differentiate as motor neurons (*Ngn2* being activated and *HES* down-regulated in the process). Later in development, *Ascl1* is activated and the newly generated cells differentiate as oligodendrocytes. Later still, *Olig* is down-regulated in the progenitors leading them to differentiate as astrocytes.

oligodendrocytes glial cells that produce processes that ensheath axons in the CNS.

reporter gene usually a 'neutral' gene that is introduced to mark the expression pattern of an endogenous gene. Well known reporter genes are *lacZ* (a bacterial gene that encodes β-galactosidase) and green fluorescent protein.

time. Progenitors in these regions are therefore **multipotent**. One of the first illustrations of this principle was found in the mouse ventral spinal cord (Fig. 5.15). Here, progenitors initially generate neurons, whereas later they produce two types of glial cell – firstly **oligodendrocytes** and finally **astrocytes**. Changes in transcription factor expression in the progenitor cells over time correlate with these different identities. The conclusion is that a neural cell's identity is influenced by the time at which the cell was generated during development (known as the cell's time of birth or **birth date**).

Multipotency of progenitors is generally demonstrated by observing the types of cell produced by progenitor divisions in two kinds of experiment. First, individual progenitor cells are labelled with a **reporter gene** by retroviral infection of entire brains (see Box 6.1, Chapter 6 for an explanation of this method). Division of the progenitor will result in a **clone** of labelled cells that can be examined subsequently to find out what cell types it contains. A second method is to culture individual progenitor cells and examine the clone of neurons that they produce. In general, mixed clones containing both neuronal and glial subtypes are observed in each type of experiment.

5.6.2 Time of birth can generate spatial patterns of neurons

An important consequence of the sequential generation of different neural cell types is that it can lead to spatial distribution patterns of these neuronal types. In some parts of the nervous system, neurons are organized or stratified into layers (also known as **laminae**) in the

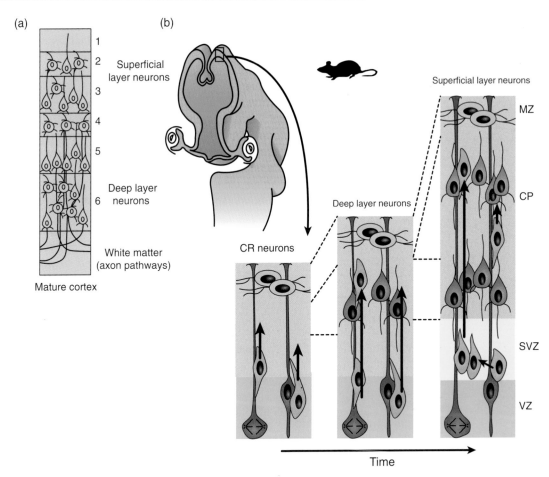

Fig. 5.16 Neurogenesis in the telencephalon generates the neuronal layers of the cortex. (a) The primary sensory cortex consists of six neuronal layers. (b) During development, cells that form the first layer migrate in from elsewhere (these are known as **Cajal–Retzius** cells (CR) and their role in controlling migration will be described in Chapter 6). Then, cortical progenitor divisions in the ventricular zone (VZ) generate a succession of neural precursors that migrate outwards to create successive neuronal layers. The migrating cells first populate deep layers (green neurons). At later stages, the migrating cells pause at the subventricular zone (SVZ). In the SVZ, these **basal progenitors** divide symmetrically before the progeny migrate outwards to form the superficial layers (blue cells). The development of connections within the cortex is considered further in Chapters 9, 11 and 12. (MZ = marginal zone; CP = cortical plate.)

ventricular-to-pial axis. The most striking manifestation of this is the mature mammalian **cerebral cortex**, which consists of six main layers of neurons. The neurons in each layer have a characteristic morphology, dendrite arborization pattern and axonal projection pattern (Fig. 5.16). For example, cells in layer 4 receive sensory input from the thalamus and project axons locally, while neurons in cortical layers 5 and 6 send axons to other parts of the brain.

The cortex develops from the dorsal telencephalon (Fig. 5.16; also Fig. 2.8 in Chapter 2). As in the spinal cord, radial glial cells divide asymmetrically to generate neural precursor cells, which migrate outwards to differentiate in the **cortical plate**. The first neural precursors generated remain close to the ventricular zone to differentiate as the deepest neuronal layers. Neurons generated later migrate past these neurons to form new, more superficial neuronal layers. Over time,

cortical plate a sheet of neural tissue in the developing mammalian brain that gives rise to most of the layers of the cerebral cortex.

more cells migrate outwards past an increasingly thick population of differentiating neurons to populate further superficial layers. The layers are therefore said to develop over time in an 'inside-out' manner. Thus, both a neuron's identity and its final location in the cortex are reflections of its time of birth.

A significant feature of cortical neurogenesis at later stages is that cells leaving the ventricular zone do not immediately become neurons. Instead, they populate a temporary **subventricular zone** (Fig. 5.16) as intermediate progenitors (also known as **basal progenitors**). These cells divide symmetrically, and after one or more further divisions their progeny cells exit the cell cycle and migrate to differentiate as superficial layer neurons (layers 2–4). Thus, basal progenitors are equivalent to ganglion mother cells in the *Drosophila* CNS. The basal progenitors represent an important cellular amplification step, which is necessary in the cortex in order to generate the huge numbers of neurons required. Indeed, in a human embryo hundreds of thousands of neurons are produced every minute at the peak of neurogenesis.

5.6.3 How does birth date influence a neuron's fate?

In the examples above, the time of birth correlates with a neural cell's identity. By what mechanism does birth date influence a neuron's fate? We saw earlier how a cell's complement of transcription factors can change over time. The question is *how* is this progression regulated? Is a neuron's fate decided directly by its birth date (a cell-intrinsic mechanism), or is the effect of birth date only indirect, with a neuron differentiating according to temporally or spatially varying environmental cues after it is born or has migrated (a cell-extrinsic mechanism)? In the former case, some mechanism intrinsic to the progenitors measures time and produces cell types appropriately. In the latter case, external signals trigger the production of different cell types over time. We shall examine the question of mechanism first in the *Drosophila* CNS and then in the mammalian cortex.

5.6.4 Intrinsic mechanism of temporal control in Drosophila *neuroblasts*

In the *Drosophila* CNS, neuroblasts divide to produce different types of neuron in sequence over time. This has proved to be a useful model for exploring temporal control of neural identity. Neuroblasts express a strict temporal sequence of transcription factor genes as they divide to produce successive **ganglion mother cells**. Thus, all neuroblasts express first the gene *hunchback* (*hb*), followed by *Krüppel*, *pdm-1* and then *castor* (note the first two played a different role in early patterning described in Chapter 4). This sequence of gene expression is tied to the first four neuroblast divisions such that the first four ganglion mother cells are marked by the expression of a different one of these 'temporal identity factors' (Fig. 5.17). Each transcription factor confers a different identity on the ganglion mother cell, causing it to produce different neurons and glia after division. In general, for all neuroblasts the first ganglion mother cells generated will produce motor neurons while later cells produce interneurons.

ganglion mother cell the daughter cell of a neuroblast in insects; it divides only once forming two neurons or a neuron and a glial cell.

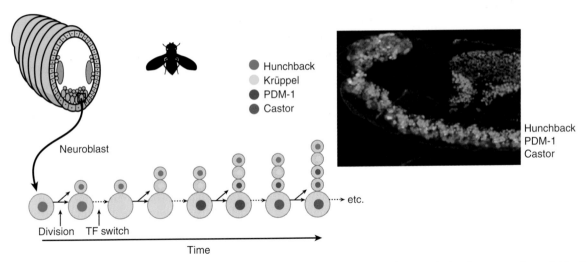

Fig. 5.17 In the *Drosophila* CNS, all neuroblasts express a common sequence of transcription factors as they divide. Each ganglion mother cell stably inherits the factor that was expressed in the neuroblast at the time at which it divided. In contrast, the neuroblast switches expression at each division to the next transcription factor (TF) in the series. The end result is that ganglion mother cells and their progeny express these factors in a spatial sequence corresponding to the order in which they are born. The image is a side view of an embryo showing the resulting spatial arrangement of Hunchback-, PDM-1 and Castor-expressing cells in the ventral nerve cord (Krüppel expression is not detected in this experiment). (Image courtesy of Thomas Brody, National Institutes of Health, USA.)

This temporal sequence gives rise to a spatial pattern reminiscent of that in vertebrate cortical layers, except that in this case neurons born later *displace* earlier neurons away from the neuroblasts. The end result is that first-born neurons (mostly motor neurons) end up on the internal side of the **nerve cord** (Fig. 5.17). It is notable that all neuroblasts exhibit the same sequence of factors despite the spatial differences in neuroblast identity due to regional patterning. Thus, the actual type of motor neuron produced by an early born cell depends on the spatial patterning information the cell inherits from its mother neuroblast. Temporal identity factors provide a general marker of ganglion mother cell birth date, which must be interpreted in conjunction with its spatial identity.

This model provides a platform for exploring questions concerning temporal identity. What causes the regular switch from one identity factor to the next? How is this coordinated with the neuroblast divisions? Can the progression be delayed or even reversed? If *hb* is experimentally reactivated in slightly older neuroblasts, they can be reprogrammed to produce more 'early' neurons. This suggests that neuroblasts retain some competence to produce early neuron fates in response to *hb* expression. However, older neuroblasts are less and less able to be reprogrammed by reactivating *hb* expression. In other words, the competence of neuroblasts to produce a range of neuronal types (their multipotency) diminishes over time.

How are the transcription factor switches regulated so that they proceed on time? Culturing single *Drosophila* neuroblasts reveals that the identity factor transitions happen normally in isolated cells – they must have an intrinsic 'clock'. For the transition from *hb* to *Krüppel* it appears that cell division itself acts as the trigger for

nerve cord the ventrally located CNS structure than runs the length of the insect; equivalent to the vertebrate spinal cord.

transcription factor switching. If cell division is inhibited, then the neuroblasts are stuck with *hb* expression. However, subsequent transitions are known to proceed on time even if later cell divisions are inhibited, showing that some other kind of internal molecular clock is at work.

5.6.5 Birth date, lamination and competence in the mammalian cortex

Returning to the mammalian cortex, the question of intrinsic and extrinsic mechanisms of temporal fate determination has been addressed by experiments that change the environment of neural precursors and examine the effect this has on their differentiation. Much use has been made of **heterochronic transplant** experiments, in which neural cells from the developing cortex are transplanted into the cortex of another embryo at a different stage of development. What is being tested is whether the transplanted cell takes on a fate that reflects the age of the animal it came from, or whether it can be reprogrammed to take on a fate appropriate to the age of the host animal. Such experiments have been performed using the ferret as a model system, because much of the ferret cerebral cortex develops postnatally, making it much easier to carry out transplant experiments. One important result is that if *migrating* neural precursors are transplanted, they always adopt fates appropriate for their age and not the age of the host. Therefore, neurons have already been assigned their fates by the time they migrate. This result rules out the possibility that they differentiate according to the environment into which they migrate.

Prior to migration, however, cells can respond differently. When early-born neural precursor cells (which would normally adopt deep-layer fates) were transplanted into older host brains, at a time when superficial cortical layers were being generated, the transplanted cells changed fates and migrated to more superficial layers (Fig. 5.18). This indicated that neural precursors can respond to environmental cues which influence their fate choice. However, when later-born cells were transplanted into younger ferrets, at the time when deeper layers are still being formed in the host, the transplanted cells still migrated to the superficial layers, suggesting that their fate had already been determined and that they could not respond to any environmental cues in the early cortex. Thus, in a manner similar to *Drosophila* neuroblasts, neural progenitors show a progressive restriction in the cell types they can produce – they lose multipotency over time. Early progenitors have the competence to produce many neural subtypes – they can adapt and 'fast-forward' according to the age of the ventricular zone; but later progenitors have much more restricted competence – they cannot 'turn the clock back'.

More recently, isolated cortical progenitor cells have been successfully cultured. These experiments have suggested that a dividing progenitor cell generates a temporal sequence of neural subtypes that reflects the sequence observed *in vivo* remarkably well. This suggests that the progenitors have an internally driven programme for neuronal subtype production, rather like *Drosophila*

in vivo pertaining to the context of the intact organism.

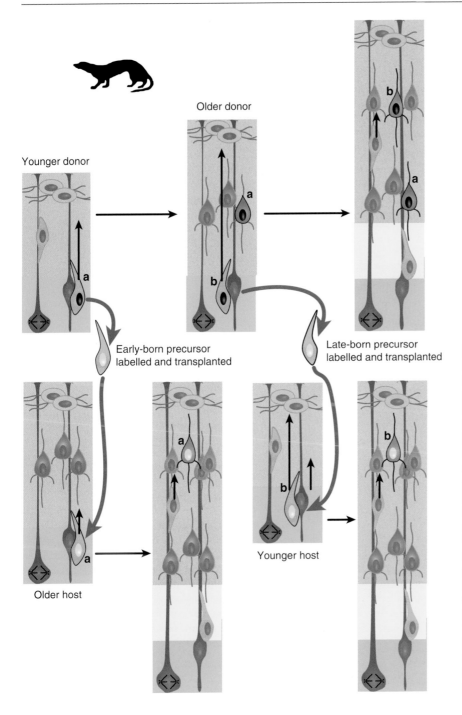

Younger donor

Older donor

Early-born precursor
labelled and transplanted

Late-born precursor
labelled and transplanted

Older host

Younger host

Fig. 5.18 Heterochronic transplantation studies in ferret. Precursor cell 'a' is extracted from a young donor (upper left), labelled (indicated by the yellow nucleus) and then transplanted into the ventricular zone of an older host (bottom left). Normally, the cell would contribute to the deep layer of early-born neurons (green cell in upper middle panel), but in the older host it is reprogrammed to contribute to the superficial layer of late-born neurons (blue). In contrast, precursor 'b' is taken from an older donor (upper middle) and transplanted into a younger host. This precursor contributes to the superficial layer of late-born neurons (lower right), just as it would have done normally (upper right). Therefore, the early-born precursor ('a') could be reprogrammed to become a late-born neuron, but the late-born precursor ('b') could not become an early-born neuron.

neuroblasts, but the physiological relevance of this remains to be explored.[6]

The picture of temporal control of neural fate that emerges, therefore, is one of an intrinsic mechanism (changes in competence over

---

[6] Details of this area can be found in Mizutani, K-I. and Gaiano, N. (2006) Chalk one up for 'nature' during neocortical neurogenesis. *Nature Neuroscience*, **9**, 717–718.

Box 5.4   Neurogenesis beyond development: adult neural stem cells

It may be supposed that neurogenesis is solely a developmental process and does not occur in the adult brain. As long ago as the 1960s, however, it became clear that new neurons are created in a few specific adult brain regions, notably the mammalian **olfactory bulb** and the **hippocampus.** In the olfactory bulb the new neurons may be required to replace worn out old olfactory sensory neurons. The hippocampus is important for formation of memories. It contains a small population of 'adult stem cells' that continue to generate new neurons during adulthood. The role of this neurogenesis in hippocampus function is not yet clear. Recent research has used genetic methods to ablate newly generated neurons in the adult mouse hippocampus. Such animals show an impairment of spatial memory. The suggestion is that new neurons must be added throughout life to maintain the ability to accumulate memories. Can these cells be manipulated in neural repair or regeneration in diseases, or even to enhance learning and memory?[7]

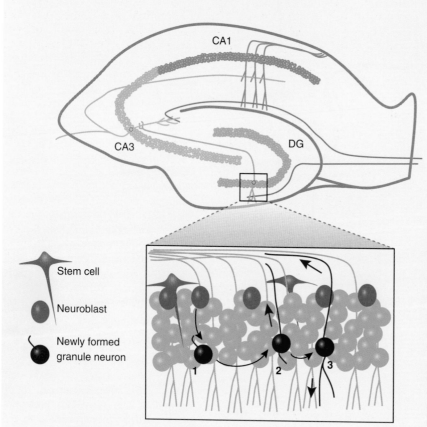

The drawing depicts neurogenesis in the adult hippocampus. A selection of nerve projections is shown to illustrate the flow of information into the hippocampus (red) to the granule neurons of the dentate gyrus (DG) (grey) and CA3 neurons (blue), and then to the CA1 neurons (green). Stem cells in the dentate gyrus divide asymmetrically to generate neuroblasts, which further divide to generate granule neuron precursors. These migrate, differentiate and make new axonal and dendritic connections with the existing network of neurons, potentially as a result of new sensory experiences.

olfactory bulb the brain region that receives input from olfactory neurons.

hippocampus a structure of the vertebrate forebrain particularly associated with learning and memory formation.

[7] Further information on adult neurogenesis can be found in Ming, G. L. and Song, H. (2005) Adult neurogenesis in the mammalian central nervous system. *Annual Review of Neuroscience*, **28**, 223–250.

time) that can be modulated or refined by extrinsic cues (the environment of the ventricular zone).

5.7 Why do we need to know about neurogenesis?

One potential future application of the knowledge obtained in the studies described in this chapter is the development of stem cell therapies to treat conditions such as neurodegenerative diseases. For this to be feasible, neural stem cells need to be manipulated to produce specific neuronal cell types. As our knowledge of the molecular mechanisms of neurogenesis expands, it will allow us to reproduce the process in culture in order to drive **embryonic stem cells** to differentiate as particular neural subtypes. At present, based on advances outlined in this chapter, conditions have been defined for the production in culture of motor neurons, cortical precursors, cerebellar granule neurons, and dopaminergic midbrain neurons. The latter are the neurons that degenerate in Parkinson's disease. In some cases these cells can even integrate successfully when injected into a developing mouse brain. Another important aspect is the discovery that neurogenesis has some limited but crucial roles to play in the adult brain (involving so-called **adult stem cells**), which may also be important for therapies (Box 5.4). A clear message is that basic research in developmental neurobiological mechanisms can help the progress of therapeutic approaches using stem cells.[8]

embryonic stem cells pluripotent stem cells that are derived from the inner cell mass of the blastocyst.

5.8 Summary

- Neurogenesis is the balance between cell proliferation and differentiation.
- Neurons are generated from progenitor cells by the action of proneural genes. This process is antagonized by Notch signalling.
- Combinations of transcription factors endow neuronal subtype identity on neural precursor cells.
- Asymmetric cell division is important in neurogenesis. Segregation of determinants such as Numb and PAR is central to this process.
- Proliferation is regulated during vertebrate neurogenesis to generate vast numbers of neurons. Extrinsic signals and variation in cell division mode are important aspects of this process.
- Progenitors can generate different subtypes of neural cells over time. This can lead to spatial patterns of neurons, such as the layers of the cerebral cortex.

---

[8] For an introduction to this area, see K. Hochedlinger, K. (2010) Your inner healers. *Scientific American*, **302**, 28–35.

Neuronal Migration

6.1 Many neurons migrate long distances during formation of the nervous system

We saw in Chapter 5 that neurogenesis results in the generation of large numbers of neurons. Different types of neurons are born in different regions of the nervous system and many of them must move away from their birthplace to reach the position in which they will function. For example, in vertebrates, cortical neurons born in the ventricular zone of the telencephalon must migrate towards the outer surface of the brain to build up the six neuronal layers of the adult cerebral cortex (see Fig. 5.16 in the previous chapter). The process by which newborn neurons move from their birthplace to their final positions, often over considerable distances, is known as **neuronal migration**, analogous to the way in which people may migrate away from their birthplace to find work in another country. In general, migration is a more significant feature of vertebrate than invertebrate neural development, mostly due to the very large numbers of cells and the large distances involved, but some neuronal migration is essential in invertebrates too.

In all cases, neuronal migration must be tightly regulated – the timing, direction, distance travelled and termination must all be controlled to ensure that appropriate numbers of cells reach the appropriate regions of the nervous system at appropriate times. A variety of strategies to regulate neuronal migration have been uncovered: some neurons migrate individually, others migrate in groups and some are guided on their journey by a scaffold provided by other cells.

6.2 How can neuronal migration be observed?

Before moving on to discuss the mechanisms that control neuronal migration, we shall first look at the various experimental techniques that have been used to visualize patterns of migration.

6.2.1 Watching neurons move in living embryos

Some organisms, such as the nematode worm *C. elegans*, have transparent embryos, allowing direct visualization of individual cells in the

Building Brains: An Introduction to Neural Development, First Edition.
David Price, Andrew Jarman, John Mason and Peter Kind.
© 2011 John Wiley & Sons, Ltd. Published 2011 by John Wiley & Sons, Ltd.

lineage the sequence of divisions that generated the cell, that is its cellular ancestry.

lateral line a sense organ found in many species of fish and amphibians that detects water movements and allows the animal to orient itself in the water.

intact, living embryo. We saw in Chapter 2 (Section 2.3.1), that the developmental **lineage** of every one of the 302 neurons in an adult hermaphrodite *C. elegans* is known. Therefore, specific neurons can be identified and their migration followed in living animals, allowing the investigation of mechanisms that control the direction of migration of individual neurons (see Section 6.5.1).

Some migrating neural cells can be visualized relatively easily in living vertebrate embryos too. For example, zebrafish embryos are also transparent, allowing scientists to follow the behaviours of individual cells in intact embryos. Migrating cells can be detected more easily if they are labelled with a specific marker, such as **green fluorescent protein** (GFP) (Box 1.4), which provides contrast and makes the cells easier to see and distinguish from their neighbours. For example, studies of how the **lateral line** forms in zebrafish have used transgenic embryos that express GFP in a specific group of migrating cells (Fig. 6.1). Formation of the zebrafish lateral line is described in Section 6.5.3.

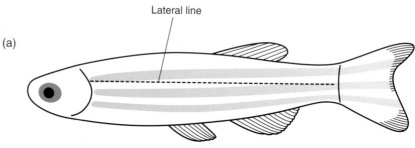

(a)

Lateral line

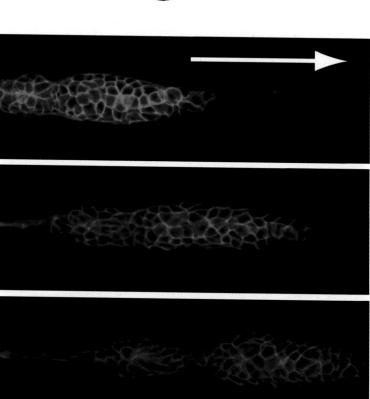

(b)

Fig. 6.1 Use of a GFP transgene to visualize migrating cells in a living zebrafish embryo. (a) In an adult zebrafish, the lateral line runs from behind the gill to just in front of the tail. (b) Three still frames taken from a time-lapse video, showing a cluster of cells migrating from left to right along the developing lateral line in a living zebrafish embryo. The cells are easy to see as the embryo contains a transgene which drives expression of GFP specifically in the migrating cells. The images in panel (b) are by Darren Gilmour, EMBL and the full-length movie can be seen at http://www.biomedcentral.com/content/supplementary/1749-8104-2-15-S1.mov (18 January 2011). Taken from Ghysen, A., Dambly-Chaudière, C. and Raible, D. (2007) Making sense of zebrafish neural development in the Minervois. *Neural Dev.*, **2**,15.

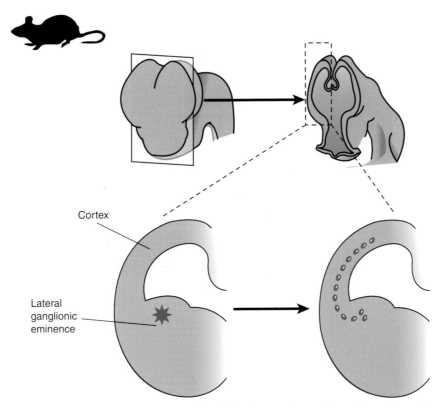

Cortex

Lateral ganglionic eminence

Fig. 6.2 Slices of embryonic mouse forebrain can be placed in tissue culture where they will continue to develop for a few days. Placing a dye crystal (red) on a specific part of the ventral telencephalon, the **lateral ganglionic eminence (LGE)**, labels a set of neurons that subsequently migrate from the lateral ganglionic eminences into the developing cortex.

6.2.2 Observing migrating neurons in cultured tissues

While direct visualization techniques are ideal for cells within small, transparent embryos or for cells that migrate along the external surface of an embryo, the pathways followed by many migrating neurons in vertebrate embryos are located deep inside the brain and so cannot be directly visualized. One way to observe the migration of individual neurons inside the brain is to place living slices of embryonic brain in tissue culture. For example, slices of mouse forebrain that contain both ventral and dorsal telencephalon can be cut from embryonic brain and placed in culture (Fig. 6.2). These slices preserve the spatial relationship between different regions of the forebrain. Placing a dye crystal on a specific region of the slice allows cells in this area to take up the dye. After one or two days in culture, labelled cells that have migrated from the area labelled by the dye can easily be identified (Section 6.8).

Recent technological advances in imaging techniques, discussed in Box 5.3 in the previous chapter, have allowed us to extend this approach. The migration of individual neurons can now be observed as it happens in living slices of embryonic brain in culture (Fig. 6.3).

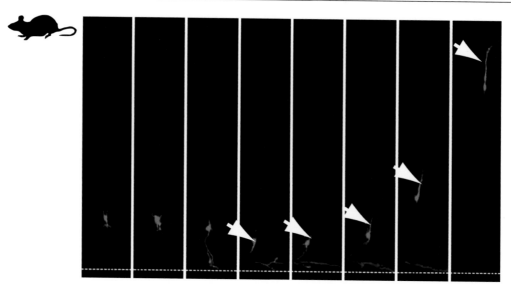

Fig. 6.3 Live imaging of migrating neurons in cultured slices of embryonic mouse cerebral cortex. A single migrating neuron has been infected with a virus that expresses green fluorescent protein (GFP). Images taken over a 96 hour time period allow us to follow the migration of the labelled cell (white arrows). Reprinted by permission from Macmillan Publishers Ltd: Nature Neuroscience. (Noctor, S. C., Martinez-Cerdeño, V., Ivic, L. and Kriegstein, A. R. (2004) Cortical neurons arise in symmetric and asymmetric division zones and migrate through specific phases. *Nature Neuroscience*, **7**, 136–144) copyright 2004.

6.2.3 Tracking cell migration by indirect methods

The relative inaccessibility of most migrating neurons in developing vertebrate brains precludes their direct visualization. For this reason, cell migration paths in vertebrate brains are most commonly tracked indirectly. Cells in an intact embryo are labelled in some way before they migrate, then the embryo is allowed to develop for a period of time before being examined to find out where the labelled cells have ended up. Although these indirect techniques do not allow us to watch the movement of cells directly, they do offer an advantage over culture-based techniques, in that migration occurs under more natural conditions and is therefore not subject to possible artefacts caused by placing tissues in culture.

Developing chick embryos are easily accessible through a hole in the egg shell (see Section 1.5.2), allowing cells to be labelled before they migrate, then the egg can be sealed and the labelled embryo left to develop normally. The labelled cells can be visualized later, after their migration. One group of migrating cells that have been extensively studied in this way using chick embryos is the **neural crest**. The neural crest comprises a set of specialized migratory cells that originate in the dorsal part of the nervous system and give rise to a wide variety of cell types including neurons of both the autonomic and peripheral nervous system (see Section 2.6.2 and Fig. 2.10).

One simple way to label neural crest cells before they migrate is to inject their **progenitors** with a dye that does not interfere with cell functions and is easy to detect (Fig. 6.4(a)). Alternatively, migration of neural crest cells can be traced in quail-chick

progenitor defined in this book as a cell that divides to give daughter cells, some of which will differentiate as neural cells. Progenitor cells are uncommitted to a particular fate and are often multipotent. Cf precursor.

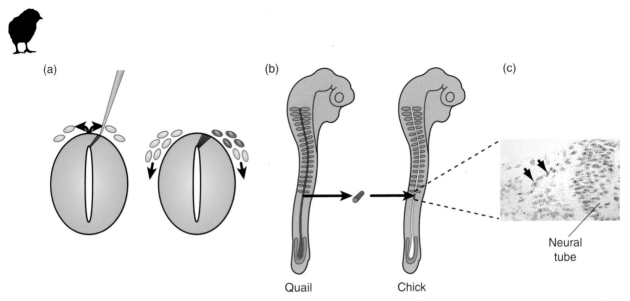

Fig. 6.4 Methods used to follow migration of neural crest cells in chick embryos. (a) Dye is injected into cells on one side of the neural tube, which is then left to develop for a few days. The dye allows easy identification of cells derived from the initial labelled cells. (b) A chick-quail chimeric embryo can be made using surgical techniques to transplant a small section of neural tube from a quail embryo (left) into a chick embryo (right). Quail cells respond to the cues in the chick embryo that control neural crest migration and therefore quail neural crest cells derived from the graft migrate in the same way as chick cells. The quail cells in such chimeric embryos can be distinguished from host chick cells by the presence of a specific nuclear marker. (c) *In situ* hybridization to detect quail-specific nuclear marker (shown in red); arrows indicate two quail neural crest cells migrating away from the neural tube. The image in panel (c) was kindly provided by Sophie Creuzet and Nicole le Douarin.

chimeras (chimeras were defined in Box 1.5). Chick and quail embryos are very similar and if a small piece of a quail embryo is grafted into a chick embryo, it will continue to develop normally and quail cells will follow their normal routes of migration. Grafted quail cells and their descendants in such chimeras can be identified subsequently by *in situ* hybridization (Box 3.4) using a quail-specific nuclear marker (Fig. 6.4(b) and (c)). The mechanisms that control the migration of neural crest cells are described in Sections 6.4.1 and 6.5.2.

Another widely used indirect technique to study cell migration in the CNS is **birth-dating**, first developed in the 1960s. In a birth-dating study, cells are tagged on the day of their birth with a specific label that is incorporated into newly-synthesized DNA (Fig. 6.5). Some embryos are then examined immediately to find out the starting positions of labelled cells born at the time of labelling. Others are left to develop normally for a time and the subsequent locations of cells born during the labelling period are revealed. Birth-dating is often used in mammals, in which direct *in vivo* visualization is impractical as their embryos are protected by extensive extra-embryonic membranes, have a large placenta and are embedded inside the uterus. Birth-dating studies were instrumental in showing that the layers of the cerebral cortex form in an inside-out manner, as described in Section 5.6.2 in the previous chapter.

chimera an individual created when cells of different genotypes come together to form an embryo.

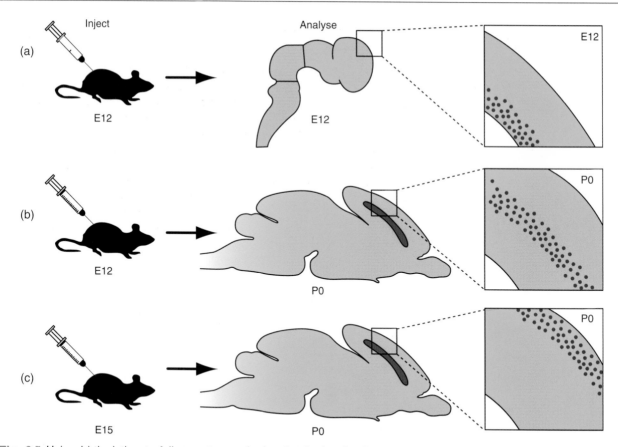

Fig. 6.5 Using birth dating to follow patterns of migration in the developing cerebral cortex. In this method, a pregnant female mouse is injected with the labelled nucleotide **bromodeoxyuridine** (BrdU). The label is taken up by the embryo, all of whose proliferating cells that are in the DNA-synthesis phase (S-phase) of the cell cycle will incorporate the label into their DNA. Labelled cells can subsequently be identified by immunohistochemistry using an antibody that recognizes BrdU. As BrdU only remains in the bloodstream for around 2 hours after injection, the labelling period is referred to as a pulse. When the embryos are subsequently processed, immunohistochemistry will reveal the positions of those cells that were in S-phase when the pulse was given. (a) In the case of the developing cerebral cortex, for example, this means when an embryo is given a pulse of BrdU at embryonic day 12 (E12), and analysed shortly afterwards, BrdU-labelled cells are found in the ventricular zone, where proliferation occurs. As neurons do not undergo cell division again after they have been born, the BrdU remains permanently incorporated in their DNA. In progenitor cells however, which keep dividing, the BrdU label becomes progressively more dilute with subsequent divisions. Thus, neurons born during the BrdU pulse retain high levels of BrdU and can readily be identified, days, weeks or even months later. (b) If BrdU is given at E12, and the embryos are then left to develop until the day of birth (P0), labelled cells are found in middle layers of the cortex, indicating that the neurons in these layers were born at E12 and subsequently migrated radially. (c) Similarly, labelling at a later stage of development (E15), followed by analysis at P0 reveals that neurons born at E15 migrate radially to occupy more superficial layers of the cerebral cortex.

bromodeoxyuridine (BrdU) a chemical analogue of the nucleotide thymidine, readily incorporated into newly-synthesized DNA.

retrovirus a small virus that inserts a DNA copy of its RNA genome into a chromosome of an infected cell.

A third indirect labelling technique that has been used to follow migration pathways in the developing vertebrate brain, involving the use of genetically-marked **retroviruses**, is described in Box 6.1.

Box 6.1   Using retroviruses to trace patterns of cell migration

Retroviruses are small, fairly simple animal viruses with an RNA genome. When a retrovirus infects a cell, a copy of its genetic material becomes stably incorporated into the cell's DNA, such that the viral genes are passed on to all of the descendants of the infected cell. Retroviruses can be modified genetically to include a **reporter gene** – a gene that encodes a foreign protein whose product is easy to detect, thus marking those cells where it is expressed. One commonly used reporter is the *lacZ* gene from the bacterium *E. coli* that encodes the protein **β-galactosidase**. β-galactosidase-expressing cells can be readily identified using an artificial substrate that stains them blue. Therefore, if a progenitor cell in the developing nervous system is infected with a genetically modified retrovirus that carries a *lacZ* reporter, the infected cell and all of its descendants (a **clone**) will express β-galactosidase and can easily be detected. As shown in the figure, this forms the basis of a technique to trace the migration paths followed by cells in the developing mouse brain. The technique can also be used to mark the progeny cells formed by the division of a progenitor cell (see Chapter 5, Section 5.6.1).

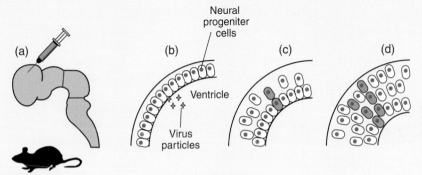

(a) *LacZ*-expressing retroviruses are injected into the forebrain ventricle of a mid-gestation mouse embryo in the uterus. Only a few virus particles are introduced, so that only a small number of neural progenitors are labelled. (b) The injected viruses (blue) infect neural progenitor cells in the ventricular zone. Viral DNA stably incorporates into the genome of each infected cell. (c) The infected cell divides, giving rise to two daughter cells, each of which expresses the *lacZ* reporter (blue). (d) After a few days, the positions of *lacZ*-expressing cells reveal the positions of all cells descended from the original infected progenitor cell.

6.3 Major modes of migration

Using a combination of these types of experimental approach, scientists have discovered three major modes of neural cell migration. Some migrating cells follow a **scaffold** that is provided by other cells. Others migrate collectively in a process known as **chain migration**. A third group migrate individually, apparently independent of close contact with other cells – often referred to as **individual migration**. We shall first look at specific examples of each of these modes of migration before going on to look at mechanisms in more detail.

6.3.1 Some migrating neurons are guided by a scaffold

Live-imaging studies of the type shown in Fig. 6.3 have confirmed that many radially-migrating neurons in the cerebral cortex move towards the **pial** surface guided by the process of a **radial glial cell**, as was predicted in pioneering observations made by Pasko Rakic in

pia a membrane that envelops the brain and spinal cord.

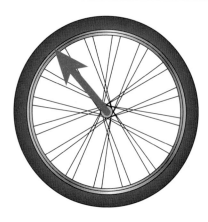

the 1970s. As the cerebral cortex approximates to a hemisphere, this is known as **radial migration**, analogous to the way in which the spokes of a bicycle wheel radiate from the hub. Despite their name, radial glia are not truly glial cells, rather they are neural progenitor cells that have long processes connected to both the ventricular and pial edges of the cortex (Section 5.3.2). The process of radial glial guided migration is shown in Fig. 6.6. Glial-guided migration is also found in other parts of the brain, for example, migrating granule cells in the developing cerebellum are guided by a scaffold provided by the processes of Bergmann glia (Box 6.2).

6.3.2 Some neurons migrate in groups

The second common mode of neuronal migration is known as collective migration or **chain migration**. One of the most studied populations of neurons that migrate in this way is the **olfactory interneurons** found in the **olfactory bulbs**. The olfactory bulbs are the first relay station for sensory information from the olfactory epithelium to the brain. In rodents, the olfactory bulbs are located at the very front of the brain, and are relatively large, reflecting the importance of the sense of olfaction for rodents. In the embryo, olfactory interneurons are derived from progenitor cells in the ventral telencephalon from where they migrate to the olfactory bulbs. Interestingly, olfactory neurons are also generated continuously during adult life, arising from a stem cell population located in the **subventricular zone** (SVZ) of the **lateral ventricle** (see also Box 5.4). Cells born here migrate to the olfactory bulb where they differentiate into neurons and integrate functionally into neural circuits. The migrating cells cover a considerable distance – in adult mice they migrate up to 5 millimeters, a distance equivalent to around 500 cell diameters (Fig. 6.7).

The path followed by migrating olfactory precursors from their birthplace in the subventricular zone to the olfactory bulb is known as the **rostral migratory stream** (Fig. 6.7). As they migrate, they form a

radial migration a mode of migration in which newborn neurons migrate from the centre of a developing structure towards its outer edge (e.g. the cortex), or vice-versa (e.g. granule cells in the cerebellum).

subventricular zone the transient layer of the forebrain neural tube that contains the basal progenitor cells.

lateral ventricle a small fluid-filled cavity within the forebrain.

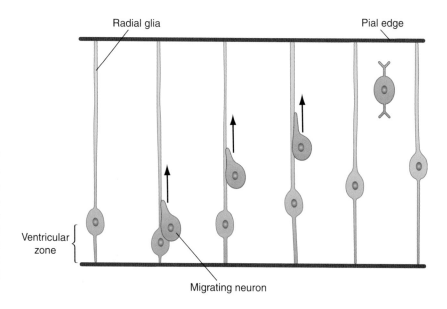

Fig. 6.6 Many newborn neurons in the cerebral cortex use the process of a radial glial cell (shown in green) to guide their outward migration. The migrating neuron (orange) forms a close association with a radial glial fibre and maintains close contact as it moves outward towards the pial edge of the cortex. The neuron dissociates from the radial glial fibre when it reaches its destination.

Box 6.2 Patterns of cell migration in the developing cerebellum

The cerebellum is part of the hindbrain and is important for regulating motor control. Mutant mice in which development of the cerebellum has been affected are often easily identified by virtue of their difficulties in motor coordination. Such mutants are often given names that reflect this poor coordination – for example, *weaver*, *shaker* and *reeler*. Study of several of these mutant mouse strains has provided valuable insight into the mechanisms of brain development (see Chapter 10, Section 10.5.3, and Section 6.7).

There are two major types of neuron in the adult cerebellum, **Purkinje cells** and **granule cells**, each of which occupies a specific layer. During development, these two types of neuron arise from neural progenitor cells in two different areas. Purkinje cells are born first, in the ventricular zone on the ventral side of the emerging cerebellum. In the mouse, this happens around embryonic day 13.5. Purkinje cells migrate towards the pial surface of the embryonic cerebellum and, by late embryonic stages, they form a broad band beneath the pial surface. The granule cells, in contrast, are born in the external granule layer (EGL) on the pial surface of the cerebellum. Vast numbers of granule cells are born, most of them during the early postnatal period. The newborn granule cells then migrate inwards, past the Purkinje cells, to form the internal granule layer. They are guided on their inward migration by the processes of Bergmann glial cells, a glial population whose cell bodies lie adjacent to the Purkinje cells. This migration appears very similar to the radial-glial guided migration of cortical neurons in the cerebral cortex. As they migrate, granule cells leave behind a bifurcated trailing process, which subsequently forms synapses with the dendrites of the Purkinje cells, creating a critical component of the circuitry of the cerebellum.

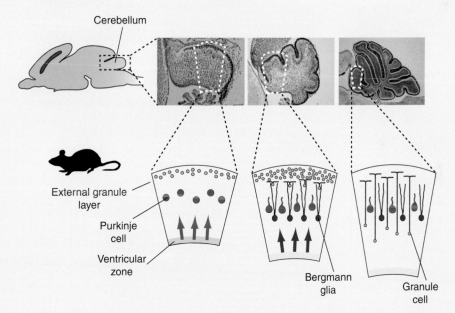

Patterns of cell migration in the developing cerebellum. The cerebellum forms in the anterior hindbrain. The top panels show the appearance of the cerebellum at three developmental stages and the schematic diagrams below show the main cell types and their migration patterns at each stage. Neural cells are born in two distinct regions of the cerebellum, the ventricular zone (pale brown) which gives rise to Purkinje cells (red) and subsequently to Bergmann glia (blue) and the external granule layer (orange circles) in which granule neurons (orange) are born. Granule neurons migrate inward, past the Purkinje cells, guided by the processes of Bergmann glia. (Photographs in the top panel are from Albert Basson, King's College, London. See Yaguchi, Y., Yu, T., Ahmed, M. U., Berry, M., Mason, I. and Basson, M. A., (2009) Fibroblast growth factor (FGF) gene expression in the developing cerebellum suggests multiple roles for FGF signaling during cerebellar morphogenesis and development. *Developmental Dynamics*, **238**, 2058–72.)

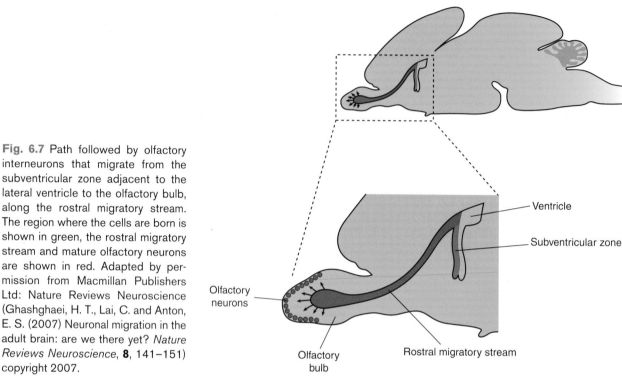

Fig. 6.7 Path followed by olfactory interneurons that migrate from the subventricular zone adjacent to the lateral ventricle to the olfactory bulb, along the rostral migratory stream. The region where the cells are born is shown in green, the rostral migratory stream and mature olfactory neurons are shown in red. Adapted by permission from Macmillan Publishers Ltd: Nature Reviews Neuroscience (Ghashghaei, H. T., Lai, C. and Anton, E. S. (2007) Neuronal migration in the adult brain: are we there yet? *Nature Reviews Neuroscience*, **8**, 141–151) copyright 2007.

continuous chain, sliding along one another to reach their destination. This type of migration is analogous to the way in which a column of ants can pass over a physical gap in their route by walking over a bridge formed by other ants, with all ants eventually reaching the other side (Fig. 6.8).

The rostral migratory stream is surrounded by a tube composed of glial cells, raising the possibility that these glia may guide migrating olfactory precursors. However, cultured olfactory neural precursors can form chains and migrate in culture in the complete absence of glial cells. This shows that olfactory precursors can migrate in the absence of a glial scaffold, at least *in vitro*, but it is not yet certain whether glia provide a scaffold for their migration *in vivo* (Fig. 6.8).[1]

6.3.3 Some neurons migrate individually

In the third major mode of neural migration cells migrate individually, without either glia or co-migrating cells to help them on their way. This mode of migration is used by neural crest cells, perhaps the best-known population of migratory cells in vertebrate embryos. The neural

---

[1] Migration in the rostral migratory stream is described in more detail by Ghashghaei, H.T., Lai, C. and Anton, E.S. (2007) Neuronal migration in the adult brain: are we there yet? *Nat. Rev. Neurosci.*, **8**, 141–51.

(a)

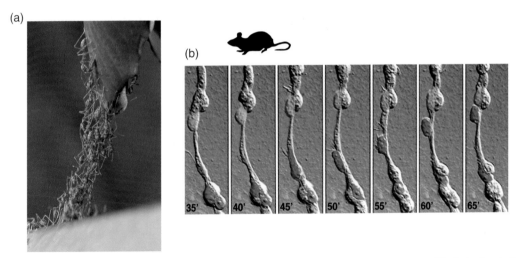

(b)

Fig. 6.8 (a) Ants cooperate with one another to form bridges, allowing them to cross over gaps. Similarly, in chain migration, migrating neurons slide over each other, using other cells for guidance and support on their journey. (b) Olfactory neural progenitor cells can form chains and migrate along one another when placed in cell culture. A set of seven frames taken from a time-lapse study over a 30 minute time-course are shown. For clarity, the migrating cell has been coloured red and two cells that do not migrate during the time-lapse study have been coloured green and blue. The red cell can clearly be seen to migrate along the chain formed by the olfactory neural progenitors. There are no glial cells in this culture, showing that migration can occur in the absence of glia. Panel (b) is reprinted from Wichterle, H., Garcia-Verdugo, J. M. and Alvarez-Buylla, A. (1997) Direct evidence for homotypic, glia-independent neuronal migration. *Neuron*, **18**, 779–91, Copyright 1997, with permission from Elsevier.

crest was introduced in Section 2.6.2. Neural crest cells arise in the dorsal part of the neural tube from where they migrate in streams of individual cells to a wide variety of destinations across the embryo (Figs 2.10 and 6.12).

Visualizing the migration of newborn neuron cells using live imaging studies on cultured slices of embryonic cortex (Fig. 6.3) has shown that some neurons migrate by **somal translocation**, apparently independent of any contact with radial glia. These somally translocating cells extend a long process to the pial surface and lose their connection to the ventricular surface (Fig. 6.9). Their leading process becomes

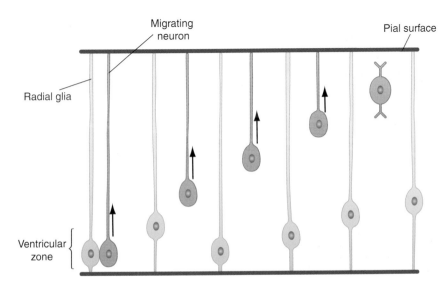

Fig. 6.9 Some newborn cells in the cerebral cortex migrate from the ventricular zone to the pial surface by somal translocation. Neurons that migrate in this way extend a single, long process towards the pial surface which shortens progressively as the neuron migrates.

progressively shorter as they move towards the pia, as if the cells were pulling themselves up on a rope.

6.4 Initiation of migration

The process of neural migration can be considered to consist of four main steps. Migration must first be *initiated* at the point when the cell starts to move (discussed in this section). The migrating cell must then be *guided* in the appropriate direction (Section 6.5). Next, the cell moves in a process commonly referred to as *locomotion* (Section 6.6). In the final step, *termination*, the cell stops once it has reached its destination (Section 6.7). Fig. 6.10 illustrates these four steps for a migrating cortical neuron being guided by a radial glial cell, but all three modes of neuronal migration that we discussed in Section 6.3 can be broken down into essentially the same four steps.

6.4.1 Initiation of neural crest cell migration

Before they migrate, neural crest cells are tightly held together with their neighbours in the **neuroectoderm**. They must therefore become less adhesive and lose their connections to neighbouring neuroectodermal cells before they can emigrate. Amongst the most important changes that occur in neural crest cells as they commence migrating are dynamic changes in expression of **cell adhesion molecules** (Box 6.3). For example, the cell adhesion molecules N-cadherin and cadherin 6 are both down-regulated as neural crest cells leave the neural tube. If down-regulation of cadherin 6 is blocked experimentally, crest cells fail to migrate away as they are stuck in the dorsal neural tube. Many of the cellular changes that occur at this early stage of neural crest cell migration are controlled by the **transcription factors** Snail1 and Snail2, which are expressed in response to bone morphogenetic protein (BMP) signalling in the dorsal neural tube (see Section 4.5.4).

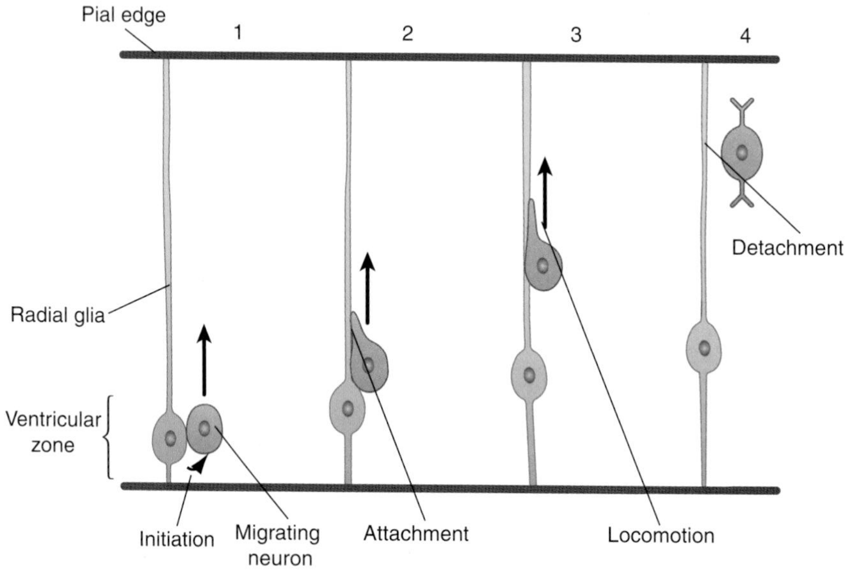

neuroectoderm the neurogenic region of the ectoderm which develops into the nervous system.

transcription factors proteins that bind to DNA to regulate gene transcription.

Fig. 6.10 Four steps in the radial migration of a newborn cortical neuron. (1) During *initiation* of movement the newborn neuron begins its outward migration. (2) The neuron forms a close *attachment* to the process of an adjacent radial glial cell that will guide it on its outward journey. (3) During *locomotion*, the cell migrates towards the pial surface. (4) Once it has reached its final position, the neuron *detaches* from the radial glial process.

Box 6.3   Cell adhesion molecules

The vast majority of cells in a multicellular organism interact intimately with their neighbours. Such cell–cell interactions are important for structural integrity within tissues and organisms, and play important roles in specific types of communication between cells. When cells migrate, they must often change the way in which they interact with neighbouring cells. Many cell–cell interactions are mediated by a class of molecules known as cell adhesion molecules. Many different types of cell adhesion molecules are known, but we shall consider only the three types that are most important during nervous system development.

The cadherins (so named as they require calcium for their adhesive activity and function in cell adherence) are a family of transmembrane proteins that span the cell's plasma membrane and bind to each other through binding sites in their extracellular domains. The cytoplasmic domain of cadherin molecules interacts with the **actin** cytoskeleton (described in Box 7.1) through a number of intracellular anchor proteins. In this way, the actin cytoskeleton of one cell is connected to that of its neighbours. Cadherins are the adhesive parts of **adherens junctions**, junctions between cells that are important for the integrity of epithelial structures, including the neuroectoderm.

Neural cell adhesion molecules (N-CAM) are widely expressed in the nervous system. Based upon structural similarity, N-CAMs are members of the immunoglobulin superfamily of cell surface proteins. Members of this large family of cell adhesion molecules most commonly form **homophilic** interactions with N-CAMs expressed on the surface of neighbouring cells. Unlike cadherins, they do not need calcium ions to mediate adhesion.

A third class of cell adhesion molecules, the integrins, mostly form connections between cells and the **extracellular matrix**, a complex network of secreted proteins and polysaccharides that surrounds most eukaryotic cells (see Box 7.2). Integrins function as **heterodimers**, composed of one α and one β subunit. Many integrins link to cytoplasmic actin, while others link to different components of the cytoskeleton. Integrins may also mediate signalling from the extracellular matrix, affecting both cell movement and shape.

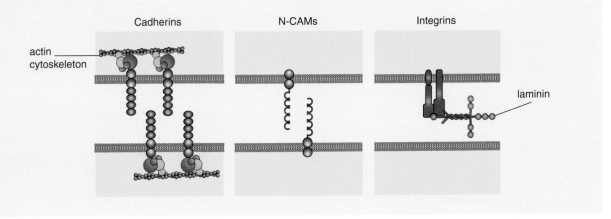

homophilic binding between molecules of the same kind.

heterodimer a protein complex consisting of two different proteins.

6.4.2 Initiation of neuronal migration

Factors that stimulate or promote the initiation of cell movement are known as **motogenic** factors. We don't yet know a great deal about the molecular mechanisms that govern the initiation of migration of cortical neurons.[2] More is known about initiation of migration by olfactory precursor cells. At the beginning of their journey, olfactory precursors move away from the subventricular zone (SVZ) where they are born and enter the rostral migratory stream (Fig. 6.7). Several secreted factors have been shown to be involved in initiating their movement. These include motogenic factors such as the secretory protein MIA (migration-inducing activity), which is produced by glial cells surrounding the migrating olfactory precursors. The secreted signalling molecules Slit1 and Slit2 are also produced by cells surrounding the SVZ. Slit proteins are best known for their involvement in axon guidance where they commonly act to repel growing axons. Their activity is discussed in more detail in Section 8.6.2. Slits are thought to be important for orienting newborn olfactory precursor cells away from the SVZ and initially directing them towards the olfactory bulb. Consistent with this, in mutant mice in which both copies of the *Slit1* gene are inactivated (i.e. *Slit1*$^{-/-}$ mice), many olfactory precursors migrate caudally instead of rostrally; in mutant mice that lack both *Slit1* and *Slit2* (*Slit1*$^{-/-}$; *Slit2*$^{-/-}$), the olfactory bulbs contain many fewer neurons.

6.5 How are migrating cells guided to their destinations?

The two major mechanisms that have so far been shown to guide the direction of migrating neurons are **chemotaxis** and guidance by a glial **scaffold**. In chemotaxis, the movement of a cell is directed by a chemical signal. Cells may either move towards such signals, known as **chemoattraction**, or away from them, known as **chemorepulsion**. Cells known to be guided by chemotaxis in the developing nervous system include specific neural precursors in *C. elegans*, neural crest cells and the cells that form the lateral line in zebrafish. In contrast, as we saw in Section 6.3.1, many migrating cortical neurons receive their directional guidance from radial glial cells.

6.5.1 Directional migration of neurons in C. elegans

We saw in Section 6.2.1 that individual cells can be identified in *C. elegans* embryos and their movement tracked under a light microscope. One pair of neural progenitors, known as the Q cells, arises at equivalent positions on either side of the *C. elegans* embryo – QL on the left side, and QR on the right (Fig. 6.11). During normal development, the Q cells and their descendants migrate in opposite directions – QL and its descendants migrate towards the posterior of the embryo while QR and its descendants migrate anteriorly, towards the head. However, in certain mutant strains of *C. elegans* in which **Wnt** signalling is defective, both QR and QL lose their directional migration and each migrates randomly along the anteroposterior axis. The Wnt signalling pathway is described in Section 3.6. Three *Wnt* genes are expressed in a gradient in the *C. elegans* embryo, with high levels posteriorly and

Wnt a highly evolutionarily conserved family of secreted proteins that regulate many different processes in developing and adult animals, including cell proliferation, differentiation and gene expression.

---

[2] For a detailed discussion of this topic, see Marín, O. and Rubenstein, J. L. (2003) Cell migration in the forebrain. *Annual Rev. Neurosci.*, **26**, 441–83.

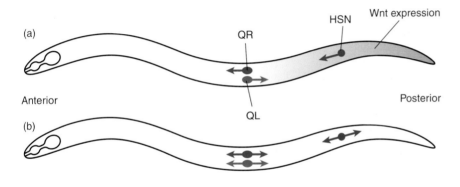

(a)

Anterior

(b)

QR

HSN

Wnt expression

QL

Posterior

Fig. 6.11 Migration of neural progenitors in *C. elegans* is regulated by Wnt signalling. (a) In the wild-type embryo, QR and HSN progenitors migrate anteriorly, while QL progenitors migrate posteriorly. Three different Wnt genes, *cwn-1*, *egl-20* and *lin-44* are expressed in a gradient (purple), with highest levels found at the posterior of the embryo. (b) In mutant embryos that lack expression of either a Wnt or the Wnt receptor *lin-17*, QL and QR cells migrate randomly along the anteroposterior axis. Many *C. elegans* genes are named for the phenotype identified during the genetic screen in which the genes were first identified. Thus, *lin* genes show defects in cell <u>lin</u>eage, while *egl* genes have defects with <u>eg</u>g <u>l</u>aying. When these genes were subsequently cloned and sequenced, it emerged that *egl-20* and *lin-44* encode Wnts, while *lin-17* encodes a Wnt receptor, frizzled. Figure modified from Salinas, P. C. and Zhou, Y. (2008) Wnt signaling in neural circuit assembly. *Ann. Rev. Neurosci.*, **31**, 339–58.

lower levels towards the anterior of the embryo (Fig. 6.11). Migrating Q cells therefore appear to be guided by responding differentially to the gradient of *Wnt* expression, although the details of the mechanism are not yet fully understood.

Wnt signalling is also required for the migration of another set of *C. elegans* neurons, the **hermaphrodite**-specific neurons or HSNs. The HSN neurons arise toward the posterior of the embryo and normally migrate anteriorly. HSNs do not migrate as far anteriorly as normal in mutants that lack Wnt activity or if Wnt is experimentally misexpressed in the anterior part of the embryo. In mutants that lack Wnt activity, there is a lack of repulsion from the posterior, while misexpression of Wnt in the anterior part of the embryo causes the HSNs to be repelled from the anterior. Thus, the anterior migration of HSNs is normally guided by repellent activity of the Wnts expressed posteriorly. As yet, it remains unclear whether Wnts play any role in vertebrate neuronal migration.

6.5.2 Guidance of neural crest cell migration

Neural crest cells express specific cell-surface receptors that allow them to respond to permissive and repulsive cues that guide them on their journey. Many neural crest cells migrate along paths that are organized segmentally. For example, in the trunk region of the embryo, migrating neural crest cells stream over the **somites** (blocks of mesodermal tissue adjacent to the neural tube that will give rise to skeletal muscle and the vertebrae, see Section 2.4.2, Fig. 2.5). While neural crest cells are generated all along the anteroposterior axis of the neural tube, they migrate only over the anterior half of each somite, avoiding the posterior half (Fig. 6.12). Migrating neural crest cells express members of the **Eph** family of **tyrosine kinase** receptors and corresponding **ephrin ligands** are expressed in posterior parts of each somite. Repulsive interactions mediated by Eph–ephrin signalling confine migrating neural crest cells to the anterior half of each somite. We have already seen how repulsive interactions mediated by Eph–ephrin signalling are important for the formation of rhombomeres in the developing hindbrain (Section 4.4.1) and we shall see later that Eph–ephrin signalling is also important for guiding axons to their targets in the developing nervous system (Section 9.5.3). Two other families of signalling molecules involved in axon guidance, the

hermaphrodite an organism with both male and female sexual characteristics and organs.

tyrosine kinase an enzyme that transfers phosphate groups (i.e. phosphorylates) onto tyrosine residues in a protein.

ligand a molecule or ion that binds to a receptor molecule, for example on the cell surface, to generate a biological response.

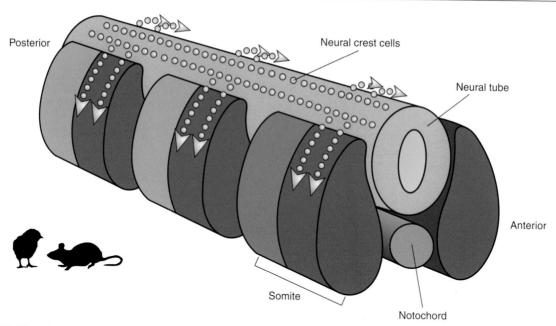

Fig. 6.12 Neural crest cells arise along the full anteroposterior extent of the neural tube but those cells that migrate over the somites are confined to the anterior half of each somite. Chemorepellent molecules, including members of the Ephrin, Semaphorin and Slit families, expressed in the posterior half of each somite (light purple) confine migrating neural crest cells to anterior regions (dark purple). Amongst other things, this gives rise to the segmentally arranged **dorsal root ganglia**, found apposed to the anterior domain of each somite.

dorsal root ganglia collections of cell bodies of peripheral sensory neurons whose axons enter the spinal cord running bilaterally along the dorsal side of the spinal cord.

semaphorins and the **Slits**, as well as their respective receptors the **neuropilins** and **Robos**, are also involved in guiding the migration of neural crest cells. These molecules are discussed in more detail in Chapter 8. Neural crest cells in the trunk region of the embryo follow inappropriate routes in mutant mice that lack either the neuropilin molecule NPN2 or the semaphorin SEMA3F. Similarly, Slit ligands expressed in somites guide Robo-expressing neural crest cells along the appropriate pathway.

In addition to these short-range interactions, neural crest cells are directed to their targets by molecules that act at longer range. For example, glial-cell-derived neurotrophic factor (GDNF) is expressed by cells in the gut where it acts to attract those neural crest cells that will form the enteric nervous system (see Fig. 2.10). (Neurotrophic factors will be discussed again in Chapter 11, in the context of programmed cell death.) In summary, a combination of short- and long-range cues act in concert to guide specific subsets of migrating neural crest cells to the appropriate destination.[3]

---

[3] For more details of the mechanisms that control neural crest cell migration, see Sauka-Spengler, T. and Bronner-Fraser, M. (2008) A gene regulatory network orchestrates neural crest formation. *Nat. Rev. Mol. Cell Biol.*, **9**, 557–68.

6.5.3 Guidance of neural precursors in the developing lateral line of zebrafish

The lateral line is a sense organ found in many species of fish and amphibians that detects water movements and allows the animal to orient itself in the water. Lateral lines are composed of a series of mechanosensory organs known as neuromasts that run lengthwise down each side of the fish between the head and the tail. In zebrafish, the cells that give rise to the lateral line neuromasts are initially derived from a **cranial placode** (placodes are discussed in Section 2.6.2). The whole placode migrates along the side of the developing fish from head to tail and periodically deposits clusters of cells that will give rise to the neuromasts (Fig. 6.13). This represents another example of collective or chain migration (Section 6.3.2).

    The migrating placode cells are guided by a **chemokine** molecule. Chemokines, or chemotactic cytokines, are a family of small, secreted signalling proteins that act to attract cells in a variety of biological situations. Signalling by cytokines is described in more detail in Box 11.4. A specific chemokine is expressed by cells along the route that the migrating placode will follow (Fig. 6.13). Cells within the placode express specific chemokine receptors and mutations that abolish

cranial placode bilateral thickenings of the ectoderm of the vertebrate head that generate sensory structures.

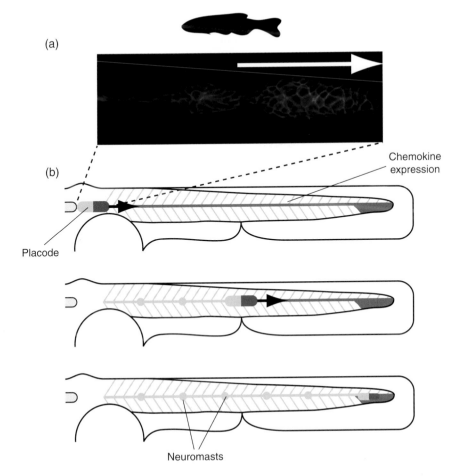

Fig. 6.13 Formation of the lateral line in the zebrafish embryo. (a) The lateral line is formed during development by a placode, composed of precursor cells that migrate along the side of the embryo, periodically leaving behind small groups of cells that will form the sensory cells of the lateral line, the neuromasts. As described in Figure 6.1, the placode cells have been engineered to express green fluorescent protein, making them easy to visualize. (b) During migration, the placode follows a line of expression of the chemokine gene *cxc12a* (green). The migrating placode cells express specific chemokine receptors that detect the chemokine. Cells at the leading edge of the placode express the receptor gene *cxcr4b* (brown) and cells further back express *cxcr7b* (blue). Image in panel (a) is by Darren Gilmour, EMBL, Germany. http:// www.biomedcentral.com/content/ supplementary/1749-8104-2-15- S1.mov%5D. Panel (b) is adapted from Aman, A. and Piotrowski, T. (2009) Cell migration during morphogenesis. *Developmental Biology*, **341**, 20–33, Copyright 2009, with permission from Elsevier.

the function of the chemokine or its receptors prevent directional migration of the placode.

6.5.4 Guidance by radial glial fibres

Many migrating cortical neurons and cerebellar granule cells are guided by the process of a radial glial cell (Section 6.3.1). The leading process of the migrating cell wraps around a radial glial cell, forming an intimate connection and suggesting that cell adhesion molecules (Box 6.3) are likely to be involved in this step of their migration. Indeed, one specific cell adhesion molecule known as **astrotactin** is critical for the attachment of migrating neurons to radial glia. Astrotactin is a cell-surface **glycoprotein** that is expressed by radially-migrating neurons both in the cerebral cortex and in the cerebellum. It does not belong to any of the major families of cell adhesion molecules. Astrotactin's importance has most clearly been shown in an experiment in which neurons and glia from the developing cerebellum were placed together in culture. The migration pathway followed by cerebellar granule cells is described in Box 6.2. In culture, isolated cerebellar granule cells (Box 6.2) attach to the processes of glial cells, and migrate along them in a similar way to that seen in the developing cerebral cortex (Fig. 6.14). When antibodies that block astrotactin are added, granule cells are unable to attach to the glia, and their rate of migration is significantly slowed down. Similarly, radial migration is abnormally slow in mutant mice that lack the astrotactin gene (*Astn1*).

Cell adhesion molecules are also important in chain migration. Optimal levels of adhesion required to allow migrating olfactory precursors to slide along one another are maintained by the neural cell adhesion molecule (N-CAM) (Box 6.3). Inhibition of N-CAM in the

glycoprotein a protein having covalently-linked carbohydrate side chains attached.

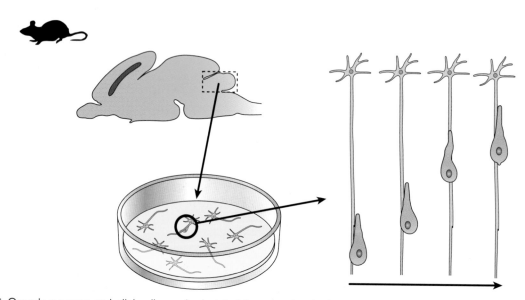

Fig. 6.14 Granule neurons and glial cells can be isolated from the developing cerebellum and plated on plastic tissue culture dishes. Under these conditions, the glial cells extend a long process, to which granule cells can attach. Once attached, the granule cell migrates along the glial fibre, mimicking the normal migration of granule cells in the developing cerebellum. Migration can then easily be followed using time-lapse microscopy.

rostral migratory stream (Section 6.3.2) leads to diminished migration and results in fewer neurons reaching the olfactory bulbs.

6.6 Locomotion

Cell movement, or locomotion, is clearly of central importance in understanding neural migration. The cell biological processes that control the locomotion of migrating neurons are probably best understood in the case of cortical neuron guidance by radial glia. These neurons migrate in a saltatory manner, that is short, rapid forward movements interspersed with relatively long stationary periods, rather like cars moving through a city, stopping and restarting at junctions.

Movement of the cell is largely driven by changes in the **cytoskeleton**, a flexible and highly dynamic network within cells that controls both cell shape and movement (see Section 7.2 for a more detailed description of the cytoskeleton). The **microtubule** component is the most important part of the cytoskeleton during neuronal migration. Microtubules grow out of a specialized structure known as the **centrosome** or microtubule organizing centre, a key player in the control of cell movement. Many migrating cells have a characteristic morphology (Fig. 6.15, see also the dye-labelled cell marked by an arrow in Fig. 6.19). A long, relatively thin protrusion, known as the leading process, projects in front of the cell in the direction of movement. The centrosome lies between the nucleus and the leading process in migrating cells, that is, in front of the nucleus. One set of microtubules emanating from the centrosome extends forward into the leading process, while another set, also connected to the centrosome, forms a cage-like structure around the nucleus. The bulk of the cytoplasm is found around the nucleus and there is often a short trailing process at the tail end of the migrating cell (Fig. 6.15).

The process of cell locomotion can be broken down into a set of repeating steps (Figure 6.16). First, the leading process extends in the direction of migration; then the centrosome moves forward, into the leading process. Next, the nucleus moves forward towards the centrosome in a process known as **nucleokinesis**, apparently being pulled forward by the connecting microtubules. Finally, the trailing process remodels, bringing it closer to the cell body. The leading process then extends again, reinitiating the cycle of steps. Clearly, the cytoskeleleton must undergo dynamic rearrangements during these changes, but the details of the mechanism by which the cytoskeleton regulates neuronal migration are not yet fully understood. One attractive model consistent with our current knowledge suggests that forces generated in the tip of the leading process act on the microtuble network to pull the centrosome forward. As the centrosome moves, it pulls in turn on the network of microtubules surrounding the nucleus, thereby pulling the nucleus forward too. At the same time, the trailing edge of the migrating cell contracts, likely driven by the **motor protein** myosin. This contraction is thought to push the nucleus forward, an effect similar to that of squeezing the bottom of a tube of toothpaste. Thus, a

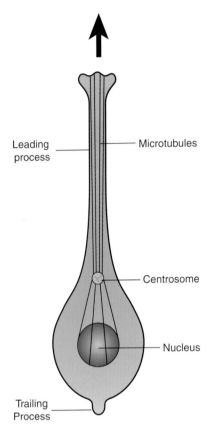

Fig. 6.15 Typical morphology of a migrating neuron. A long, thin, leading process extends forwards in the direction of migration and a shorter trailing process is found at the rear end of the cell. A network of microtubules emanating from the centrosome extends forward into the leading process and backward to enmesh the nucleus.

microtubule a major component of the cytoskeleton, composed of tubulin protein.

centrosome the intracellular organelle that organizes the microtubules of the cytoskeleton.

motor protein a protein that propels itself along intracellular filaments.

(a)   (b)   (c)   (d)

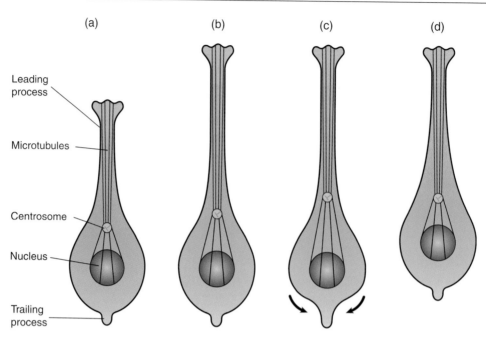

Fig. 6.16 Stages of cell migration. (a) Shows the location of key cellular components as the cell is beginning to migrate. (b) In the first stage, the leading process extends, likely driven by microtubule extension. (c) Next, the centrosome moves forward into the leading process. At the same time, the trailing end of the cell contracts (arrows), driving the rear of the cell forward. (d) Finally, the nucleus moves forward towards the centrosome and the trailing process retracts. The cell repeats these steps until it reaches its destination.

combination of pulling and pushing forces are likely act to propel the migrating cell forward.

Microtubules are very dynamic and their behaviour is regulated by a number of different types of proteins. For example, some proteins that bind to microtubules can make them more or less stable, while others cause microtubules to grow or to shrink. Intriguingly, mutations have been found in genes that encode two different microtubule binding proteins, *LIS1* and *DCX*, in patients with a birth defect known as lissencephaly, in which neuronal migration is severely abnormal (Box 6.4).

6.7 Journey's end – termination of migration

So far we have seen how neural migration is initiated, how migrating neurons are guided towards their destination, and how changes in the cytoskeleton drive locomotion in migrating neurons. In the fourth and final step in their journey, neurons must terminate their migration once they have reached their destination. How do cells know when they have reached the correct position? Again, this is probably best understood for glial-guided neurons in the cerebral cortex and cerebellum. An important clue came from analysis of a mutant strain of mice known as **reeler** mice. The *reeler* mutant arose in a colony of laboratory mice in Edinburgh, Scotland, in the late 1940s. As indicated by the name, these mutant mice have poor motor coordination causing them

Box 6.4 Studying lissencephaly gives insight into cell migration mechanisms

Important clues concerning the mechanisms that control radial migration in the emerging cerebral cortex have come from studies that identified the genes underlying a rare birth defect in humans, known as lissencephaly. Classical lissencephaly (meaning 'smooth brain') is a severe developmental brain disorder in which the folds of the cerebral cortex, known as sulci and gyri, are either greatly diminished or completely absent (see figure). In addition, the grey matter of the cortex is much thicker in lissencephalic brains, has only four layers instead of the usual six, and the majority of neurons are found in the deepest layers. Taken together, these features indicate that lissencephaly is due to the failure of cortical neurons to migrate normally.

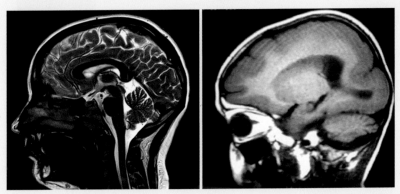

An MRI scan of the brain of a lissencephalic patient (right). Note the almost complete absence of the characteristic folds normally found in the human cortex (left panel shows scan of normal brain). Adapted by permission from Macmillan Publishers Ltd: Feng, Y. and Walsh, C.A. (2001) Protein-protein interactions, cytoskeletal regulation and neuronal migration. *Nature Reviews Neuroscience*, **2**, 408–16, copyright 2001.

Mutations in a number of different genes have been found in patients with lissencephaly. In most of these cases, the normal protein products of the mutant genes are associated with microtubule function. Individuals with heterozygous mutations in the *LIS1* gene have classical lissencephaly. LIS1 protein is thought to act with microtubules and the motor protein dynein to regulate migration.

Another subset of lissencephalies are caused by mutations in the *doublecortex* gene (*DCX*). It seems that cells that lack DCX protein are unable to migrate normally to form the upper layers of the cortex. DCX is another microtubule binding protein that acts to promote microtubule bundling.

A third group of lissencephalies is due to mutations in the genes *TUBA1A* and *TUBB2B*, which encode α- and β-tubulin respectively, the protein subunits of which microtubules are composed. Given the widespread importance of microtubules, it may seem surprising that mutations in tubulin genes would only cause problems in the developing brain. It turns out that most of the mutations found in tubulin-encoding genes in lissencephalic patients are point mutations that affect conserved amino acids involved in interactions with microtubule binding proteins. It is possible that such mutations could affect interactions between microtubules and regulatory proteins which are expressed only in the cerebral cortex, thus accounting for the cortex-specific deficits.

A number of knock-out mouse models have been made to investigate the mechanisms by which *Lis1* or *Dcx* mutations may lead to lissencephaly. However, as the mouse cerebral cortex lacks both sulci and gyri, direct comparisons with human phenotypes are tricky. The phenotypes of *Lis1* and *Dcx* knock-out mice are generally much less severe than those seen in human patients, indicating that mice are less sensitive to loss of LIS1 or DCX than are humans.

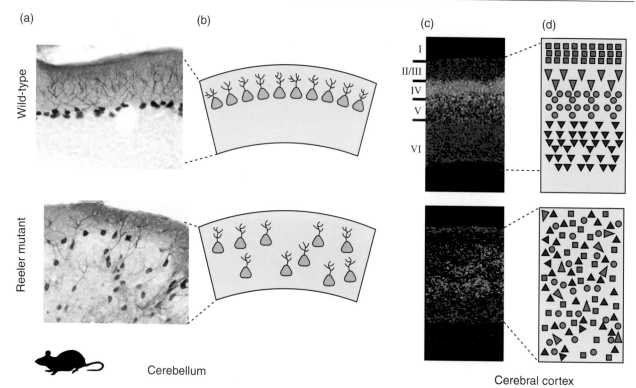

Fig. 6.17 Defective migration in cerebellum and cerebral cortex of *reeler* mutant mice. (a) Immunohistochemistry on wild-type and *reeler* mouse brains, using an antibody that specifically recognizes Purkinje cells. In wild-type cerebellum (top panel), Purkinje cells are arranged in a one-cell thick layer. In *reeler* mutants (lower panel), this regular arrangement is highly disturbed and Purkinje cells are more widely distributed in the cerebellum. (b) Cartoons summarizing the findings shown in panel (a). (c) Lamination is also highly abnormal in the cerebral cortex of *reeler* mutants. The composite images show *in situ* hybridizations which reveal the expression of four different genes, each expressed by a specific class of neuron that is normally found in a specific layer of the mature cortex. In this experiment, each *in situ* hybridization was conducted separately and given a different false colour. The composite images were made by combining the four separately-coloured images together. In a wild-type mouse (top panel) neurons expressing each of the four genes are neatly separated into clearly-recognizable layers. However, in *reeler* cortex (lower panel) the cells are much less organized and no clear pattern of layers is visible. (d) Cartoons summarizing the findings shown in panel (c). (Pictures in panels (a) and (c) are reprinted from Katsuyama, Y. and Terashima, T. (2009) Developmental anatomy of reeler mutant mouse. *Develop. Growth Differ.*, **51**, 271–286, and Dekimoto, H., Terashima, T. and Katsuyama, Y. (2010) Dispersion of the neurons expressing layer specific markers in the reeler brain. *Develop. Growth Differ.*, **52**, 181–193.)

to 'reel' around in their cages. The scientist who first characterized the *reeler* mutants, Douglas Falconer, evocatively described their gait as 'remarkably suggestive of inebriation'.[4] The motor deficits are likely due to abnormalities in the structure of the cerebellum, which controls aspects of motor coordination. In *reeler* mutants, the characteristic laminar structure of the cerebellum (see Box 6.2) doesn't form correctly because newborn neurons are unable to migrate to their appropriate positions. For example, the Purkinje cells, normally found in an organized layer one cell thick, form disorganized clumps in *reeler* mutants (Fig. 6.17). Other mutations that affect the development of the cerebellum are discussed in Section 10.5.3.

---

[4] Falconer, D. S. (1951) Two new mutants, 'trembler' and 'reeler', with neurological actions in the house mouse. *J. Genet.* **50**, 192–201.

The cerebral cortex also develops abnormally in *reeler* mutant mice. The specific cell types that are normally confined to individual layers of the cerebral cortex are instead scattered throughout the depth of the cortex (Fig. 6.17). In *reeler* mutant cortex, many radially migrating neurons do not pass earlier-born cells as they normally would (see Fig. 5.16) so later-born cells accumulate inappropriately at deeper positions. Some published descriptions of the *reeler* cortex suggest that the cortical layers are inverted, with deeper layer neurons found superficially and superficial layer neurons found at deeper levels, but this likely represents an oversimplification of the phenotype. The gene whose function is lost in *reeler* mutants is named **reelin** and is conserved in humans. Mutations in the human homologue (named *RELN*) cause a form of lissencephaly, consistent with a role in regulating migration.

The *reelin* gene encodes a large secreted protein that associates with the extracellular matrix. *reelin* is expressed abundantly by **Cajal–Retzius cells**, a population of specialized neurons found in the most superficial layer of the developing cerebral cortex. Exactly how *reelin* controls the laminar position of migrating cells in the developing cerebral cortex is not well understood. One possibility is that Reelin protein acts as a chemoattractant, attracting migrating neurons towards the pial surface. Alternatively, it could act as a stop signal, instructing migrating neurons to detach from the radial glial scaffold once they have reached the correct position. As successive waves of migrating cells use the same glial fibres as guides, failure of early-migrating cells to detach in *reeler* mutant cortex could lead to a log-jam, physically preventing later-born cells from migrating past their predecessors that remain attached to the radial glial scaffold.[5]

6.8 The mechanisms that govern migration of important populations of cortical neurons remain unknown

Although radially migrating cells make a major contribution to the developing cerebral cortex, not all cortical cells follow this route and additional migratory pathways in the developing mammalian forebrain have been discovered. Important evidence for the existence of additional migration pathways came from experiments using genetically marked retroviruses to track the fates of cells descended from neural progenitors in the mid-gestation mouse forebrain (Box 6.1). As can be seen in Fig. 6.18, many **clones** of *lacZ*-expressing cells were organized in radial columns. These clones most likely arose from progenitor cells in the ventricular zone that gave rise to daughter cells that subsequently migrated radially

Cajal–Retzius cell a specific subtype of neuron found near the pial edge of the marginal zone of the developing cerebral cortex. Named after their co-discoverers, Santiago Ramon y Cajal and Gustaf Retzius.

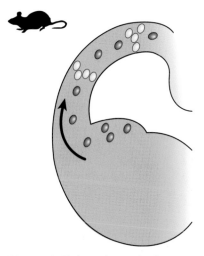

Fig. 6.18 Embryonic cerebral cortex contains both radial- and tangentially-migrating cells. Progenitor cells were infected at around embryonic day 12.5 (E12.5) and after a few days of development in the uterus, infected cells and their progeny were traced (see Box 6.1 for details of the method). Many *lacZ*-expressing cells are found in clonally related groups. Many clones were composed of radially-migrating neurons (shown in yellow). Cells in these clones are likely to be born near the ventricular surface, then migrate radially. Other clones were composed of tangentially-migrating neurons (shown in blue and by arrow) that had migrated parallel to the ventricular surface.

---

[5] For more detail about *reelin*'s role in regulating neuronal migration, see Soriano, E. and Del Río, J. A. (2005) The cells of Cajal-Retzius: still a mystery one century after. *Neuron.* **46**, 389–94.

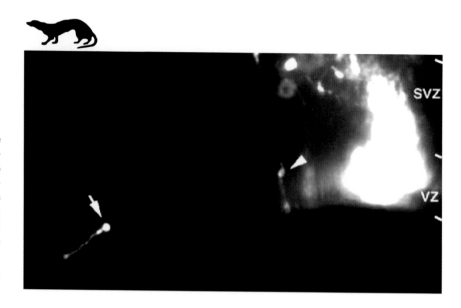

Fig. 6.19 Tangential migration in the developing cerebral cortex. A dye-labelled neuron migrating parallel to the ventricular surface (arrow). A single, labelled radial glial cell is also shown (arrowhead). Reproduced from O'Rourke, N. A., Chenn, A. and McConnell, S. K. (1997) Postmitotic neurons migrate tangentially in the cortical ventricular zone. *Development*, **124**, 997–1005.

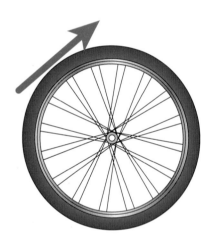

interneurons neurons within the central nervous system that function as connectors between other neurons.

projection neurons a general term for neurons that project axons over a distance, rather than locally.

ganglionic eminences ventral regions of the embryonic telencephalon.

towards the pia. Other clones, however, contained cells that were dispersed at considerable distances in a tangential direction, suggesting that some cells in the developing telencephalon migrate long distances in this direction.

More evidence that some cells in the embryonic cerebral cortex migrate tangentially came from experiments in which the migration of individual fluorescently labelled cells in cultured slices of cortex was followed by time-lapse microscopy (Fig. 6.19).

We now know that many of the tangentially-migrating neurons in the developing cerebral cortex migrate into the cortex from ventral parts of the telencephalon. Clear evidence for this was obtained in experiments again using cultured slices of mouse forebrain, as shown in Fig. 6.2. Analysis of neurons that migrate tangentially from the ventral telencephalon into the cortex showed that most of them are inhibitory **interneurons** that express the neurotransmitter GABA (γ-aminobutyric acid), usually referred to as **GABAergic neurons**. In contrast, most of the radially-migrating neurons in the cortex were excitatory **projection neurons** that expressed the neurotransmitter **glutamate**. In slice cultures where embryonic cortex is cultured separately from the ventral telencephalon, the cortex has many fewer GABAergic interneurons at the end of the culture period, showing that this tangential migration from the ventral part of the telencephalon is a major source of the interneurons normally found in the cortex (Fig. 6.20).

Thus, the two main types of neurons required for the establishment of cortical circuits are born in separate areas. Excitatory neurons are born in the cortex itself, and migrate radially outward to their final destinations in the cortical layers. In contrast, cortical GABAergic interneurons arise in ventral parts of the telencephalon, the **ganglionic eminences**, and many of them then migrate along a tangential trajectory into the developing cortex. Details of the

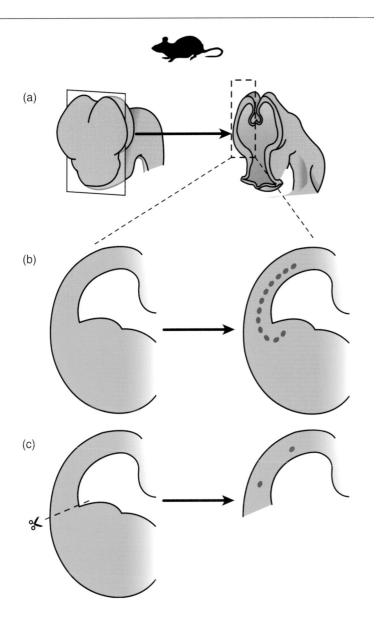

Fig. 6.20 Many GABAergic neurons migrate tangentially from the embryonic ventral telencephalon into the cortex. (a) Slices were cut from an E12.5 embryonic mouse forebrain and placed in culture. (b) Intact slices were left to develop for 2 days then stained with an antibody that detects GABAergic neurons. Many such neurons (red) were found in the cerebral cortex. (c) Dorsal and ventral parts of the telencephalon were separated before being placed in culture. In this case, the cultured dorsal telencephalon contained many fewer GABAergic neurons, indicating that these neurons usually migrate from ventral to dorsal telencephalon.

mechanisms that control this tangential migration have not yet been worked out.[6]

6.9 Summary

- Different types of neurons are born in different regions of the developing nervous system and many of them must then migrate to reach the area where they will function. Correct assembly of functional circuits depends critically on the correct number of neurons getting

---

[6] For more detail on tangential migration in the forebrain, see Marín, O. and Rubenstein, J. L. (2001) A long, remarkable journey: tangential migration in the telencephalon. *Nat. Rev. Neurosci.*, **2**, 780–90.

to the right place at the right time, and if the process goes wrong the effects on the brain are severe.

- Three major modes of neuronal migration have been found. Migrating neurons may be guided by a scaffold provided by other cells, they may migrate collectively or they may migrate as individual cells.

- Migration in each of these modes can be broken down into four steps – initiation, guidance, locomotion (movement) and termination.

- Changes in cell adhesion are required to allow cells to migrate.

- The movement of migrating cells is driven by dynamic changes in the cytoskeleton.

- Many of the molecules involved in controlling migration have been identified and we are beginning to understand some of the mechanisms.

- There are still many unanswered questions. One major challenge currently facing researchers in this field is to determine the extent to which the molecular mechanisms worked out using cultured cells and tissues also apply *in vivo*.

How Neurons Develop Their Shapes

7

7.1 Neurons form two specialized types of outgrowth

Newborn neurons undergo various cell-shape changes during development. As we saw in the previous chapter, many neural precursors initially make temporary shape changes during migration. Once they reach their final destination, they then must attain their characteristic final morphologies by growing long cellular extensions or **neurites**. This process is known as **neurite outgrowth**. Neurites are differentiated into two structural and functional types – **axons** and **dendrites**. Owing to the different structures and functions of axons and dendrites, neurons are said to be polarized cells. This **neuronal polarity** is fundamental to neuronal function, since it determines the ability of neurons to receive and send electrical signals in a directed way. Classically, dendrites integrate incoming information for the neuron, whereas axons carry information away from the cell body in the form of an **action potential**. In this chapter we examine how neurons produce outgrowths during differentiation. We also look at the mechanisms that lead to the distinction between axons and dendrites.

neurite a collective term for axons and dendrites, especially applied to the immature stages during outgrowth.

neuronal polarity cell polarity refers to morphological asymmetries across a cell. In the case of neurons, neuronal polarity refers to the fact that neurites are differentiated into axon and dendrites.

action potential the self-propagating voltage change across the cell membrane as a nerve impulse is transmitted along axons and dendrites.

7.1.1 Axons and dendrites

Axons and dendrites are morphologically, molecularly and functionally distinct. Neurons vary enormously in the morphology of their axons and dendrites (Figure 7.1). However, as a simplification, axons are generally long and uniformly thin, and their termini contain neurotransmitter-loaded vesicles and form synapses with the dendrites of other neurons or with muscles. Dendrites are usually shorter, become thinner with distance and are often highly branched to form a **dendritic tree**, which allows the neuron to have many contacts with other neurons. For example, each **Purkinje cell** of the cerebellum has a huge dendritic tree that receives an estimated 100 000 synapses (Fig. 7.1(e)). The role of dendrites is to integrate synaptic activity to produce a varying electrical output that may result in an axonal action potential (as addressed in Chapter 12, Section 12.2.1). In vertebrates, dendrites of some neurons are also covered with tiny outgrowths called **dendritic spines**, which are

Building Brains: An Introduction to Neural Development, First Edition.
David Price, Andrew Jarman, John Mason and Peter Kind.
© 2011 John Wiley & Sons, Ltd. Published 2011 by John Wiley & Sons, Ltd.

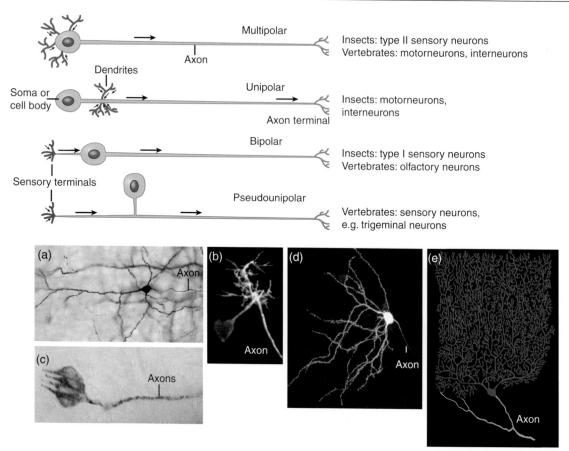

Fig. 7.1 Neurons can be classified according to the number of processes that extend from the cell body (also called the **soma**). The majority of CNS neurons are unipolar in invertebrates but are multipolar in vertebrates. Sensory neurons tend to be of varied types and they have sensory terminals rather than true dendrites. It should be emphasized that there are many variations on these classes, and also that axons can be branched. For instance some neurons are unusual in having an elaborately branched axon and very simple dendrites (e.g. basket cell neurons in the cortex). The images show some representative neurons: (a) Pyramidal neuron from the mouse sensory cortex (multipolar); (b) *Drosophila* motor neuron (unipolar) (image courtesy of Alex Mauss, University of Cambridge); (c) group of five *Drosophila* sensory neurons (bipolar); (d) spiny stellate neuron from the mouse sensory cortex (multipolar) (image courtesy of Lasani Wijetunge, University of Edinburgh); (e) Purkinje neuron of the cerebellum (image courtesy of Matthias Landgraf, University of Cambridge). The last image is a colour tracing based on an original drawing made by the influential neuroanatomist Santiago Ramón y Cajal in 1899.

soma the neuronal cell body (as opposed to the neurites).

the receiving sites for their synapses. These contain receptors for neurotransmitters and all their associated signal transduction apparatus. The formation of synapses and dendritic spines is addressed in Chapter 10.

The polarized neuron actively maintains the molecular distinctiveness of its axon and dendrites. Experiments have studied the ability of proteins to move laterally within the plasma membrane by using optical tweezers (a laser beam) to pull individual proteins from one region of a neuron to another. Proteins could be pulled around the **soma** and dendrites with ease, but they could not be pulled into the axon. There appears to be a barrier to diffusion at the base of the axon, but not the dendrites. Such experiments show that the membrane of the axon forms a separate domain from the membrane of the dendrites and soma (the

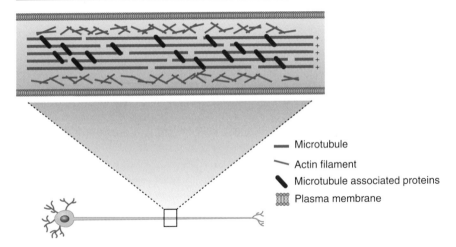

— Microtubule

— Actin filament

— Microtubule associated proteins

▦ Plasma membrane

Fig. 7.2 The cytoskeleton of an axon. Parallel bundles of orientated microtubules form its core, stabilized by microtubule associated proteins (MAPs). Actin filaments form a surrounding gel-like meshwork under the plasma membrane.

somatodendritic domain), helping to maintain the axon's distinctiveness and neuronal polarity.[1]

7.1.2 The cytoskeleton in mature axons and dendrites

At the core of the neurite is its **cytoskeleton**, which gives structure, shape and stability (Fig. 7.2). The cytoskeleton also provides a highway along which molecules are transported from the cell body to the neurite tip. Important cytoskeletal components are the filamentous protein **polymers** called **microtubules** and **actin filaments** (Box 7.1). As well as constituting the mitotic spindle of dividing cells, microtubules form a dynamic network in non-dividing cells that radiate out from the **centrosome**. Mature axons contain a core of aligned microtubules, all of which are orientated in the same direction with their 'plus' ends pointing towards the axon terminal (Fig. 7.2). This array is stabilized by the binding of accessory proteins, which crosslink the separate strands and inhibit depolymerization. These are generally known as **microtubule-associated proteins** (MAPs), and Tau is one such protein that is characteristic of axons. Dendrites are also filled with microtubules, but they are less ordered and have mixed orientations. Dendrite microtubules have different accessory proteins, including MAP2. In experiments, these different MAPs are often used as molecular markers to distinguish axons and dendrites (as seen in Fig. 7.13).

In most cells, actin filaments form a meshwork directly under the plasma membrane giving shape and resilience. This is true also of both axons and dendrites. A third class of cytoskeletal component are the intermediate filaments. These give strength to an axon and determine its diameter. It is currently believed, however, that they play little role in neurite formation and so are not discussed further.

cytoskeleton the subcellular network of protein polymers within cells that gives them their shape and robustness and underlies their ability to move or change shapes. Its main components are microtubules, microfilaments and intermediate filaments.

polymer a molecule composed of many similar subunits.

centrosome the intracellular organelle that organizes the microtubules of the cytoskeleton.

---

[1] To read about these interesting experiments, see Winckler, B., Forscher, P. and Mellman, I. (1999) A diffusion barrier maintains distribution of membrane proteins in polarized neurons. *Nature*, **397**, 22.

Box 7.1   Component molecules of the cytoskeleton

The intracellular meshwork of protein filaments that comprises the cytoskeleton plays a central role in the morphology of all cells. As might be expected, cytoskeletal structures are also important in both the formation and function of axons and dendrites. Cytoskeletal filaments are linear polymers of subunit proteins. **Microtubules** consist of α- and β-**tubulin** protein subunits. **Actin** subunits (G-actin) polymerize to form actin filaments (F-actin or **microfilaments**). An important characteristic of these polymers is that their two ends are distinct – they have polarity. Under certain cellular conditions, microtubules and actin filaments can grow by the addition of extra subunits. In the case of microtubules, α- and β-tubulin heterodimers are added to the so-called 'plus' end. Actin filaments can grow through the binding of additional G-actin subunits to either end of the filament, but preferentially binding to the so-called 'barbed' end. In both cases the dissociated subunits exist in dynamic equilibrium with the polymeric states and the stabilization and destabilization of the polymeric state is a major target of mechanisms that control neurite outgrowth and retraction.

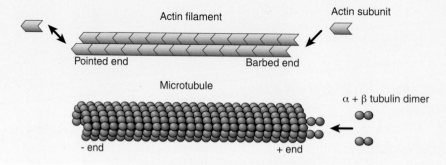

7.2 The growing neurite

7.2.1 A neurite extends by growth at its tip

Axons and dendrites have many similarities in their mode of growth, but also some important differences, which will be addressed later. One might imagine that a growing neurite extends by stretching out. However, most of the neurite is rigid; it grows instead by the addition of new cellular components to its tip (Fig. 7.3). Thus, a neurite is assembled rather like the way in which a railway track or a pipeline is

Fig. 7.3 A growing axon is characterized by a growth cone at its tip, which is the site of axon construction and extension. Behind the growth cone, the axon is a rigid structure with a stable cytoskeletal core. The microtubules of the cytoskeleton radiate into the axon from the centrosome. The axon extends by the addition of new material in the growth cone (as indicated by the paler section in the lower neuron).

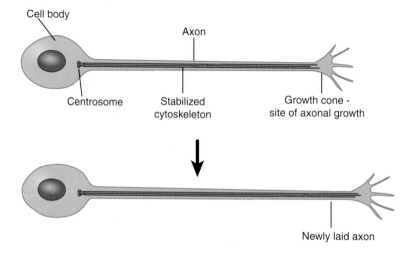

laid down. The growing point of an extending neurite is called the **growth cone**. This is the site at which the cytoskeleton is assembled to lay down the growing neurite. It is also the part of the developing neurite that senses its environment, allowing it to respond to signals that promote or inhibit outgrowth. Some of these are spatial signals that guide the direction of growth. The guidance of axon growth is addressed in the next chapter.

7.2.2 Mechanisms of growth cone dynamics

First described by Santiago Ramón y Cajal as long ago as 1890, the growth cone is the business end of the growing neurite. It has two major regions, known as the central and the peripheral zones (Fig. 7.4). The central zone contains bundled microtubules, giving structural support to the neurite. The peripheral zone is characterized by the presence of thin sheet-like protrusions, or **lamellipodia**, that are pushed out by the growth cone in an amoeba-like fashion. As the growth cone moves forward, long finger-like processes, named **filopodia**, sprout

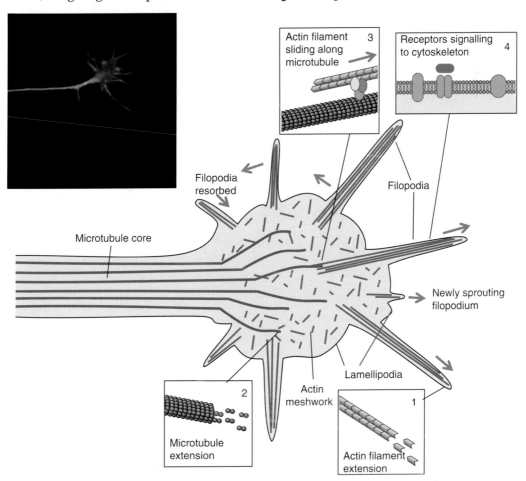

Fig. 7.4 The growth cone. [1] Actin polymerization drives the formation and extension of filopodia at the tip. Lamellipodia are pushed out between the filopodia. [2] Within the central zone, microtubules of the axon core are extended as the growth cone moves forward. [3] Motor proteins push actin filaments along microtubules. [4] The plasma membrane is studded with numerous receptor proteins that allow the growth cone to respond to environmental signals. The image shows a growth cone of a cultured neuron with microtubules (green) and actin filaments (red) (reproduced courtesy of Monica Hoyos Flight, Imperial College London).

from its leading edge, exploring the environment through which it is passing and helping it to move forward.

Lamellipodia and filopodia both contain a highly dynamic actin cytoskeleton. Actin filaments undergo rapid cycles of elongation and retraction. During growth, actin monomers polymerize to form actin filaments at the leading edges of the growth cone (Inset 1 in Fig. 7.4). Conversely, depolymerization of actin filaments leads to retraction of filopodia. Behind the filopodia, the microtubules also extend and retract dynamically (Inset 2). As the growth cone advances, microtubule growth predominates to form the axon core in the wake of the growth cone. In addition to actin and microtubule polymerization, motor proteins like myosin cause actin filaments to slide outward along the microtubules in the central zone, rather like an extendable ladder (Inset 3). This helps to push out the filopodia and lamellipodia.

The plasma membrane of the growth cone is studded with a variety of proteins that mediate interactions with other cells and the environment through which the growth cone is passing (Inset 4). These include receptors for specific molecular cues that influence outgrowth. Inside, the growth cone is packed with molecules that transduce signals from activated receptors to trigger changes in actin and tubulin polymerization dynamics. We shall return to these molecular mechanisms later in the chapter.

It should be apparent that there is a lot of resemblance between cell movement during neuronal migration (Chapter 6) and growth cone movement during outgrowth. In fact, one can think of axon growth as being a specialized form of cell migration in which the cell body doesn't follow the growing point.

7.3 Stages of neurite outgrowth

7.3.1 Neurite outgrowth in cultured hippocampal neurons

So far we have looked mainly at what happens in a *growing* neurite. There are, however, other steps to consider before this. Experiments studying neuronal outgrowth and polarity often use cultures of dissociated neurons derived from the rat embryonic **hippocampus**. In such cultures, outgrowth occurs in several steps over a number of days (Fig. 7.5). Initially, the neural precursor cell is spherical (Stage 1). The gel-like meshwork of actin filaments under its plasma membrane maintains this shape and acts as a barrier to the formation of outgrowths. The first step of neuronal differentiation, therefore, requires that this filament meshwork is disrupted at specific points, which allows penetration by microtubules leading to the formation of filopodia or lamellipodia (Stage 2). Initially these 'sprouts' are very dynamic – they grow and retract repeatedly, but some of them subsequently expand to form neurites (Stage 3). Next, the cell becomes polarized: one neurite extends rapidly and becomes the future axon (Stage 4). Then, the remaining neurites stop their cycles of growth and retraction, develop branches and mature into dendrites (Stage 5). For certain neurons, these dendrites eventually establish their typical morphology by developing dendritic spines (Stage 6). We shall see that all these steps require coordinated regulation of cytoskeletal structure and dynamics.

hippocampus a structure of the vertebrate forebrain particularly associated with learning and memory formation.

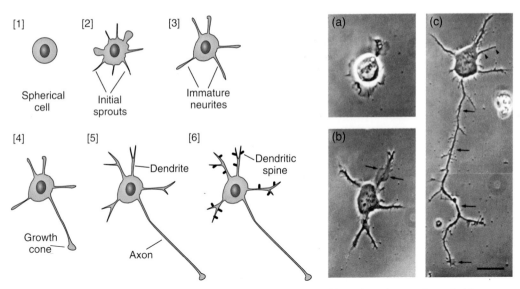

Fig. 7.5 Stages in neurite outgrowth and neuronal polarization as observed in cultured rat embryonic hippocampal cells. [1] Initially the neuronal cell is spherical; [2] appearance of initial sprouts of filopodia and lamellipodia; [3] expansion of sprouts to form immature neurites; [4] specification of one rapidly growing neurite as the axon; [5] remaining neurites form branches to become dendrites; [6] maturation of dendrites and axons. (a)–(c) show cells at stages 2, 3 and 5 respectively and are reproduced from the research paper that originally characterized this culture system. (Images from Dotti, C.G., Sullivan, C.A. and Banker, G.A. (1988) The establishment of polarity by hippocampal neurons in culture. *Journal of Neuroscience*, **8**, 1454–1468, copyright. The Society of Neuroscience.)

7.3.2 Neurite outgrowth in vivo

Cultured hippocampal neurons provide an excellent *in vitro* system for studying the mechanisms underlying neurite outgrowth and the acquisition of polarity, as we shall see later. It is apparent, however, that many neurons *in vivo* follow a somewhat different course of differentiation. For example, in many neurons only a single neurite grows out first and this usually becomes the axon. Only later are further neurites formed that become dendrites. This is observed, for instance, in some *C. elegans* motor neurons. It is also seen in vertebrate **Purkinje** neurons and **retinal ganglion cells**. Thus, there are several ways in which a neuron can attain its polarity. Either the axon is specified from among a number of immature neurites, as in the case of hippocampal neurons, or it derives from the first outgrowth to emerge. A common link between these processes is the need to designate a single neurite as the axon whereas all other neurites later become dendrites by default.

in vitro pertaining to experiments conducted outside the organism.

in vivo pertaining to the context of the intact organism.

retinal ganglion cells neurons in the retina that transmit visual information through the optic nerve, optic chiasm and optic tract to their targets in the thalamus and the tectum or the superior colliculus in mammals.

7.4 Neurite outgrowth is influenced by a neuron's surroundings

7.4.1 The importance of extracellular cues

When cultured in isolation many neurons will spontaneously grow neurites, suggesting that outgrowth is dependent on a neuron's intrinsic differentiation programme. Exogenous signals or cues, however, also play a central role in promoting and shaping outgrowth. As a consequence, the morphology of a cultured neuron rarely mimics completely that of the equivalent neuron *in vivo*. For instance, cerebellar Purkinje neurons have hugely elaborate dendritic trees (Fig. 7.1(e)). Cultured Purkinje cells, on the other hand, do not form such elaborate trees. They can nevertheless be induced to form more highly branched dendrites if they are cultured along with the neurons they would normally synapse with (called granule cells), showing that the neurons are responding to cues secreted by their partners. Thus, the *in vivo* environment is important for the acquisition of mature neuronal morphology.

7.4.2 Extracellular signals that promote or inhibit neurite outgrowth

What is the molecular nature of these environmental cues? Many diffusible and contact signals are known to promote outgrowth in different types of neuron. These derive from both surrounding cells and the intervening **extracellular matrix** (ECM, Box 7.2). A common assay

---

Box 7.2   The extracellular matrix

The extracellular matrix is the gel-like material that provides structural support between cells in many tissues and organs. It consists of fibrous proteins and **polysaccharides** that are secreted by the cells. Important extracellular matrix proteins include collagens, fibronectin and laminin. Collagens form a structural framework. Laminin is a large multidomain **glycoprotein** consisting of three separate chains. Laminin and fibronection bind both to collagens and to a cell membrane receptor called integrin (see Chapter 6, Box 6.2), thereby allowing growth cones to adhere to and move through the ECM. **Proteoglycans** are proteins decorated with attached polysaccharide chains, which are responsible for the gel-like nature of the ECM and also affect cells by binding to several cell membrane proteins. Two major groups of such molecules involved in neuronal development are heparan sulphate proteoglycans (HSPGs) and chondroitin sulphate proteoglycans (CSPGs).

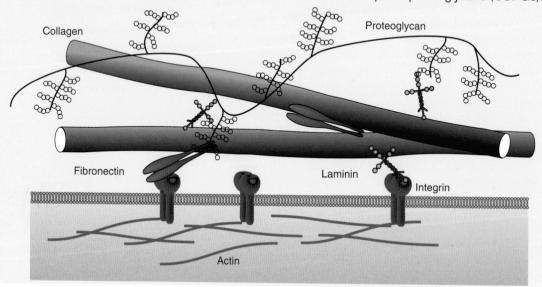

---

polysaccharide a polymer of sugar (carbohydrate) subunits.

glycoprotein a protein having covalently-linked carbohydrate side chains attached.

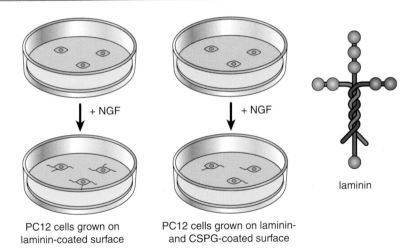

PC12 cells grown on laminin-coated surface

PC12 cells grown on laminin- and CSPG-coated surface

laminin

Fig. 7.6 Investigations of neurite outgrowth often use PC12 cells – an immortalized cell line derived from the rat **adrenal medulla** that can be induced to undergo neuronal differentiation in culture by the addition of **nerve growth factor** (NGF). In this instance, coating the culture dish with the ECM protein, laminin, promotes both the number and length of outgrowths produced by the cells (blue dishes). Addition of the proteoglycan, CSPG, inhibits this (orange dishes). A cartoon of the multi-subunit laminin protein is shown on the right. The different parts of the protein bind to various components of the ECM and to integrin receptors on cells.

to test the effect of molecules on neurite growth is to follow outgrowth in cultured neural precursor cells. The ECM protein laminin is a potent inducer of neurite outgrowth in such an assay (Fig. 7.6). Experiments in *Xenopus* have highlighted the role of laminin in neurite outgrowth *in vivo*: when expression of laminin's receptor, integrin, is disrupted in neurons then defects are observed in the initiation of axon formation.

Other ECM molecules inhibit outgrowth. Chondroitin sulphate proteoglycans (CSPGs) inhibit laminin-induced outgrowth of cultured cells (Fig. 7.6). Consistent with this, CSPGs are expressed in areas of the developing CNS known to be inhibitory to axon crossing, such as the roof plate of the neural tube (Chapter 4, Fig. 4.14). Interestingly, there appears to be enhanced expression of growth-inhibiting CSPGs after CNS lesions. This is one of the factors that limits axon regeneration after spinal cord damage. We shall see later that CSPGs also play roles during axon guidance (Chapter 8) and the plasticity of neuronal connectivity (Chapter 12).

Besides the ECM, diffusible signals secreted by surrounding cells are also important in shaping outgrowth. These include various growth factors, such as vascular endothelial cell growth factor (VEGF) and **neurotrophins** (e.g. nerve growth factor, see Chapter 11, Section 11.4.1). Other cues that affect the *direction* of axon growth are discussed in the next chapter (Chapter 8).

7.5 Molecular responses in the growth cone

7.5.1 Key intracellular signal transduction events

Extracellular cues bind to their cell surface receptors on the growth cone to cause changes in neurite growth. Formation of filopodia and lamellipodia requires cytoskeletal rearrangements and the recruitment of new membrane components to the growing site. These effects are achieved via a highly complex network of **intracellular signalling** molecules and **second messengers**, which link the cell surface receptors to the proteins (effectors) that directly alter membrane and cytoskeleton dynamics. As an example of these

intracellular signalling molecules the process (and molecules) that mediate a cell's response to an extracellular signal.

second messengers intracellular molecules that act as relays for extracellular signals bound to cell surface receptors; they include cyclic AMP, PIP3 and Ca^{2+}.

Fig. 7.7 The small G protein molecular switch as exemplified by Rac. When bound to a molecule of GDP, Rac is in its inactive conformation. Signals that promote neurite outgrowth lead to the activation of a GEF (Guanine-nucleotide exchange factor). GEF facilitates the swapping of Rac's GDP for GTP, thereby activating Rac. Rac can then influence the function of effector proteins. Inhibitory signals, or the absence of signal, act via a GAP (GTPase activating protein), which causes Rac to hydrolyse its bound GTP to GDP, thereby inactivating it.

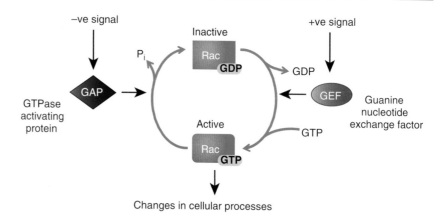

processes, here we focus on one important class of intracellular signalling molecules, the **small G proteins**.

7.5.2 Small G proteins are critical regulators of neurite growth

G proteins (guanine nucleotide binding proteins) constitute a large family of intracellular proteins found in all cells. They are involved in transducing extracellular signals into intracellular responses, such as changes in gene expression, cell shape and protein secretion. Some G proteins are linked closely to the surface receptors themselves but others are small cytosolic proteins. These **small G proteins** (also known as small GTPases) act as molecular switches that can be flipped between their active and inactive conformational states by the binding of GTP or GDP, respectively, in response to receptor activation (Fig. 7.7). Some receptors activate a **GEF** (Guanine-nucleotide exchange factor), which facilitates the swapping of bound GDP for GTP, thereby causing G protein activation. The active protein can then bind to effector proteins to influence their function (e.g. proteins that directly alter cytoskeletal stability). Other signals act via a **GAP** (GTPase activating protein) to promote the **hydrolysis** of bound GTP to GDP, thereby returning the G protein to its inactive conformation.

hydrolysis the breaking of a covalent chemical bond by a water molecule.

The archetypal small G protein is **Ras**. Ras has a wide variety of roles in regulating cell behaviour and gene expression, and is also activated by various growth factors to promote neuronal survival and plasticity (Chapters 11 and 12). The best-known members of this family for cell shape regulation are Rho, Rac and Cdc42 (Fig. 7.8). Each small G protein is activated differently by extracellular cues (via their own dedicated GEFs and GAPs) and each has different effectors to alter different cellular processes, although there is also much crosstalk between the pathways (refer back to Chapter 3, Section 3.7 for a reminder of key principles concerning signal transduction). In neurons, activation of Rho inhibits axon elongation, whereas activated Rac promotes elongation. It is largely the balance between these activities that regulates neurite growth or retraction.

G protein involvement in neurite growth is studied by manipulating their activity in cultured neurons and *in vivo*. This is achieved either

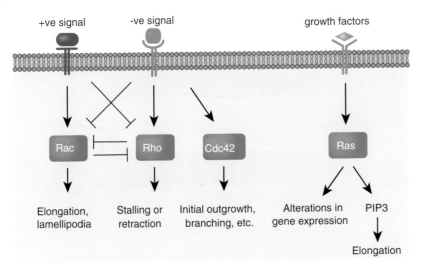

Fig. 7.8 Several small G proteins are at the heart of regulating neurite outgrowth. Axon growth is largely determined by the balance between Rac and Rho activities. Cdc42 plays important roles in other aspects of neurite outgrowth. Ras is a target of many growth factors and has several roles related to outgrowth. It affects gene expression in response to cues received by the axon. It also promotes elongation via the **PIP3** signalling pathway (discussed later in this chapter).

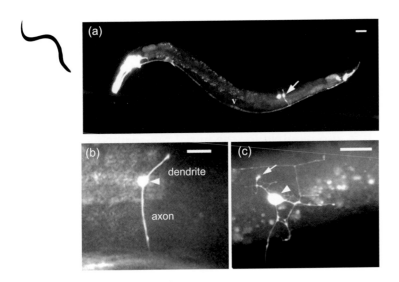

Fig. 7.9 Axon growth of *C. elegans* neurons has been used to study small G protein functions *in vivo*. (a) A single bipolar sensory neuron has been labelled by **green fluorescent protein** (GFP) expression. (b) The same at higher magnification. (c) When this neuron expresses a hyperactive Rac protein it produces extra outgrowths from both its axon and dendrite. (Images from Struckhoff, E. C. and Lundquist, E. A. (2003) The actin-binding protein UNC-115 is an effector of Rac signaling during axon pathfinding in *C. elegans*. *Development*, **130**, 693–704.

by mutating the GAPs and GEFs that regulate their activity, or by expressing mutant forms of the small G proteins that are inactive or hyperactive. In *Drosophila*, inactivating Rac *in vivo* inhibits axon outgrowth in certain neurons of the CNS **mushroom body**. Inactivation of a Rac-specific GAP in the same neurons (thereby hyperactivating Rac) causes axon over-extension. *C. elegans* has also proved a useful *in vivo* model for such studies (Fig. 7.9).[2]

mushroom body a structure in the insect brain that is the seat of olfactory learning and memory.

7.5.3 Effector molecules directly influence actin filament dynamics

Among the small G proteins, Cdc42 activation particularly promotes the actin polymerization and bundling that leads to filopodium

---

[2] Further information on small G proteins in neurite outgrowth can be found in Hall, A. and Lalli, G. (2010) Rho and Ras GTPases in axon growth, guidance, and branching. *Cold Spring Harb. Perspect. Biol.*, **2**, a001818.

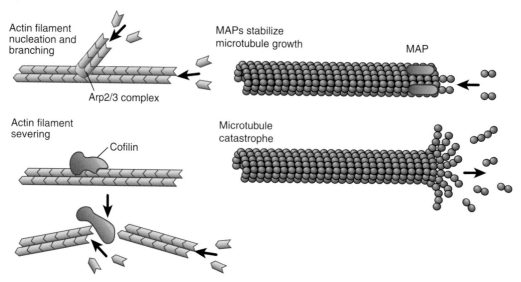

Fig. 7.10 Examples of effector proteins that alter actin and microtubule dynamics. The Arp2/3 complex nucleates the formation of new actin filaments. It also promotes branching of existing filaments (as shown here). Cofilin severs actin filaments and also increases the rate of actin subunit dissociation from the pointed end. Paradoxically, such activity is required for axon growth since it 'loosens' the actin filament meshwork, provides new barbed ends for extension and also frees up actin subunits for such extension. Microtubule associated proteins (MAPs) are involved in microtubule stabilization in the wake of the growth cone. Other factors (not depicted) cause the dissociation of tubulin from the plus end, resulting in rapid shortening of the microtubule (so-called microtubule catastrophe).

formation. It is also required for the initial remodelling of the actin meshwork that is required for initial outgrowth. Rac activation plays a similar role in promoting the actin meshwork in lamellipodia. Rho tends to inhibit these processes. These effects are achieved via the regulation of numerous target or effector proteins such as the Arp2/3 complex (Arp = actin related protein) and cofilin (Fig. 7.10). Like the G proteins themselves, most of these effectors are not specific to the nervous system – they are required for cytoskeletal dynamics in all cells. In response to activated Cdc42, the Arp2/3 complex can nucleate (initiate) the formation of new actin filaments. Acting with other proteins, it can also cause filament branching, a characteristic of the actin meshwork in lamellipodia. Many of these effector proteins are regulated by **phosphorylation** (see Chapter 3, Section 3.7). For instance, cofilin is inhibited by phosphorylation in response to activated Rho.[3]

phosphorylation the addition of a phosphate group to a molecule often causing its activation or deactivation.

7.5.4 Regulation of other processes in the extending neurite

While actin dynamics drive neurite outgrowth via filopodium and lamellipodium formation, other processes are also regulated. Microtubule dynamics are regulated in order to extend the microtubule core in the wake of the advancing growth cone. Similarly to actin, this is achieved through the activation of proteins that promote microtubule

---

[3] For more detail on regulation of actin dynamics during neurite outgrowth, see Da Silva, J.S. and Dotti, C.G. (2002) Breaking the neuronal sphere: regulation of the actin cytoskeleton in neuritogenesis. *Nature Reviews Neuroscience*, **3**, 694–704.

extension at their plus ends and the inhibition of proteins that cause **microtubule catastrophe** (i.e. rapid dissociation of subunits from the plus ends) (Fig. 7.10). In the axon, microtubule extension is enhanced by the binding of proteins such as MAP1B. Other effector proteins promote the movement of membrane vesicles to the plasma membrane and their subsequent fusion to allow outgrowths to extend. Conversely, during retraction, excess plasma membrane is resorbed by **endocytosis**.

endocytosis the process by which a cell absorbs extracellular molecules by engulfment to form intracellular vesicles. Also a way for plasma membrane and its constituents to become internalized.

7.6 Active transport along the axon is important for outgrowth

Neurite extension requires the movement of cellular building blocks such as cytoskeletal proteins and membrane vesicles from the cell body to the sites of neurite growth. Simple diffusion of these components would be too slow to support growth. Instead they are carried into the neurite via **active transport** (Fig. 7.11). In this process, microfilaments and especially microtubules act as tracks to guide the transport. Proteins and other components to be transported are known as

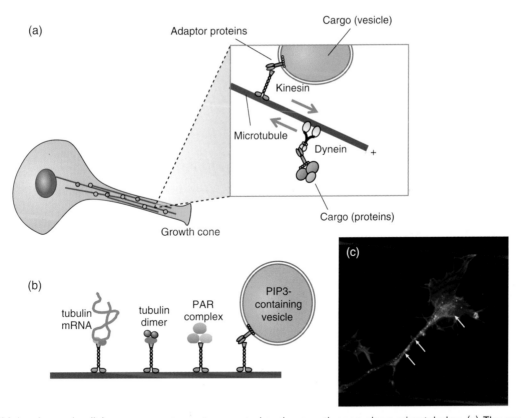

Fig. 7.11 Molecules and cellular components are transported to the growth cone along microtubules. (a) The motor protein kinesin moves components towards the growth cone whereas dynein move them back to the cell body. Many adaptor proteins are involved in tethering specific cargoes to the motor proteins. (b) Some examples of the wide variety of cargoes that are transported to the growth cone. PIP3 and PAR are important regulators that will be discussed later in this chapter. (c) Transport of fluorescently labelled vesicles (seen as dots) visualized in a growing hippocampal axon in which microtubules (blue) and actin (red) are also detected. Some of the vesicles are indicated by arrows. (Image shown by kind permission of Monica Flight Hoyos, Imperial College London.)

cargoes. A wide variety of cargoes are transported, including proteins required for the building of axon (such as tubulin), as well as some of the proteins that themselves regulate outgrowth, such as the **PAR complex** (discussed in the next section). Moreover, vesicles and organelles are also transported, such as mitochondria and **endosomes**. Recently it has emerged that even messenger RNAs and ribosomes are transported into the growth cone. Actin and tubulin mRNAs are examples of such molecules. This allows the local translation of specific proteins within the tip of the growing axon to facilitate rapid growth (see Section 8.10 in the next chapter for further detail).

The cargoes transported initially are concerned with neurite growth. Subsequently, components are transported that must be localized to the synapses for neuronal function. Transport can be observed in live neurons by using microscopy to track fluorescently labelled vesicles as they move through the axon (Fig. 7.11).

Cargoes are moved along cytoskeletal tracks by molecular motor proteins (Fig. 7.11). These motors move along cytoskeletal filaments using energy derived from ATP hydrolysis. Myosin motor proteins transport cargoes along actin filaments while proteins of the kinesin and dynein families are the motors that use microtubules. Dynein moves to the minus end of microtubules, whereas kinesin moves to the plus end. Since microtubules are all aligned in an axon with their plus ends pointing towards the terminal, kinesin is responsible for transport away from the cell body (**anterograde** transport) while dynein transports towards the cell body (**retrograde** transport).

7.7 The development of neuronal polarity

7.7.1 Signalling during axon specification

In Section 7.3, we saw that neuronal polarity is achieved by the specification of one neurite as the axon, while all other neurites become dendrites. The mechanism by which a neurite becomes an axon is therefore a key step in the acquisition of neuronal polarity. Important signalling events occur in the tip of a neurite when it becomes an axon, followed by its rapid extension. Many signalling molecules are involved, but a critical early event appears to be the activation of the **PIP3** signalling pathway. Levels of PIP3 are observed to be high in the tips of actively growing axons. This triggers axon elongation via the localized inactivation of a **protein kinase** called GSK-3β (Fig. 7.12).

The PAR complex is important for axon initiation in a variety of vertebrates. As we saw in Chapter 5 (Section 5.5.5), this highly conserved protein complex is associated with asymmetric cell division in *Drosophila* and *C. elegans*. It is perhaps not surprising, therefore, that the PAR complex is also important for neuronal polarity. In cultured neurons, the complex has been observed to become concentrated in the axonal tip, and experimental inhibition of the complex can prevent axon specification.

Much evidence suggests that a key step in axon initiation downstream of these signalling processes is the recruitment of stabilized

endosomes an intracellular organelle transporting material away from the plasma membrane.

PIP3 (phosphatidylinositol 3,4,5-trisphosphate) – a membrane-associated phospholipid second messenger involved in regulating many cellular processes, including cell shape changes, migration and neuronal polarity.

protein kinase an enzyme that transfers a phosphate group to a protein (usually from ATP), thereby regulating the protein's function.

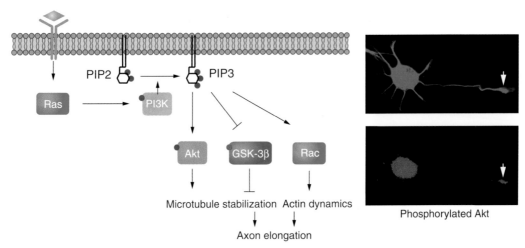

Fig. 7.12 Signalling events in axon specification. When activated, PI3 kinase (PI3K) catalyses the formation of PIP3. PIP3 regulates growth cone dynamics via the activation of protein kinase Akt, inhibition of protein kinase GSK-3β and activation of Rac. PI3K, Akt and GSK-3β are all regulated by phosphorylation (attachment of phosphate is represented by the small dots: green phosphates denote activation, red ones inhibition). On the right is a cultured hippocampal neuron visualized in green using an antibody specific for tubulin. In red is the distribution of the phosphorylated (activated) form of Akt, which reflects the local presence of PIP3. Note that expression is concentrated at the tip of the future axon (arrow) but not the other neurites. (Images adapted from Shi, S-H., Jan, L. Y. and Jan, Y-N. (2003) Hippocampal neuronal polarity specified by spatially localized mPar3/mPar6 and PI 3-Kinase activity. *Cell*, **112**, 63–75 copyright (2003), with permission from Elsevier.)

microtubules to the neurite. This was demonstrated in experiments on cultured hippocampal neurons in which one neurite was treated with taxol, a drug that prevents microtubule dissociation. The treated neurite inevitably became the axon of the neuron (Fig. 7.13). *In vivo*, microtubule stabilization is achieved by the recruitment of axon-specific MAPs (including MAP1B and Tau proteins) in response to signalling events.

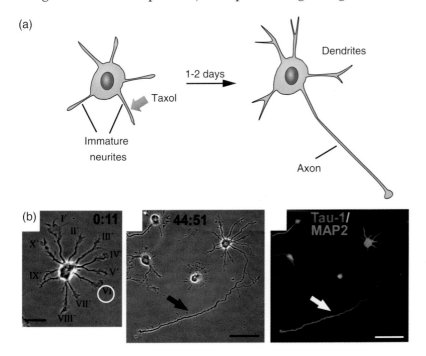

Fig. 7.13 Experiment demonstrating the importance of stabilizing microtubules in specifying the axon. (a) Taxol is administered to one neurite, resulting in transient stabilization of its microtubules. A few days later, that neurite has elongated dramatically, while the lengths of untreated neurites have not changed. (b) A single neurite of this cultured neuron was treated with taxol (circled). After two days, this neurite has extended. Fluorescence microscopy shows that this neurite accumulated an axon-specific MAP (Tau-1, in red), whereas the other neurites accumulate a dendrite-specific MAP (MAP-2, in green). (Images from Witte, H., Neukirchen, D. and Bradke, F. (2008) Microtubule stabilization specifies initial neuronal polarization. *J. Cell Biol.*, **180**, 619–632. Rockefeller University Press.)

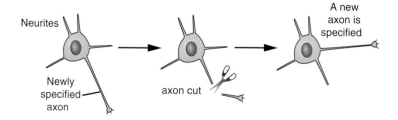

Fig. 7.14 Specifying a single axon. If the axon of a cultured hippocampal neuron is cut, a second neurite elongates to form a replacement axon.

7.7.2 Ensuring there is just one axon

In cultured hippocampal cells, only a single neurite becomes the axon, the remainder later becoming dendrites. If this axon is cut off, then another neurite can differentiate to take its place (Fig. 7.14). This gives a clue as to how neurons become polarized to produce just one axon. One suggestion is that all the neurites compete for a limited amount of a growth-permitting molecule(s) produced in the cell body. One neurite wins this competition to become the axon, which then extends rapidly. If the axon is removed, then the remaining neurites can compete once more for this molecule. The nature of this axon-promoting factor is as yet unknown but PIP3 and the PAR complex are strong candidates. Both these axon regulators are known to be transported as cargoes to the growing tip of the axon (Fig. 7.11). This model also suggests how microtubule stabilization leads to axon specification and rapid extension: it may enhance the transport of signalling components into the neurite, allowing it to monopolize the cellular pool.[4]

Why is this interesting? Injury or disease can cause axon degeneration leading to paralysis, and this tends to be permanent since CNS axons rarely regenerate *in vivo*. If the mechanism behind the process of axon specification is understood, then perhaps axon regeneration could be promoted therapeutically.

7.7.3 Which neurite becomes the axon?

stochastic random, unpredictable, occurring by chance.

In cultured neurons many neurites grow and they all appear capable of becoming an axon (as shown, for instance, by the taxol and axon cutting experiments). So which one does? As neurites dynamically extend and contract, it is possible that small **stochastic** differences in the accumulation of signalling molecules or in microtubule stabilization may be enough to trigger axon formation in any one of the neurites. However, unlike these cultured cells, imaging of differentiating neurons *in vivo* shows that the axon emerges in a highly orientated manner relative to a neuron's surroundings. For instance, in Purkinje cells, the axon grows out of the cell on the side facing the ventricular (inner) surface of the cerebellum whilst dendrites project from the pial (outer) side (see Chapter 6, Box 6.2). It is highly likely, therefore, that extracellular signals determine the specification of the axon. For instance, one side of a cell may experience a signal that activates the PIP3 pathway on that side only. This scenario can be replicated in cultured

---

[4] Further information on neuronal polarity can be found in Arimura, N. and Kaibuchi, K. (2007) Neuronal polarity: from extracellular signals to intracellular mechanisms. *Nature Reviews Neuroscience*, **8**, 194–205.

hippocampal neurons: when one immature neurite is treated with a laminin-coated bead, a rapid rise in PIP3 is observed at the neurite tip followed by its sudden elongation as an axon.

It is also likely that the centrosome plays a role in determining where the axon will appear on the neuron. Since microtubules radiate from the centrosome into the axon, it has been suggested that the location of the centrosome within the cell favours a neighbouring neurite to become the axon. *In vivo*, we saw earlier that many neurons of the vertebrate CNS initially form only a single neurite, which becomes the axon. This first appears while the neuronal precursor cell is still in the **ventricular zone**, and it initially forms the leading process of the migrating neuron (Chapter 6, Section 6.6). Only once the neuron has reached its destination are further neurites formed. One suggestion is that different cues stimulate axon and dendrite formation: initially the cell senses an early axon-promoting signal and only becomes exposed to a dendrite-promoting cue upon reaching its destination.

ventricular zone the inner side of the neural tube closest to its lumen in the developing vertebrate brain. This transient layer contains neuronal progenitor cells.

7.8 Dendrites

7.8.1 Regulation of dendrite branching

Much of what has been discovered about neurite outgrowth applies both to axons and dendrites. Dendrites have growth cones and extrinsic signals promote dendrite growth: for instance, **neurotrophin** signalling increases dendrite length and complexity when applied to the developing ferret visual cortex. Such dendrite-promoting signals act via small G proteins, as has been shown in a variety of neuronal systems, including Purkinje cells, hippocampal pyramidal neurons and retinal ganglion cells. As with axons, Rac and Cdc42 promote dendrite growth whereas Rho inhibits growth. A major difference, however, is that different proteins and mRNAs are transported into growing dendrites and axons, giving them their different characteristics.

neurotrophin a family of proteins including brain derived neurotrophic factor (BDNF) and nerve growth factor (NGF) that induce the survival, development and function of neurons.

Dendrites of most neurons are characterized by complex branching. Observation of live neurons in rat hippocampal slices in culture suggests that the major mechanism of branching is the formation of protrusions that sprout from the sides of existing branches (so-called interstitial branching). As might be expected, these first appear as individual filopodia on the sides of dendrites. Many of these filopodia subsequently retract, but some are invaded by microtubules, thereby stabilizing them as branches, which then develop their own growth cones. The initiation of branch sprouting requires the local destabilization of the actin gel lining a dendrite segment, and Cdc42 seems particularly associated with the special actin dynamics required for this. On those neurons that have dendritic spines, the formation of such spines appears to involve a similar mechanism to branching. For instance, Rac is required in Purkinje cells for both dendrite branching and spine formation. Spine formation (**spinogenesis**) and regulation of spine shape is revisited in detail in Chapters 10 and 12.[5]

---

[5] For more reading on dendrite formation, see Scott, E.K. and Luo, L. (2001) How do dendrites take their shape? *Nature Neuroscience*, **4**, 359–365.

Fig. 7.15 Self-avoidance in *Drosophila* sensory neurons. The body wall of a *Drosophila* larva has multipolar sensory neurons for touch and pain reception. The dendritic trees of these neurons contain numerous branches that never cross each other. (a) and (b) show a class of these neurons with highly branched dendrites. Neurons in (c) and (d) belong to a less branched class. In (d) expression of the *Dscam* gene has been disrupted, resulting in many branches crossing each other. This indicates a failure in dendrite branch self-avoidance. (a = axon; s = soma). The neurons here are visualized because they have been engineered to express green fluorescent protein. (Images on the left are reproduced with kind permission of K. Emoto, Osaka Bioscience Institute, Japan; images on the right are adapted from Hughes, M. E., Bortnick, R., Tsubouchi, A., Bäumer, P., Kondo, M., Uemura, T. and Schmucker, D. (2007) Homophilic Dscam interactions control complex dendrite morphogenesis. *Neuron*, **54**, 417–427, copyright (2007), with permission from Elsevier.)

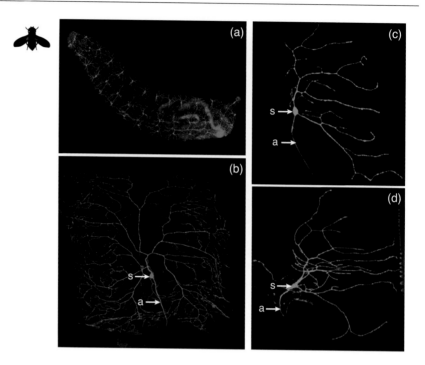

spontaneous electrical activity electrical activity that arises from the endogenous properties of a neuronal or a neural network.

isoform different forms of a protein often produced from the same gene by use of different combinations of exons.

DSCAM Down's Syndrome Cell Adhesion Molecule; a member of the immunoglobulin superfamily. The *Drosophila* gene can produce many thousands of isoforms, rather reminiscent to antibody variation in the immune system.

7.8.2 Dendrite branches undergo self-avoidance

A neuron's dendrites fill a space known as its **dendritic field**. A key characteristic of such fields is that dendrite branches evenly fill the space without touching or overlapping, which ensures even sampling of the receptive area by the neuron. In contrast, the dendritic fields of neighbouring neurons can overlap extensively. This phenomenon whereby dendrite branches especially avoid contact with each other if they originate from the same neuron is known as **dendrite self-avoidance**. It arises by mutual repulsion between growth cones during outgrowth; but how can dendrite branches recognize that they arise from the same neuron? Two types of mechanism have been proposed. First, if the neuron has matured to the stage that it has **spontaneous electrical activity**, this activity will be synchronized between its dendrites, but not necessarily with dendrites of other neurons. Secondly, differences in cell surface molecules between neurons may be involved.

The latter mechanism has been demonstrated for a class of *Drosophila* body wall sensory neuron that has highly branched dendrites (Fig. 7.15). In this case, each neuron expresses a different **isoform** of a cell adhesion molecule called **DSCAM** (for further information on cell adhesion molecules, see Chapter 6, Box 6.3). This is ensured because the *Drosophila Dscam* gene has the capacity to produce up to 100 000 different isoforms of the protein but only one is produced (randomly) within each neuron. Thus, neighbouring neurons are very unlikely to express the same isoform. Mutual repulsion only occurs between branches if they express the same isoform (i.e. if they arise from the same neuron).[6]

---

[6] For more information on DSCAM, see Hattori, D., Millard, S.S., Wojtowicz, W.M. and Zipursky, S. L. (2008) Dscam-mediated cell recognition regulates neural circuit formation. *Annu. Rev. Cell Dev. Biol.*, **24**, 597–620.

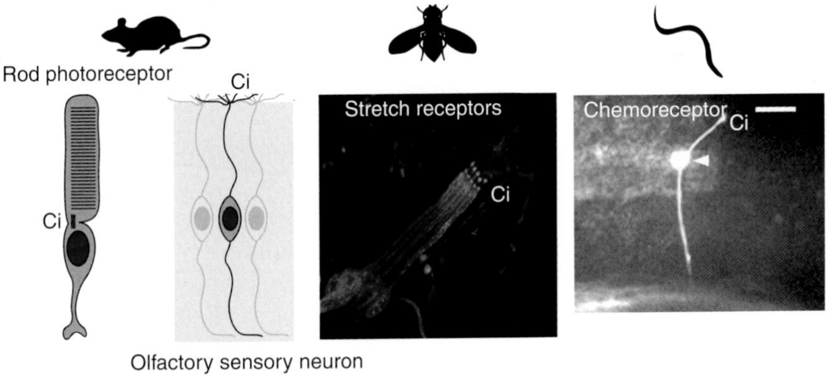

Fig. 7.16 A modified cilium (Ci) forms the basis of the receptive apparatus of many sensory cells. From left to right: mouse rod photoreceptor, mouse olfactory sensory neuron, *Drosophila* stretch receptor neurons, *C. elegans* sensory neuron. (Fourth image from Struckhoff, E. C. and Lundquist, E. A. (2003) The actin-binding protein UNC-115 is an effector of Rac signaling during axon pathfinding in *C. elegans*. *Development*, **130**, 693–704.

7.8.3 Dendrites and other sensory structures based on modified cilia

Many sensory cells in the PNS have specialized outgrowths for sensory transduction that are based on modified **cilia**. Cilia are highly structured cellular protrusions with a core of microtubules called the axoneme, which extends from a modified centrosome called the basal body. Cilia are best known as the beating organelles that make certain **protozoa** and sperm cells motile (the sperm's flagellum is actually a long cilium). In vertebrates, ciliated neural cells include cone and rod photoreceptors, olfactory sensory neurons and inner ear hair cells (Fig. 7.16). The major sensory neurons of *Drosophila* and *C. elegans* also have cilia-based sensory dendrites (Fig. 7.16). The cilium is a complex structure with up to 1000 proteins associated with its construction or function. During outgrowth (ciliogenesis), proteins and membrane vesicles must be transported along the axoneme to the tip of the growing cilium. This process uses a specialized transport process called **intraflagellar transport** (IFT), which requires dynein and kinesin motors and specialized adaptor proteins (IFT proteins). Defects in this process can cause a variety of genetic diseases (Box 7.3).

protozoa a group that includes most unicellular eukaryotic organisms, such as *Amoeba* and *Paramecium*.

Box 7.3 Sensory dendrites, cilia and ciliopathies

In addition to sensory cells, cilia are found on many specialized cell types in humans, including the kidney and lung airway. Most embryonic cells also have a so-called primary cilium, which performs a receptive function in SHH signalling (Chapter 4, Box 4.4). Given the cilium's complexity and diversity of functions, it is not surprising that a heterogeneous range of human disorders are now known to be the result of defects in genes required for ciliogenesis. These are known as **ciliopathies** and are characterized by cystic kidneys, CNS developmental defects, polydactyly (extra digits), degeneration of photoreceptors, anosmia (inability to smell) and defective mechanoreception and thermoreception – all of which result from defects in ciliated cells.

7.9 Summary

- Newly formed neurons grow neurites, which differentiate into axons and dendrites.
- The growth cone is the site of neurite growth. It responds to signals to extend or retract.
- Extracellular signals modulate intracellular processes in the growth cone such as cytoskeletal and membrane dynamics.
- Signal transduction involves many intracellular regulators, including small G proteins. In turn these regulate effector proteins that alter cytoskeletal dynamics.
- Active transport of vesicles, proteins and mRNAs is important for facilitating rapid neurite growth. Transport proceeds along microtubule tracks.
- Neurons acquire polarity whereby neurites differentiate into axons and dendrites.
- Polarity entails the specification of a single neurite as an axon, the rest become dendrites by default.
- Dendrites undergo branching and self-avoidance.

In this chapter, we have looked at the mechanisms underlying the formation and extension of dendrites and axons. In the next chapter, we focus on how these mechanisms are harnessed to guide growing axons along the long and often tortuous paths that they must travel in order to reach their correct destinations.

Axon Guidance

8.1 Many axons navigate long and complex routes

In the preceding chapters, we have seen how different types of neurons are specified during embryogenesis, how they migrate to the appropriate place in the developing brain and how they produce an axon that will enable them to form connections with appropriate synaptic partners. In this chapter we shall discuss the mechanisms by which axons reliably and reproducibly carry out the remarkable feats of navigation that make connections with their appropriate partners possible. A wiring diagram of the adult human brain would contain more than 10^{11} neurons each making connections with an average of 1000 target cells. While some of these connections are made between cells that lie close together, many are between cells that are separated by considerable distances – for example, a motor neuron in the human spinal cord may synapse with a muscle in the big toe. Much of the wiring pattern of the CNS is laid down during embryogenesis, presenting the embryo with an extraordinarily complex task. Understanding how this task is achieved is a fascinating and important challenge that has occupied many developmental neurobiologists around the world for decades.

8.2 The growth cone

There are many similarities between axon pathfinding and the process of cell migration, which was discussed in Chapter 6. The main difference is that in axon pathfinding, the cell body remains in place as the tip of the growing axon moves further away. The most important part of the axon for navigation is the **growth cone,** which was discussed in some detail in Section 7.2 (see Fig. 7.4). To recap briefly, as the growth cone moves toward its target, it actively explores the areas that lie ahead and on either side by continuously extending **filopodia** and **lamellipodia.** The plasma membrane of the growth cone is studded

filopodia (singular filopodium) a finger-like cellular outgrowths associated with cell shape changes. They are important for migrating cells, growth cones and dendritic spine formation.

lamellipodia (singular lamellipodium) sheet-like cellular outgrowths associated with cell shape changes. They appear on migrating cells and growth cones.

Building Brains: An Introduction to Neural Development, First Edition.
David Price, Andrew Jarman, John Mason and Peter Kind.

Fig. 8.1 Changes in the cytoskeleton cause growth cones to change direction. The growth cone is very sensitive to the presence of guidance cues in its environment, and can change direction in response to such cues. In the example shown here, the growth cone is initially travelling towards the top of the page (a). As it moves forward, it encounters an attractive cue, shown in green. The cue is present in a gradient, with highest levels in the top right corner. Those filopodia on the right-hand side of the growth cone are exposed to a higher concentration of the attractive cue than those on the left. As a result, (b) the actin filaments (red) within the filopodia on the right-hand side of the growth cone form a stabilizing interaction with microtubules coming from the axon shaft (purple). This is known as microtubule capture. Conversely, actin filaments within filopodia on the left-hand side do not capture microtubules and the filopodia subsequently retract. Thus, filopodia on the right-hand side are stabilized, those on the left-hand side are not, with the net result that the growth cone turns to the right.

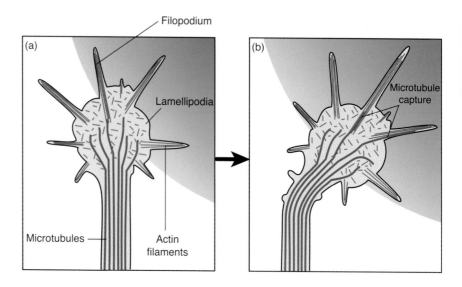

with a variety of receptor molecules that act as exquisitely sensitive sensors for the presence of environmental cues that direct movement of the axon. Signals transduced by these receptors trigger changes in actin and tubulin dynamics in the underlying **cytoskeleton**, leading to directed movement (Fig. 8.1).

Although the precise details of the mechanisms involved are not fully understood, it is likely that the key changes to the cytoskeleton that cause growth cones to turn in response to an attractive cue are as follows. The dynamic extension and retraction of each filopodium is driven by **polymerization** and **depolymerization** of actin filaments (see Box 7.1). When a filopodium encounters an attractive cue, a signal is relayed towards the central domain of the growth cone. In the central domain, microtubules extend dynamically from the stable microtubule core in the axon shaft. In response to the incoming signal, some of these microtubules form an interaction with actin filaments in the filopodium that is being stimulated. This process is known as **microtubule capture** (Fig. 8.1). Once captured in this way, the microtubules become stabilized, thus reinforcing the direction of growth cone turning. Conversely, cues that repel growing axons trigger a response in the filopodium that leads to rapid depolymerization of the filaments, thereby causing the growth cone to collapse.[1]

8.3 How might axons be guided to their targets?

Before going on to discuss the precise nature of the cues that guide navigating axons, it may first be helpful to consider an analogy. The problem facing a newborn neuron sending out an axon to find a distant target cell can be compared to that of a tourist arriving in an unfamiliar environment and having to find their way to a specific

polymerization the process by which monomers are assembled to generate a polymer.

depolymerization the process by which a polymer is broken into monomers.

---

[1] More details on the role of the growth cone cytoskeleton during axon guidance can be found in Lowery, L. A. and Van Vactor, D. (2009) The trip of the tip: understanding the growth cone machinery. *Nature Reviews Molecular Cell Biology*, **10**, 332–343.

destination. The magnitude of the problem facing the tourist varies, depending on the environment which they must navigate through. To take an extreme example, a tourist finding themselves in the Scottish mountains during a white-out snowstorm and having to find their way across featureless terrain to a safe refuge would only be able to get there successfully if they had full information on every detail of the route. They would have to know how many steps to take, which direction to head in, where to turn to avoid obstacles and so on. Clearly, such precise navigation while effectively blind to external cues would be extremely challenging. In the developing nervous system, pre-programming of this sort would require navigating axons to hold a very large amount of diverse information, given the vast number and complexity of possible routes open to them. Full pre-programming therefore seems an unlikely mechanism to control axon guidance during wiring of the nervous system.

On the other hand, if the tourist arrived in the centre of an unfamiliar city and had to find their way to a large stadium on the city outskirts, many more options would be available to help them find their way (Fig. 8.2). In this situation, they could use landmarks as intermediate points on their journey – for example, turning left after

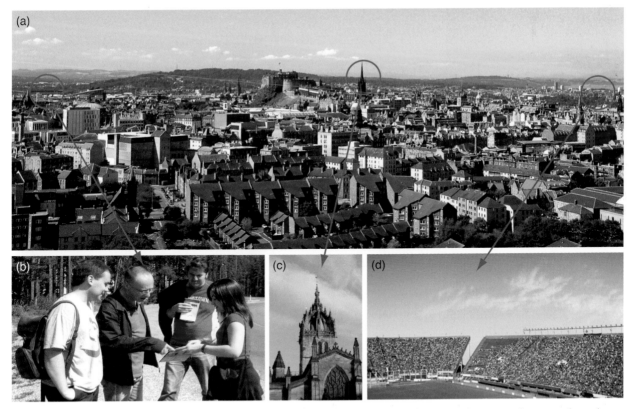

Fig. 8.2 (a) The prospect faced by the axon of a newborn neuron setting out to find an appropriate synaptic partner is analogous to that faced by tourists visiting an unfamiliar city and having to find their way to a specific destination, such as a sports stadium. Such visitors may use a variety of strategies to help them locate the stadium. For example, they may consult a map and memorize the route beforehand (b). They may rely on distinctive landmarks to help them recognize the route (c). They may rely on other cues in the environment, such as the noise generated by a crowd already present in the stadium (d). In practice, people would most likely use a combination of such strategies. (Photo in panel (b) courtesy of Tian Yu).

reaching a particular church. By breaking the route down into a series of shorter steps, each marked by a particular landmark, the task of memorizing the route becomes much easier. Other environmental cues could help the tourist find the stadium. For example, they could be guided by noise made by the crowd already there. In this case, they would simply head in the direction from which the crowd noises came. The sound would become progressively louder as they got closer to the stadium, giving them confidence that they were moving in the right direction and ultimately leading them to their destination. Thus, by recognizing and following appropriate cues in the environment, tourists can successfully navigate complex environments.

In a similar way, the axons of newborn neurons could be guided to their targets by cues in their environment. In this case, each navigating axon would require only enough pre-programming to allow it to recognize and respond appropriately to specific environmental cues. Possible types of cue include **intermediate target cells** and specific molecules (**axon guidance molecules**) that could instruct the axon which direction to take. Such molecular cues could act either at short range or over a distance. As we shall see, in practice, navigating axons are guided to their destinations by a combination of such mechanisms.

8.4 Breaking the journey – intermediate targets

The overall routes travelled by developing axons are often long and complex, so the task of working out how patterns of wiring are first established seems daunting. However, it turns out that in many cases complete journeys are composed of a series of smaller steps. In other words, axons navigate toward one or more intermediate targets on their way to their final destination (Fig. 8.3). This is analogous to our city tourist using specific landmark buildings to help them find their way to the stadium. One well-studied example of this is seen in the grasshopper embryo, where **guidepost cells** act as intermediate targets for the axons of neurons in the developing leg (Fig. 8.4). Axons that originate from the Ti1 neurons in the distal part of the developing grasshopper limb make contact with a series of three guidepost cells on their journey towards the body. After making contact with the second guidepost cell, they make a 90° turn and continue growing until they come into contact with a third guidepost cell, whereupon they turn once more and head towards the body. If the third guidepost cell is experimentally ablated, the navigating axons fail to make the 90° turn; instead they stall and then move on in apparently random directions. This clearly shows that the guidepost cell is essential for these axons to navigate correctly. In other words, the intermediate target is crucial in allowing the axon to navigate correctly towards its final target in the CNS. In vertebrate embryos, specific groups of cells or anatomical structures may act as intermediate targets for navigating axons. For example, as described later in this chapter the **floor plate** of the spinal cord acts as an intermediate target for certain axons (Section 8.7).

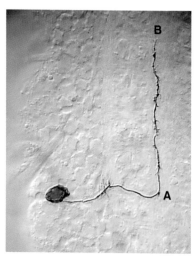

Fig. 8.3 Long journeys made by navigating axons often consist of a series of shorter steps. The photograph shows a single labelled neuron in a *Drosophila* embryo. Its axon has projected in one direction then taken a 90° turn. This strongly suggests that the axon initially projected towards point A then, upon reaching A, it changed its behaviour to grow towards B. (Image courtesy of Keri-Lee Harris, University of Melbourne.)

floor plate the most ventral region of the neural tube.

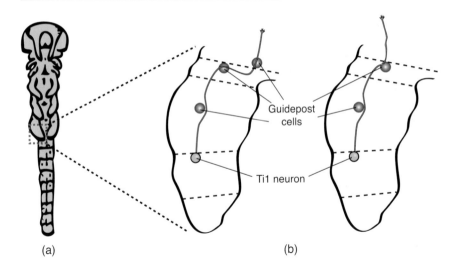

(a)

(b)

Fig. 8.4 Guidepost cells act as intermediate targets in the developing grasshopper limb. (a) A view of a grasshopper embryo from its ventral surface, with anterior at the top. The cell body of the Ti1 pioneer neuron (orange) lies near the distal tip of the developing limb and projects its axon towards the body. As it goes, it interacts with several cells that act as guideposts (green). After reaching the second guidepost cell, it makes a 90° turn toward the third guidepost. (b) If the third guidepost cell is experimentally ablated, the axon fails to turn and appears to lose its way. (Adapted by permission from Macmillan Publishers Ltd: Nature. Bentley, D. and Caudey, M. (1983) Pioneer axons lose directed growth after selective killing of guidepost cells. *Nature*, **304**, 62–65) copyright 1983.)

8.5 Contact guidance

In many situations, navigating axons are given instructions by molecular cues that they encounter on their journey. These cues can be subdivided into two major groups. One group of cues are *secreted*, and are therefore able to act at a distance from the point where they are produced – these cues will be discussed later, in Section 8.6. Another group of guidance cues are found *on the surface* of cells, such that close physical contact is necessary between the navigating axon and the cell that expresses the guidance cue. This type of interaction is referred to as **contact guidance**. Common types of contact guidance cues include molecules present on the surface of other cells or **extracellular matrix**. Contact guidance may serve either to attract or to repel growing axons, referred to as **contact attraction** and **contact repulsion**, respectively (Fig. 8.5). The guidepost cells in the developing grasshopper leg that were discussed in the previous section provide an example of contact guidance – they express a specific guidance cue on their surface.

extracellular matrix the gel-like meshwork of protein and carbohydrate polymers that surrounds cells and gives structural support in most organs and tissues.

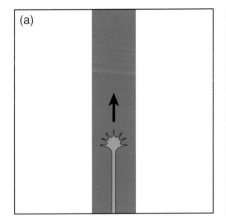
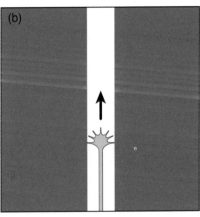

(a)

(b)

Fig. 8.5 Contact guidance: some guidance cues require the navigating axon to come into physical contact with the cue and therefore act over a short range. Such guidance cues may either attract or repel growing axons. (a) In contact attraction the migrating axon follows a route demarcated by an attractive cue, shown in green. (b) In contact repulsion the axon is confined to a particular trajectory, minimizing its contact with the repellent cue, shown in red.

8.5.1 Contact guidance in action: pioneers and followers, fasciculation and defasciculation

Returning to our analogy of a tourist attempting to find their way to a stadium on the outskirts of an unfamiliar city, one potential strategy open to them would be to follow other people who knew the way. They may be able to recognize others bound for the same stadium by the way they were dressed (this would be a good strategy if heading for a sports match where fans display their allegiance by wearing clothing in their team's colours). Similarly, while all axons must somehow find their way to the correct destination, this task is simplified for some axons because they reach their target by following the paths of others that have already made the journey. Thus, a relatively small number of **pioneer neurons** first find their way to the correct target region and other axons, sometimes referred to as follower axons, follow behind. We shall explore the mechanisms that guide pioneer axons later in the chapter. Follower axons follow the route laid down by the pioneers by associating tightly with the pioneer axons, forming bundles of axons known as **fascicles** in a process known as **fasciculation**. This is therefore a form of contact guidance. An example of this is seen in the ventral nerve cord of *Drosophila* (Fig. 8.6). Two thick bundles of axons run longitudinally along either side of the ventral midline in the *Drosophila* embryo, each composed of a number of axon fascicles. The association between bundled axons in each fascicle is mediated by **homophilic** interactions between **cell adhesion molecules** (**CAM**s, see Box 6.3 in Chapter 6) on the axon surface. For example, axons that express the CAM fasciclin I (fasI) will preferentially associate with other fasI-expressing axons while those expressing fasII will fasciculate with other fasII-expressing axons. This provides evidence in support of the **labelled pathway hypothesis**, which states that axons join specific fascicles based on the type of cell adhesion molecules that they express. At each step on its journey, the axon expresses different cell adhesion molecules on its surface, allowing it to associate with specific sets of axons to guide it on its way.

Once they have joined an appropriate fascicle, axons will grow along it until they reach the point at which they must leave, for example when they reach an intermediate target. In other words, axons must **defasciculate** from the contralateral longitudinal pathway at the appropriate point. Defasciculation is regulated by BEAT proteins, named after the *beaten path* mutant, in which axons fail to defasciculate correctly. BEAT proteins act by disrupting the homophilic interactions between cell adhesion molecules, thereby promoting defasciculation (Fig. 8.7).

8.5.2 Extracellular matrix provides a substrate for navigating axons

Axons do not grow just anywhere in the developing nervous system, they require a specific type of substrate to grow along. Usually, this comprises either cell adhesion molecules (Box 6.3 in Chapter 6) present

homophilic binding between molecules of the same kind.

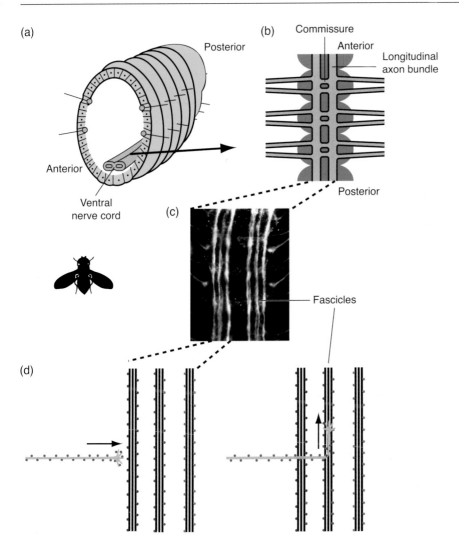

(a)

Posterior

Anterior

Ventral
nerve cord

(b) Commissure

Anterior

Longitudinal
axon bundle

Posterior

(c)

Fascicles

(d)

Fig. 8.6 Major axon pathways in the *Drosophila* ventral nerve cord. (a) The *Drosophila* ventral nerve cord, shown in orange, lies over the ventral midline of the embryo. The ventral nerve cord was described in more detail in Fig. 2.2. (b) The nerve cord resembles a ladder, with two thick bundles of axons running longitudinally along the anteroposterior axis, one on either side of the midline and joined by a number of regularly spaced commissures, like the rungs of a ladder. The commissures contain bundles of axons that cross from one side of the embryo to the other. (c) Immunostaining with an antibody that recognizes a specific cell surface protein labels just three specific parallel fascicles on either side of the ventral midline, highlighting the fact that the thick longitudinal pathways are composed of multiple fascicles. (d) The labelled pathway hypothesis suggests that axons join specific fascicles based on the type of cell adhesion molecules that they express. A growing axon, expressing a specific cell adhesion molecule (red) approaches a group of three fascicles, each of which expresses a different cell adhesion molecule on its surface (shown in blue, red and green). The incoming axon specifically joins the fascicle that expresses the same cell adhesion molecule.

on the surface of neighbouring cells or extracellular matrix molecules such as laminin (Box 7.2 in Chapter 7). Specific receptors in the growth cone membrane recognize and bind to these molecules, some of which provide an environment that allows axons to grow through that area, while others serve to prevent growth cones entering a particular area. Somewhat confusingly, these molecules are not usually considered to be true axon guidance molecules because they act by providing a permissive or non-permissive environment for axons in general, rather than by providing a specific instruction to a particular growth cone to change its direction of movement.

8.5.3 Ephs and ephrins: versatile cell surface molecules with roles in contact guidance

One family of cell surface proteins that are important for contact guidance of navigating axons are the **ephrins** and their receptors the **Ephs**. We already encountered Ephs and ephrins in Chapter 4, where their role in forming **rhombomeres** in the hindbrain was

rhombomeres anatomically distinguishable tissue blocks formed in the hindbrain (or rhombencephalon).

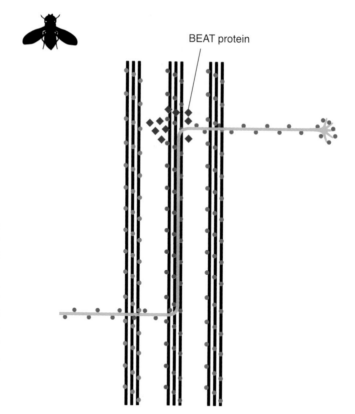

BEAT protein

Fig. 8.7 BEAT proteins can cause defasciculation. An incoming commissural axon (orange) joins the fascicle that expresses the same CAM (red) and grows along it. BEAT protein (purple diamonds) is expressed near the point at which the axon exits the fascicle, and promotes defasciculation by disrupting homophilic adhesion between the CAM molecules expressed on the axon and the fascicle, allowing the axon to leave the fascicle.

tyrosine kinase an enzyme that transfers phosphate groups (i.e. phosphorylates) onto tyrosine residues in a protein.

ligand a molecule or ion that binds to a receptor molecule, for example on the cell surface, to generate a biological response.

retinotopic map the map of retinal ganglion cell position in a target brain structure.

described (see Section 4.4.1, Fig. 4.11). These large families of cell surface molecules play important roles in a wide variety of developmental processes. Ephrins are cell-surface proteins that fall into two classes, ephrinAs, which are attached to the plasma membrane by a lipid anchor, and ephrinBs, which have a transmembrane domain. The Eph family of **tyrosine kinase** receptors act as receptors for ephrins and also fall into two classes, EphAs and EphBs. In general, the EphAs are receptors for ephrinAs while EphBs are receptors for ephrinBs, although there are some exceptions (for example, ephrinA4 binds to EphBs). Altogether, mammals have eight ephrins and 13 Eph receptors. As cell surface proteins, they mediate contact guidance. Interestingly, although mainly regarded as **ligands**, Ephrins are also able to act are receptors and can transduce signals in some situations. This means that bidirectional signalling can occur through Eph–ephrin interactions. Although they are not diffusible molecules, gradients of Ephs and ephrins, and other surface-bound molecules, are found across some tissues due to differences in expression levels in the cells across that tissue. As described in detail in Chapter 9, Section 9.5.3, gradients of Eph receptor expression in the retina and complementary gradients of ephrin expression in the tectum (their target structure in the midbrain) allow the formation of **retinotopic maps**, specific patterns of connection that are important for vision.

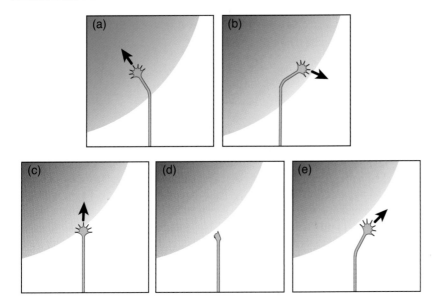

Fig. 8.8 Major forms of chemotropism. (a) Chemoattraction: the navigating axon senses a gradient of an attractive cue (green) and moves towards its source. (b) Chemorepulsion: the axon senses a gradient of a repulsive cue (red) and turns to move down the gradient, away from the source. ((c)–(e)) Growth cones can also respond to repulsive cues by collapsing. In the example shown here, the growth cone first becomes exposed to a chemorepellent cue (c), causing it to withdraw all filopodia and collapse (d). The growth cone can then start to move forward again, but in a different direction (e).

8.6 Guidance of axons by diffusible cues – chemotropism

So far, we have seen how axons can be guided by short-range interactions requiring direct cell–cell contact. Like our tourist using the noise generated by a crowd of spectators as a cue to guide him towards a stadium, axons may also be guided by cues that act over longer distances. This process, known as **chemotropism**, involves the directed growth of axons in response to a diffusible factor. Diffusible chemotropic cues may either attract growing axons (**chemoattraction**) or repel them (**chemorepulsion**) (Fig. 8.8).

It is easy to imagine how a diffusible molecule released by target tissues (whether final or intermediate targets) could form a molecular concentration gradient across a tissue. Growth cones that are sensitive and attracted to the particular cue could then follow the concentration gradient, leading the axons towards their target, the source of the chemoattractant. Similarly, growth cones can move down concentration gradients of chemorepellent molecules, leading them away from the source (perhaps deflecting them towards their correct target). Observations of growth cones in culture have shown that some respond to repulsive cues by turning smoothly away from them (Fig. 8.8(b)). Others respond more dramatically by collapsing and then, after a short pause, re-growing in a direction that might be more permissive; this process can be repeated many times allowing the growth cone to find the correct path by a process of trial and error (Fig. 8.8(c)–(e)). Growth cones are extraordinarily sensitive to small concentration differences across them, allowing them to detect and respond to the gradients generated in developing organisms, although there are limits to their ability if the gradients are not steep enough, e.g. a long way from their source.[2]

[2] More information about the theoretical considerations of how growth cones detect gradients can be found in Mortimer, D., Fothergill, T., Pujic, Z., Richards, L.J. and Goodhill, G.J. (2008) Growth cone chemotaxis. *Trends in Neurosciences*, **31**, 90–98.

8.6.1 Netrin – a chemotropic cue expressed at the ventral midline

Although chemotropism was first suggested as a possible mechanism for axon guidance by Ramón y Cajal more than 100 years ago, it was not until the mid-1990s that specific chemotropic cues were identified. **Netrin**, the first chemotropic axon guidance molecule to be described in vertebrates, was found by virtue of its ability to attract a specific group of axons, known as **commissural axons**, in the developing neural tube (Box 8.1). The cell bodies of vertebrate spinal cord commissural neurons lie in the **dorsal** part of the spinal cord. Their axons first project ventrally, towards the floor plate, where they cross over the midline into the contralateral spinal cord. Commissural axons are guided on this first step of their journey by netrin-1, a chemotropic cue expressed in the floor plate (Fig. 8.9).

Since the discovery of netrins, rapid progress has been made in identifying additional axon guidance molecules. At present, the best understood families that include secreted axon guidance molecules are the netrins, Slits and semaphorins (Fig. 8.10). The Slits and semaphorins are discussed below. Many axon guidance molecules and their receptors are highly evolutionarily conserved. Our understanding of axon guidance mechanisms has benefited greatly from the ability to investigate the actions of these molecules in **genetically tractable organisms**, in particular *Drosophila*.

genetically tractable organism an organism whose genetic make-up can be manipulated relatively easily.

8.6.2 Slits

Slits are large secreted proteins that were first shown to act in axon guidance through genetic screening experiments in *Drosophila* (see Box 1.1 in Chapter 1). Slit proteins act through a transmembrane receptor named ROBO (short for Roundabout, which was also first identified in a genetic screen). The roles played by Slit and ROBO in guiding axons at the ventral midline of the nervous system in *Drosophila* and in vertebrates are described in detail in Section 8.7.2. Like their fly counterpart, vertebrate Slit homologues are important for guiding axons at the ventral midline of the nervous system where they act as chemorepellant molecules, preventing inappropriate crossing of the midline. This role is strongly conserved evolutionarily – Slit also regulates midline crossing in *C. elegans*. Slits are involved in the formation of numerous other axon tracts; for example, they help guide the axons of **retinal ganglion cells** through the **optic chiasm** in vertebrates (Section 8.8.1).

optic chiasm structure on the ventral surface of the brain composed of the axons of retinal ganglion cells. These axons cross the midline at this point, creating the chiasm's characteristic X-shape.

8.6.3 Semaphorins

The semaphorins are a large and diverse family of cell surface and secreted proteins. The first semaphorin to be described, initially called fasciclinIV and subsequently renamed semaphorin-1A (SEMA1A), was identified through its expression on specific axon fascicles in *Drosophila*. The first vertebrate semaphorin to be described was purified by virtue of its potent activity in promoting growth cone collapse (the process shown in Fig. 8.8(c)–(e)) – this molecule was initially named

Box 8.1   Netrins

The chemoattractive activity that guides commissural axons to the floor plate of the vertebrate spinal cord was purified in Marc Tessier-Lavigne's laboratory in an heroic set of biochemical experiments that required the use of 1000s of embryonic chick brains (Serafini, T., Kennedy, T. E., Galko, M. J., Mirzayan, C., Jessell, T. M. and Tessier-Lavigne, M. (1994) The netrins define a family of axon outgrowth-promoting proteins homologous to *C. elegans* UNC-6. *Cell*, **78**, 409−24). The novel protein was given the name **netrin**, derived from the Sanskrit for 'one who guides'. There are two members of the netrin family in vertebrates, netrin-1 and netrin-2. In mutant mice that lack netrin-1, commissural projections are completely absent. Netrins are highly evolutionarily conserved molecules and a homologue of netrin was identified in a genetic screen set up to identify genes involved in coordinating movement in the nematode worm *C. elegans*. This *C. elegans* netrin is encoded by the gene, *unc-6*, where *unc* is short for <u>unc</u>oordinated. The poorly coordinated movement seen in *C. elegans unc-6* mutants is a consequence of axon guidance defects, demonstrating that netrin's axon guidance role is conserved during evolution. Genetic screens in *C. elegans* also led to the identification of two types of netrin receptor molecules, encoded by the genes *unc-40* and *unc-5*. Both are evolutionarily conserved trans-membrane proteins. The *Drosophila* homologue of *unc-40* is known as *frazzled*. Mammals have two proteins homologous to UNC-40, named DCC (<u>d</u>eleted in <u>c</u>olon <u>c</u>ancer) and neogenin, and four UNC-5 homologues, named UNC5H1-4. It is thought that UNC-40/DCC mediates attractive responses to netrin while UNC-5 mediates repulsion by netrin. Therefore, although first described as a chemoattractant, netrin can in fact act either to attract or to repel axons, depending on the type of receptors that they express.

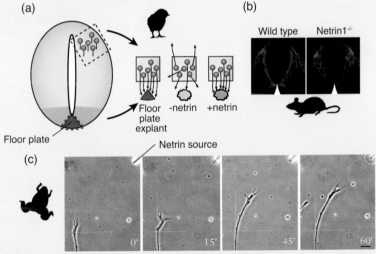

(a) Cell bodies of commissural interneurons are located in the dorsal region of the neural tube. Their axons project ventrally, toward the floor plate, attracted by netrin-1. When placed together in culture, axons will grow out from an **explant** of dorsal neural tube towards an explant of floor plate (red wedge). Dorsal neural tube axons are not attracted by non-neural cells that do not express netrin-1 (grey) but if such cells are genetically modified to produce high levels of netrin-1 (purple), axons are strongly attracted towards them. (b) In the spinal cord of wildtype mice, commissural axons can be seen projecting towards the floor plate and crossing to the other side (white arrowhead). However, in mutant mice lacking netrin-1 (*netrin1^{-/-}*), axons do not project toward the floor plate and fail to cross at the floor plate. (Panel (b) is reprinted from Serafini, T. *et al.* (1996) Netrin-1 is required for commissural axon guidance in the developing vertebrate nervous system, *Cell*, **87**, 1001−1014 Copyright 1996, with permission from Elsevier.) (c) Isolated axons growing in culture are attracted towards a source of netrin. The four panels show frames from a time-lapse study of *Xenopus* retinal axons growing on a glass microscope slide that has been coated with a cell adhesion molecule. In the series shown here, netrin has been released from the pipette tip just visible in the top right-hand corner of each panel. Note how the growth cone changes direction to head towards the netrin source. (Panel (c) is reprinted from de la Torre, J. R. *et al.,* (1997) Turning of retinal growth cones in a netrin-1 gradient mediated by the netrin receptor DCC, *Neuron*,**19**, 1211−24 Copyright 1997, with permission from Elsevier.)

explant part of an organism that has been excised and cultured in isolation.

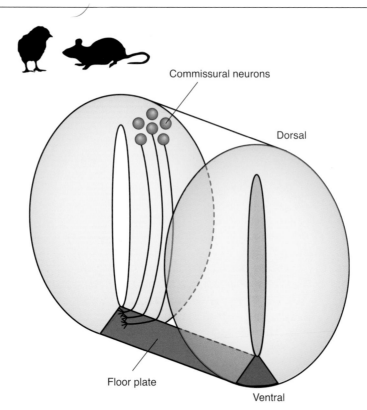

Fig. 8.9 The axons of dorsally-located commissural neurons in the vertebrate spinal cord start their journey by projecting axons towards the floor plate. Netrin-1 expressed in the floor plate (red) acts as a chemoattractant, directing the growing axons toward the floor plate. This is just the first step in these axons' journey; it will continue in Fig 8.12.

Fig. 8.10 Four major families of guidance molecule and their receptors. The growth cones at the tips of growing axons contain cell surface receptors specific for a variety of guidance cues. Some cues, such as Slits and netrins are secreted and can therefore form extracellular gradients. Other cues, such as ephrins are located at the cell surface and can only provide guidance signals to growth cones that make physical contact with the cells which express the cue molecule. The semaphorins are produced in different forms, some are secreted while others are found on the cell surface. Gradients of surface molecules across a region arise where cells within the region express an ordered range of levels on their surfaces.

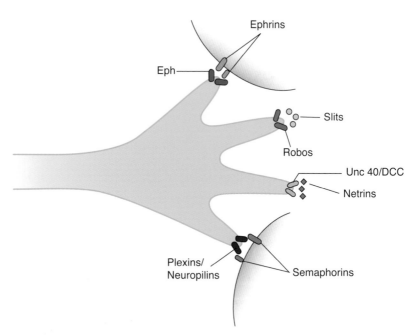

multimeric proteins that consist of more than one subunit.

collapsin but is now known as SEMA3A. Some semaphorins have transmembrane domains, others are linked to the membrane by a lipid anchor and some are secreted.

Semaphorins signal through **multimeric** receptor complexes whose precise composition is not fully understood but at least two types of semaphorin receptor have been identified – plexins and neuropilins. Semaphorins seem to act mostly as chemorepulsive cues in axon guidance. Semaphorins are widely expressed outside the nervous system and have roles in the development and normal function of a wide range of tissues.

8.6.4 Other axon guidance molecules

A number of molecules that were first identified by virtue of entirely different functions can also act as axon guidance cues. These include members of the Wnt, Hedgehog and bone morphogenetic protein (BMP) families of intercellular signalling molecules. Multiple roles for Wnts in axon guidance have been uncovered in *C. elegans*, in *Drosophila* and in mammals. Wnt activity mediates axon repulsion in both the *Drosophila* nerve cord and the vertebrate **corticospinal tract**. Wnt signalling is also required to guide the axons of commissural neurons towards the brain after crossing the vertebrate spinal cord (see Section 8.7.3). BMPs and SHH are both involved in guiding commissural axons to the ventral midline of the vertebrate spinal cord (see Chapter 4, Section 4.5.5, for a recap of where these signals are produced in the neural tube). BMPs appear to push commissural axons away from dorsal neural tube through a chemorepulsive mechanism while SHH cooperates with netrin-1 to attract these axons to the ventral midline.

corticospinal tract a collection of axons that connect the cerebral cortex to the spinal cord.

8.7 How do axons change their behaviour at choice points?

We have already seen that long journeys made by navigating axons are often broken up into a series of smaller steps with intermediate targets. This suggests that the axon must alter its response to specific cues once it reaches an intermediate target, such that it is no longer guided towards the intermediate point, but towards the next target on its journey instead. Consequently, intermediate targets are sometimes called choice points. To discuss the types of molecular mechanisms that underlie such changes in axon behaviour, we shall now return to the commissural axon pathway in the vertebrate spinal cord, which has been particularly well studied.

8.7.1 Commissural axons lose their attraction to netrin once they have crossed the floor plate

Given that commissural axons are initially attracted to soluble netrin expressed in the floor plate, why don't they stop once they reach the source of the netrin cue? It turns out that once commissural axons reach the midline, a switch occurs such that they lose their attraction to netrin. This was first demonstrated by studying the behaviour of navigating commissural axons in explanted pieces of spinal cord in tissue culture. To make it easier to visualize the axons, the spinal cord was first cut open along the dorsal surface, then the tissue laid flat in

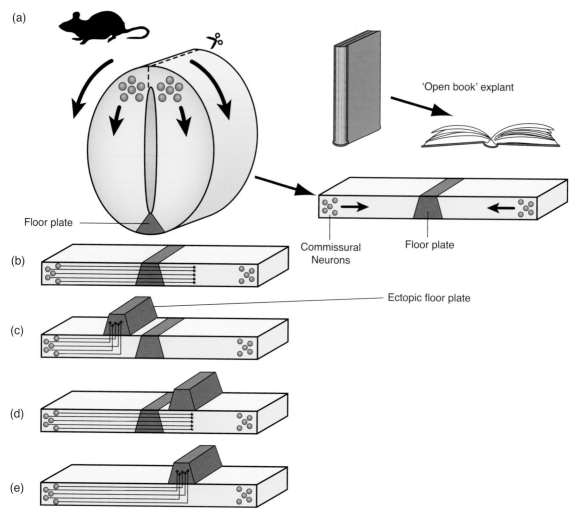

(a)

'Open book' explant

Floor plate

Commissural Neurons

Floor plate

(b)

Ectopic floor plate

(c)

(d)

(e)

Fig. 8.11 'Open book' cultures demonstrate that commissural axons lose their attraction to netrin once they have crossed the ventral midline (floor plate). (a) An open book culture is made by cutting along the dorsal edge of the neural tube and opening it up. The tissue is then laid flat, such that the dorsalmost parts of the neural tube lie at the outside edges of the explant, while the floor plate is in the middle. The effect is similar to that of opening a book and laying it on a flat surface. (b) Axons grow towards the floor plate and cross over to the other side. (c) If an extra piece of floor plate is placed beside the explant, on the same side as the labelled axons, they head towards the ectopic floor plate, attracted by the netrin that it produces. (d) However, if the extra floor plate is placed on the other side of the explant, such that the commissural growth cones have already crossed over the floor plate before becoming exposed to netrin produced by the ectopic floor plate tissue, they are no longer attracted to it. (e) If floor plate tissue is excised from the explant, commissural axons are now attracted to the extra floor plate tissue. This shows that commissural axons lose sensitivity to netrin upon encountering floor plate tissue, rather than losing sensitivity after travelling a specific distance. (Adapted from Shirasaki, R., Katsumata, R. and Murakami, F. (1998) Change in chemoattractant responsiveness of developing axons at an intermediate target. *Science,* **279,** 105–107 and Sanes, D. H., Reh, T. A. and Harris, W. A. (2004) *Development of the Nervous System* 2nd edn, Academic Press).

the culture dish, creating a so-called 'open book' explant (Fig. 8.11). By placing a crystal of the lipophilic dye DiI (see Box 8.2) on the explant, over the cell bodies, the paths followed by commissural axons can easily be visualized. Before they have reached the floor plate, commissural axons can be lured off-course if they are presented with an ectopic source of netrin, demonstrating that they are attracted to netrin (Fig. 8.11). However, as soon as they have crossed to the other side of the floor plate, they no longer respond to an ectopic netrin source.

Box 8.2 Axon pathways can be labelled using fluorescent carbocyanine dyes

One particularly useful tool that has been developed to allow the visualization of axon pathways within an embryo is the use of **lipophilic** fluorescent dyes. A number of such dyes are available, but perhaps the best known and most widely used is **DiI** (pronounced 'dye-eye', short for 1,1'-dioctadecyl-3,3,3',3'-tetramethylindocarbocyanine perchlorate). Due to their lipophilic nature, these dyes readily incorporate into the plasma membrane of a neuron, and can diffuse along the full length of axons. Labelling can be either **anterograde**, in which case dye that is initially taken up by cell bodies diffuses along axons until it reaches the growth cone, or **retrograde**, where dye taken up by axons diffuses back towards the neuronal cell bodies.

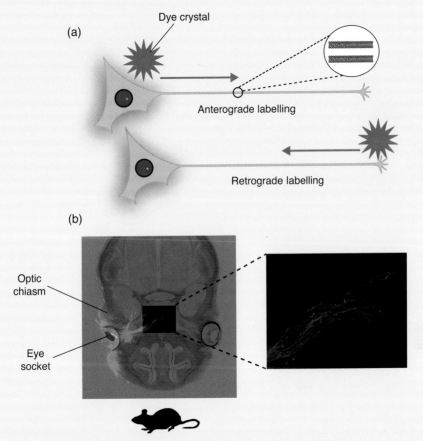

(a) In anterograde labelling a crystal of DiI (shown in red) is placed over the cell bodies of a group of neurons. The dye diffuses along the neuronal plasma membrane, fluorescently labelling the entire axon. Similarly, in retrograde labelling, placing a dye crystal near the end of a set of axons fluorescently labels the cell bodies from which the axons project. (b) Shows a section cut through the head of a mouse embryo in which a DiI crystal was placed in one of the eye sockets and allowed to diffuse. The dye has diffused along the axons projected by the retinal ganglion cells (RGCs) through the optic nerve towards the optic chiasm. The optic nerve is clearly labelled red. The panel on the right shows a high-power magnification of the area in the black box and demonstrates that individual axons can be clearly identified using this method. (Photographs in panel (b) courtesy of Matthew Down, University of Edinburgh, UK.)

lipophilic having affinity for lipids.

This indicates that commissural axons are able to cross the midline as a result of losing sensitivity to the midline attractant netrin. This example neatly illustrates a principle of axon guidance mechanisms – the behaviour of navigating axons often changes at choice points, mediated either by a change in the expression of receptors or alterations in signal transduction pathways.

8.7.2 Putting it all together – guidance cues and their receptors choreograph commissural axon pathfinding at the ventral midline

While the loss of attraction to netrin is an important step in allowing commissural axons to cross the midline, it is insufficient to account for the whole process of midline crossing. Additional factors must be involved. It turns out that many of the proteins involved in controlling midline crossing are highly conserved between *Drosophila* and vertebrates. For example, netrin expressed at the ventral midline in *Drosophila* acts as a chemoattractant for commissural axons. As can be seen in Fig. 8.6, neurons on either side of the *Drosophila* nerve cord project axons that cross over the midline by joining a **commissure** then joining the longitudinal pathway on the opposite side (referred to as the **contralateral** pathway) and heading anteriorly towards the brain. Just like commissural axons in vertebrates, these *Drosophila* commissural neurons project axons from one side of the nervous system to the other and are important for neural coordination between the two sides of the animal. Such axons are a common feature of animals with bilateral symmetry. The similarities in the paths followed by commissural axons in the *Drosophila* ventral nerve cord and those followed by vertebrate commissural axons in the neural tube are shown in Fig. 8.12.

Three of the key molecules that control commissural axon guidance were first identified using forward genetic screens in *Drosophila*

commissure a bundle of axons **(commissural axons)** that extends across the midline to connect structures on either side of the nervous system. Commissures are important for coordinating neural activity on the two sides of the animal.

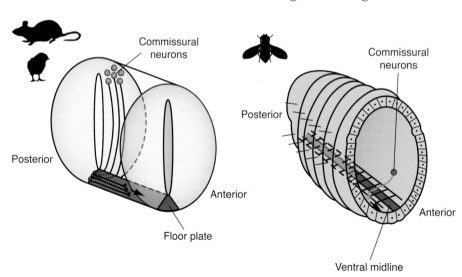

Fig. 8.12 Commissural axons follow similar paths in vertebrate and *Drosophila* embryos. In the vertebrate spinal cord (left panel), commissural axons first project to the floor plate, attracted by netrin. They then cross over to the other side and turn anteriorly, towards the embryo's head. Similarly, in *Drosophila* (right panel), commissural axons cross over the ventral midline before turning anteriorly. In each case, guidance cues expressed at the ventral midline play a crucial role in guiding axons of commissural neurons.

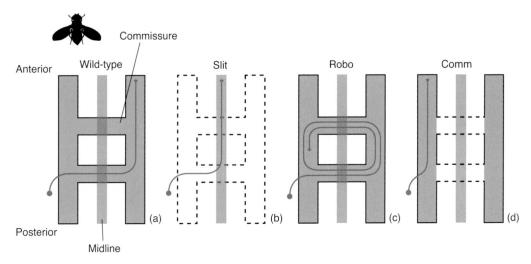

Fig. 8.13 Phenotypes of *Drosophila* mutant embryos that lack key axon guidance molecules at the ventral midline. (a) In wildtype flies, commissural neurons (red) project an axon towards the midline. The axon joins a commissure to cross the midline. On reaching the opposite side of the nerve cord, the axon enters a longitudinal fascicle and heads anteriorly. (b) In *slit* mutant flies, commissural axon tracts collapse onto the ventral midline, giving the ventral nerve cord a slit-like appearance. (c) In *robo* mutants, commissural axons that should cross the midline only once instead cross and recross multiple times, giving rise to the roundabout appearance that gave the gene its name. (d) In *commissureless* (*comm*) mutants, commissural axons fail to cross the midline at all, instead they remain in the longitudinal fascicle on the same side as the cell body.

(see Box 1.1). The genes encoding these molecules were named *slit*, *robo* (*roundabout*) and *comm* (*commissureless*), based on the appearance of the ventral nerve cord in mutant flies. Flies lacking each of these genes exhibit distinct axon guidance defects in the ventral nerve cord (Fig. 8.13).

As described in Section 8.6.2 above, *slit* encodes a secreted protein that is expressed by the midline glia and acts as a chemorepellent signal. An important role for Slit at the ventral midline is to repel commissural axons from the midline once they have crossed it. In *slit* mutant flies, axons are attracted to the midline by netrin as normal but fail to move away from midline on the other side. Rather, they appear to become stuck at the midline, collapsing into a single large bundle, giving rise to the slit-like appearance of the axon bundles that gave the gene its name.

The *robo* genes encode receptors for Slit, so axons in *robo* mutant flies are unable to respond normally to Slit's chemorepellent activity. There are three *robo* genes (*robo1-3*): in *robo1* mutants, commissural axons are less sensitive to Slit-mediated chemorepulsion but they still retain some sensitivity due to expression of the other two genes. In *robo1* mutants, commissural axons that have crossed the midline are not sufficiently repelled by Slit, allowing them to cross and recross the midline multiple times and leading to the distinctive appearance that gave rise to the name *roundabout*.

If commissural axons are repelled by Slit, how are they able to move to the midline in the first place? It turns out that commissural axons are insensitive to Slit's chemorepellent activity before crossing but then become sensitive to it after they have crossed. This is another example of an axon growth cone changing sensitivity to a guidance cue at a

Fig. 8.14 The combined activities of Slit and netrin guide commissural axons at the ventral midline. (a) Commissural axons approach the ventral midline, attracted by the netrin gradient (blue dots) emanating from the midline. At this stage, ROBO protein is not present on the surface of the growth cone, so the axon is insensitive to the repellent activity of Slit (red circles). In *Drosophila*, COMM prevents ROBO reaching the growth cone surface at this stage. In vertebrates, RIG1 prevents growth cones from responding to Slit at this stage. (b) Once the commissural growth cone reaches the ventral midline, ROBO protein is permitted to reach the growth cone surface. This renders the growth cone sensitive to Slit, driving it away from the midline and preventing it from recrossing. At the same time, the growth cone becomes insensitive to netrin's chemoattractive activity. (c) After crossing the midline, Robo remains present in growth cones, rendering them continuously sensitive to the midline repellent activity of Slit. Growth cones remain insensitive to netrin at this stage.

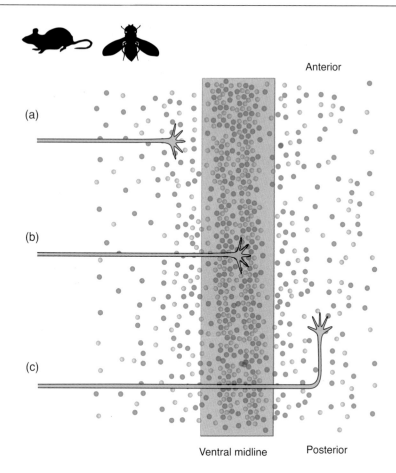

choice point. The key to understanding this change in sensitivity to Slit came from analysis of mutant flies lacking the third gene, *comm*. In *comm* mutant flies, ventral nerve cord commissures are completely absent because axons that lack *comm* activity are unable to cross the midline. COMM protein is found only in commissural axons before they cross the midline. Its expression is down-regulated during crossing such that COMM protein is absent from the post-crossing segments of commissural axons. COMM is thought to act by preventing ROBO protein reaching the surface of the growth cone. Thus, before growing axons reach the midline, COMM prevents ROBO from reaching growth cones. The axons are therefore insensitive to Slit, allowing them to approach the midline in response to netrin. After crossing, COMM expression decreases, allowing ROBO to reach the growth cone surface. Thus, the axon becomes sensitive to Slit and is actively repelled from the midline, allowing it to move to the other side and preventing it from recrossing. In *comm* mutants, ROBO is always present in growth cones, so they are always sensitive to Slit and are therefore unable to cross the midline at all. This mechanism is summarized in Fig. 8.14.

Like their *Drosophila* counterparts, the vertebrate homologues of Slit and ROBO play important roles in controlling the behaviour of commissural axons at the ventral midline of the spinal cord. Just as in *Drosophila*, netrin and Slit are both expressed at the ventral midline in vertebrate embryos. We saw above that vertebrate commissural axons are attracted to the floor plate of the spinal cord by netrin but become insensitive to netrin's chemoattractive activity upon crossing the midline. Vertebrate commissural axons are insensitive to the chemorepellant activity of Slit before reaching the ventral midline but become sensitive to it after crossing, preventing them from recrossing. However, vertebrates do not have a homologue of the *comm* gene and it is important to remember that while there are strong similarities between the mechanisms operating at the ventral midline in vertebrates and *Drosophila*, they are not identical. In vertebrates, the role played by *Drosophila* COMM protein seems to be taken on by a divergent member of the Robo family, known as RIG1. The full details of RIG1's mechanism of action are not yet understood but it appears to render commissural axons insensitive to Slit before crossing the ventral midline and allows them to become sensitive to Slit after crossing.[3]

Before they reach the midline, vertebrate commissural axons express the netrin receptor DCC, which mediates attraction to netrin. As we have already seen, ROBO is inhibited at this stage, and the axons are insensitive to Slit activity. Once they reach the midline, however, down-regulation of RIG1 allows ROBO to reach the growth cone surface. In growth cones that express both ROBO and DCC, binding of Slit to ROBO is thought to block the activity of DCC. This may account for the finding that commissural axons lose their sensitivity to netrin upon reaching the midline. After crossing the midline, DCC expression is down-regulated so axons remain insensitive to netrin.

8.7.3 After crossing the midline, commissural axons project towards the brain

Once commissural axons have safely negotiated the ventral midline, they must turn again and head rostrally, toward the brain. During this stage of their journey in vertebrate embryos, they are guided by a member of the **Wnt** family, WNT4. Wnts are best known for their activity as signalling molecules, in a wide variety of developmental situations. However, they can also act as axon guidance molecules. WNT4 is expressed in a gradient in the ventral neural tube, with high levels at the rostral end and lower levels caudally. The growth cones of commissural axons move up the WNT4 concentration gradient, taking them towards their ultimate targets in the brain (Fig. 8.15).

8.8 How can such a small number of cues guide such a large number of axons?

It seems surprising that the relatively small number of guidance cues identified so far is sufficient to generate the enormous complexity of the wiring of the mammalian brain. One explanation for this apparent paradox is that cues may act in combination, thereby increasing the

---

[3] A more detailed account of our current understanding of the regulation of commissural axon guidance at the ventral midline can by found in Evans, T. A. and Bashaw, G. J. (2010) Axon guidance at the midline: of mice and flies. *Current Opinion in Neurobiology*, **20**, 79–85.

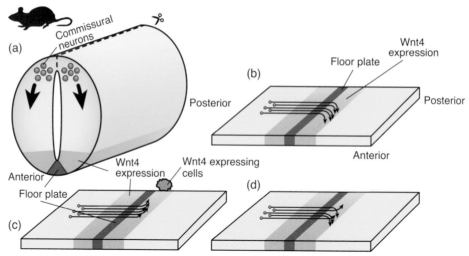

Fig. 8.15 After crossing the midline, vertebrate commissural axons follow an anteroposterior gradient of WNT4, directing them toward the brain. (a) Commissural neurons in the dorsal spinal cord project axons ventrally, toward the floor plate, guided by netrin-1 (red). WNT4 is expressed just dorsal to the floor plate in an anteroposterior gradient, with highest levels found anteriorly (orange). (b) Cutting the spinal cord open along the dorsal surface and laying it flat results in an 'open-book' preparation that can be placed in tissue culture (as shown in Fig. 8.11). The trajectories followed by commissural axons can be visualized by placing a crystal of a lipophilic dye, such as DiI (Box 8.2), over the cell bodies. In these cultures, axons follow the same trajectories as they would in the intact neural tube, crossing the midline then making a 90° turn and heading anteriorly. (c) If a clump of cells expressing high levels of WNT4 is placed against the posterior edge of an open-book culture, commissural axons navigate towards the source of WNT4, in the opposite direction to normal. (d) In an open-book culture of neural tube taken from a mutant mouse that lacks the Wnt receptor, Frizzled-3, commissural axons project randomly along the anteroposterior axis. (Adapted from Lyuksyutova, A. I., Lu, C. C., Milanesio, N., King, L. A., Guo, N., Wang, Y., Nathans, J., Tessier-Lavigne, M. and Zou, Y. (2003) Anterior-posterior guidance of commissural axons by Wnt-frizzled signalling. *Science*, **302**,1984–8.)

possible number of responses to particular cues. For example, we saw above that commissural axons at the ventral midline are guided by a combination of netrin and Slit. The full range of mechanisms employed to maximize the potential information provided by guidance cues remains to be discovered but we do know of at least two more strategies which are outlined below.

8.8.1 The same guidance cues are deployed in multiple axon pathways

We have already seen that Slit–Robo signalling guides commissural axons at the floor plate of the spinal cord. However, mutant mice that lack one or more *Slit* or *Robo* gene also have defects in many other axon pathways. For example, the visual pathway, which carries information from the retina into the brain, is defective in *Slit* and *Robo* mutant mice as a result of many retinal ganglion cell axons misnavigating. Similarly, axon tracts that connect the two halves of the forebrain, such as the **corpus callosum** and the **hippocampal commissure**, do not form normally in these mutants.

There are many other examples of the same guidance cues being deployed to direct navigation of different types of axons. One reason that this is possible is that these cues act only over fairly short distances, perhaps a few millimetres for a diffusible cue, and much less for contact guidance cues. Thus, there is little likelihood that cues produced in

corpus callosum major fibre tract composed of axons connecting the cerebral hemispheres.

hippocampal commissure a large axon bundle that connects the two hippocampi across the midline of the brain.

one part of the developing CNS could interfere with development of pathways in other regions.

8.8.2 Interactions between guidance cues and their receptors can be altered by co-factors

In the last few years, it has become clear that some extracellular molecules can influence the binding of guidance cues to their receptors and alter the way in which a growth cone responds to a particular cue. The best characterized of these are the **heparan sulphate proteoglycans** (**HSPG**s), cell surface proteins that have long, complex carbohydrate side chains (see Box 7.2). HSPGs are found on the surface of all animal cells. Their presence is required for several growth factors (such as FGFs and Hedgehogs) to activate their receptors – a **ternary complex** is formed between the growth factor, its receptor and the HSPG. Similarly, some guidance cues, including the Slits, require HSPGs to activate signalling. Mutant mice that lack HSPGs throughout their CNS lack most commissural axon pathways, showing that HSPGs are needed for these pathways to form. Interestingly, the side chains of HSPGs are very variable, giving them the potential to encode a very large amount of information. It seems that specific HSPG modifications can differentially influence the way that an axon responds to a particular guidance cue. For example, axons appear to respond differently to Slit signalling depending on the specific subtype of HSPG present in their environment.[4]

ternary complex a complex containing three proteins bound together.

8.9 Some axons form specific connections over very short distances, likely using different mechanisms

Throughout this chapter we have focused on mechanisms that guide axons on relatively long journeys. However, it should not be forgotten that some connections form over much shorter distances, for example many interneurons in the cerebral cortex synapse with cells that lie only a few cell diameters away. These cells most likely use quite different types of mechanism to find their targets. To return to our analogy of a tourist navigating an unfamiliar environment, if they were in a shopping mall looking for a specific type of shop, they would be surrounded by potential targets, laid out in a highly accessible pattern. Simply by sampling shops at random, they would very likely find a suitable shop quickly. In the same way, axons of cortical interneurons searching for local targets could send out their axons essentially randomly with a high probability of finding their synaptic partners. Such random axon outgrowth would lead to many inappropriate connections being attempted, so there would have to be additional processes by which appropriate connections were selected and inappropriate attempts withdrawn (see Chapter 10, Section 10.4.5). Such a process might appear inefficient but it does have the advantage that it likely requires the cells to carry less information for their guidance – all they

---

[4] More details on this emerging mechanism can be found in Holt, C. E. and Dickson, B. J. (2005) Sugar codes for axons? *Neuron,* **46**,169–72.

would have to know is what they are looking for. In a rapidly evolving structure such as the cerebral cortex, this might allow connectivity patterns to change more flexibly as more neurons were added during the course of evolution. It has been known for decades that overproduction of axons followed by pruning of inappropriate ones occurs in development but there is still little known about the molecular mechanisms; for further reading on this topic see Innocenti, G. M. and Price, D. J. (2005) Exuberance in the development of cortical networks. *Nature Reviews Neuroscience*, **6**, 955–65.

8.10 The growth cone has autonomy in its ability to respond to guidance cues

8.10.1 Growth cones can still navigate when severed from their cell bodies

As we have seen throughout the book, a cell's response to an intercellular signal is often mediated by the activation of specific patterns of transcription. Obviously, a prerequisite for such a response is that a nucleus must be present. Surprisingly, as first shown in the 1970s and 1980s, axons can continue to grow and navigate correctly even after they have been surgically separated from their cell bodies. This shows that the navigating growth cone does not necessarily need to communicate with a nucleus in order to respond normally to guidance cues.

8.10.2 Local translation in growth cones

Research over the last few years has uncovered an intriguing novel mechanism for guiding axons – the localized translation of mRNAs within navigating growth cones. This allows the growth cones to synthesize new proteins in response to a guidance cue without the need to transmit information to the nucleus. As we saw in the previous chapter (Section 7.6), the ability of growth cones to synthesize proteins counters the historical belief that all of the proteins found in growth cones were made within the cell body and then transported along the axon to the growth cone. Local translation seems to be essential for some types of axon to respond to certain guidance cues, but does not appear to be a universal mechanism.

Evidence for local translation in growth cones first emerged from studies on the developing visual system in *Xenopus* (Fig. 8.16). Retinal ganglion cells (RGCs) can be cultured on glass slides coated with

Fig. 8.16 A retinal axon growing across a glass slide that has been coated with a cell adhesion molecule (a) will change direction to head towards a source of a chemoattractant (green) (b). However, if the axon is exposed to a compound that blocks protein synthesis, it no longer responds to the chemoattractant (c).

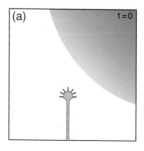
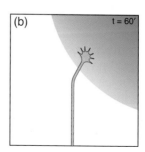
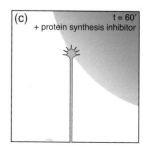

laminin. Cultured RGCs extend axons that will grow towards attractive cues such as netrin-1 or SEMA3A. If RGC axons in such cultures are cut, severing the connection between the navigating axons and their cell bodies, the axons are still able to turn towards the chemoattractant source. As they do so, new proteins are synthesized in the growth cone, as shown by the incorporation of radiolabelled amino acids. When a protein synthesis inhibitor is added to the growing axons, they lose the ability to turn towards the source of the attractive cue, but are still able to grow. Similarly, growth cones of cultured RGC axons collapse in response to application of a chemorepellent cue, but collapse is prevented if a protein synthesis inhibitor is added first, showing that local translation is required for these axons to respond to chemorepellent cues.

mRNAs for a variety of types of protein have been shown to be locally translated in growth cones. It turns out that several of these encode either components of the cytoskeleton (such as actin) or proteins that regulate cytoskeleton dynamics (such as cofilin, see Chapter 7, Section 7.5.3). β-actin mRNA molecules contain a short sequence in their 3′ **untranslated region**, known as a 'zipcode', which instructs the cell to transport them to the growth cone.[5]

> **laminin** a protein component of the extracellular matrix.

> **untranslated region** 3′ or 5′ regions of mature RNA that do not code for proteins.

8.11 Transcription factors regulate axon guidance decisions

For most of this chapter, we have focused on cell surface and extracellular molecules that are needed for axon guidance. However, it should not be forgotten that region-specific expression of **transcription factors** also plays an important role in many axon guidance mechanisms. There are at least two main ways in which transcription factors contribute to axon guidance decisions. First, transcription factors are required for setting up correct expression patterns of axon guidance cues, including cell adhesion molecules. For example, as described in Chapter 4, Section 4.4.3, graded expression of engrailed transcription factors in the developing tectum is believed to set up gradients of ephrin expression, which will subsequently guide the axons of incoming retinal ganglion cells (Chapter 9, Section 9.5.3). Secondly, just as specific combinations of transcription factors specify neuronal identity (Chapter 5, Section 5.4.3), they can both determine the initial pathway that an axon selects and influence the choices it makes at subsequent points, for example by controlling the expression of specific receptor molecules in the axon.

In general, the roles played by transcription factors in axon guidance are less well understood at present than those played by axon guidance cues. However, the role of specific transcription factors in controlling choices made by retinal ganglion cell (RGC) axons at the optic chiasm has been studied in some detail. In rodents, the vast majority of RGC axons cross the midline at the optic chiasm and enter the

> **transcription factors** proteins that bind to DNA to regulate gene transcription.

---

[5] For a more detailed discussion of the significance of local translation for axon guidance, see Lin, A. C. and Holt, C. E. (2008) Function and regulation of local axonal translation. *Curr. Opin. Neurobiol.*, **18**, 60–8.

Fig. 8.17 Axons of retinal ganglion cells (RGCs) pass through the optic nerve to the optic chiasm before moving on to their targets in the brain. In rodents, the vast majority of RGC axons, shown in magenta, cross the midline at the optic chiasm and enter the contralateral optic tract. A small number, whose cell bodies lie in the ventrotemporal crescent (shown in blue), do not cross over at the optic chiasm, rather they enter the ipsilateral optic tract. Axons of RGCs in the ventrotemporal crescent express EphB1 and are repelled by ephrinB expressed at the chiasm (grey). Other RGCs do not express EphB1 and are therefore free to pass through the ephrinB expression domain at the chiasm and enter the contralateral optic tract. EphB1 expression is under the control of the transcription factor ZIC2.

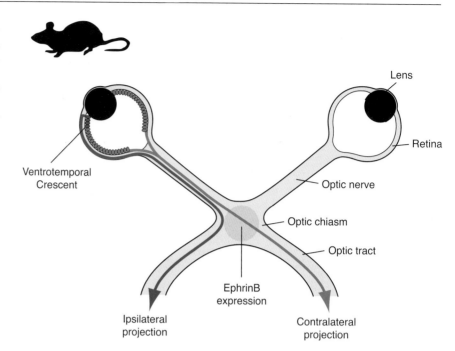

ipsilateral on the same side.

contralateral optic tract. However, a small number of RGCs located in the **ventrotemporal crescent** of the retina project axons that do not cross the midline, instead entering the **ipsilateral** optic tract. These are responsible for the limited degree of binocular vision experienced by rodents. The mechanisms that control whether or not an RGC axon crosses the midline at the optic chiasm are complex, but one key player is ephrinB, which is expressed at high levels at the optic chiasm.

The zinc finger transcription factor ZIC2 is expressed only in RGCs in the ventrotemporal crescent. ZIC2 activates the expression of EphB1; therefore RGCs in this part of the retina contain high levels of EphB1 in their growth cones and consequently are repelled by ephrinB expressed at the chiasm. This causes them to project ipsilaterally rather than cross the midline. Another transcription factor, islet2, is expressed only by retinal ganglion cells that lie outside the ventrotemporal crescent. Islet2 represses the expression of ZIC2, therefore ZIC2 expression is absent in RGCs outside the ventrotemporal crescent. Consequently, EphB1 expression is not activated in these cells so their growth cones are insensitive to the ephrinB expressed at the chiasm and they can therefore cross to the contralateral side (Fig. 8.17).[6]

In this chapter, we have encountered a wide variety of molecular mechanisms that permit the basic wiring pattern of the CNS to be laid down during embryogenesis. Once this basic pattern is established, the detailed circuit that allows the nervous system to function can begin to be established. In Chapter 9, we shall discuss the mechanisms that govern this next phase of nervous system development.

---

[6] More details on the mechansims that guide axons at the optic chiasm can be found in Petros, T. J., Rebsam, A. and Mason, C. A. (2008) Retinal axon growth at the optic chiasm: to cross or not to cross. *Annual Rev. Neurosci.*, **31**, 295–315.

8.12 Summary

- Navigating axons are tipped with growth cones that can detect the presence of specific guidance cues in the environment.
- Guidance cues may either attract or repel growing axons. Some guidance cues act locally, others act at a distance.
- Although the routes followed by navigating axons can be long and tortuous, they are often broken up into smaller stages. Axons often change their sensitivity to specific cues at intermediate targets or choice points on the journey.
- The same axon guidance molecules are deployed in multiple axon guidance pathways.
- Many axon guidance molecules and their receptors are evolutionarily conserved and genetic approaches in *Drosophila* have been instrumental in working out molecular mechanisms.
- A comparatively small number of axon guidance cues are able to direct very complex wiring patterns.

Map Formation

9

9.1 What are maps?

A **map** can be defined as a spatially ordered representation of a given area or physical feature of an object. In the nervous system, features of the external world are represented in a highly structured manner. Perhaps the most recognizable examples of maps in the human brain are the homunculi in the cerebral cortex (Fig. 9.1). A **homunculus** is simply defined as any representation of the human body. The **somatosensory homunculus** is the representation or map of the sensory input from various body parts on the **somatosensory cortex**. It was first described in the 1930s by Wilder Penfield, a neurosurgeon working in Canada. While conducting surgery on patients who were awake to treat epilepsy and brain tumours, Penfield stimulated the sensory cortex and asked the patient to report the location of the sensations. He conducted similar experiments to define the **motor homunculus** in an adjacent region of the cortex (called the motor cortex) by asking patients to report on muscle twitches/movements. By systematically moving the stimulating electrodes, Penfield drew the first maps of the body as they were represented in the brain and in the process became known as the first brain cartographer.[1]

somatosensory cortex cortical region(s) that processes touch, proprioception, temperature and pain.

9.2 Types of maps

In their simplest form, brain maps are very similar to geographical maps, that is two-dimensional pictorial representations of a given geographic area. For example, Penfield's homunculus is a two-dimensional picture of the body plan in the cerebral cortex of humans. However, before continuing we need to broaden the discussion and identify the various types of maps located throughout the nervous system that reflect more than just the spatial layout of features in the body's external environment.

There are two broad subdivisions of maps: those that represent the arrangement of brain areas that can be defined by their

---

[1] For a further reading on Wilder Penfield see http://scienceblogs.com/neurophilosophy/2008/08/wilder_penfield_neural_cartographer.php [20 November 2010].

Building Brains: An Introduction to Neural Development, First Edition.
David Price, Andrew Jarman, John Mason and Peter Kind.
© 2011 John Wiley & Sons, Ltd. Published 2011 by John Wiley & Sons, Ltd.

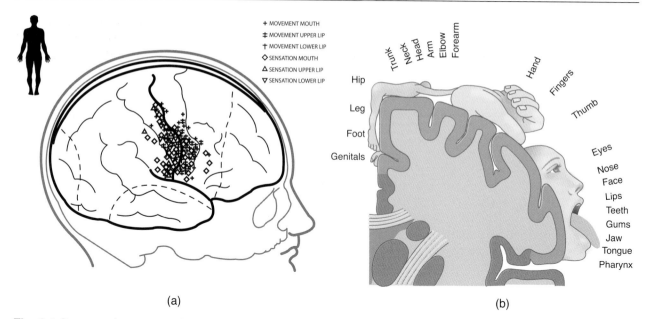

(a)

(b)

Fig. 9.1 Somatotopic representation or homunculus in the primary somatosensory cortex. (a) A drawing of the human brain from one of Penfield's experiments showing the stimulation sites from which Penfield subsequently drew a map of human movement and sensation on the cortex. Reproduced from Penfield, W. and Boldrey, E. Somatic motor and sensory representation in the cerebral cortex of man as studied by electrical stimulation. *Brain*, **37**, 389–433 by permission of Oxford University Press. (b) A schematic diagram of a representative **coronal** section through the brain of a man showing the somatosensory cortex with the location of each body part superimposed on the cortical surface. Two important features to note are: (1) adjacent regions of the body are generally represented in adjacent parts of the cortex, and (2) not all regions of the body are represented equally. Instead body parts with more sensory receptors (e.g. the finger tips, tongue and lips) have a disproportionately larger representation in the cortex than body parts with fewer sensory receptors (e.g. the chest, back and legs). This is referred to as the *magnification factor* of maps.

cytoarchitecture the appearance of a structure in the nervous system that results from the shape or distribution of its cells or clustering of cells.

topographic map two-dimensional representation of the spatial position of stimuli on a sensory surface.

cytoarchitectural differences, which we will term **coarse maps**, and those that functionally subdivide a brain area and process the spatial location or other feature of a stimulus, which we will call **fine maps**. Fine maps can be further subdivided into **topographic** and **feature** maps. Because the sensory homunculus is a map of the spatial relationship between the sensory receptors in the skin, it is an example of a topographic map. As we shall see, map formation is critically linked with precise connectivity between brain structures and is a common feature of sensory and motor systems in most animals, from invertebrates to primates. It is beyond the scope of this chapter to provide a detailed description of map formation in all systems or species so we have chosen specific examples to illustrate key points about the mechanisms by which maps form.[2]

9.2.1 Coarse maps

In all brains from invertebrates to primates, different regions are highly specialized for different functions. Previously we learned that the major

---

[2] For more detail see Price, D. J. and Willshaw, D. J. (2000) *Mechanisms of Cortical Development*, Oxford University Press; Hubermann, A. D. Feller, M. B. and Chapman, B. (2008) Mechanisms underlying development of visual maps and receptive fields. *Annual Review of Neurosciences*, **31**, 479–509.)

brain regions are patterned in the **neuroectoderm** (e.g. forebrain, midbrain, hindbrain). At later stages these brain regions become further specialized into distinct nuclei (in this context, a nucleus means a collection of cells) or areas with particular functions. This can be seen as an extension and refinement of the patterning processes described in Chapter 4.

For example, the **neocortex** of humans can be subdivided into more than 50 distinct areas based on their appearance or cytoarchitecture as well as by their connections with other brain regions and by their function. The map of human cerebral cortical areas is known as **Brodmann's map** (Fig. 9.2) after a German neuroscientist, Korbinian Brodmann, who first used cytoarchitectural landmarks to describe them in 1901. Rodents have fewer cortical areas but the mechanisms

neuroectoderm the neurogenic region of the ectoderm that develops into the nervous system.

neocortex the part of the cerebral cortex that has expanded massively in the evolution of higher mammals.

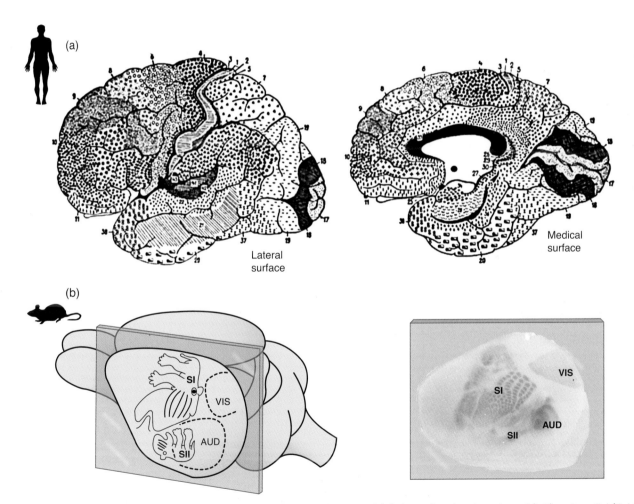

Fig. 9.2 Example of coarse maps in the cortex of the human and mouse. (a) Schematics showing a lateral (left) and medial (right) view of a human brain with Brodmann areas superimposed. (Taken from Ranson, S. W. (1920) *Anatomy of the Nervous System*, W. B. Saunders.) (b) Schematic of the mouse brain showing the visual (VIS), auditory (AUD) and somatosensory (SI and SII) cortical areas indicated. The grey translucent panel represents the tangential plane of section with an image of a brain slice through layer 4 depicted.

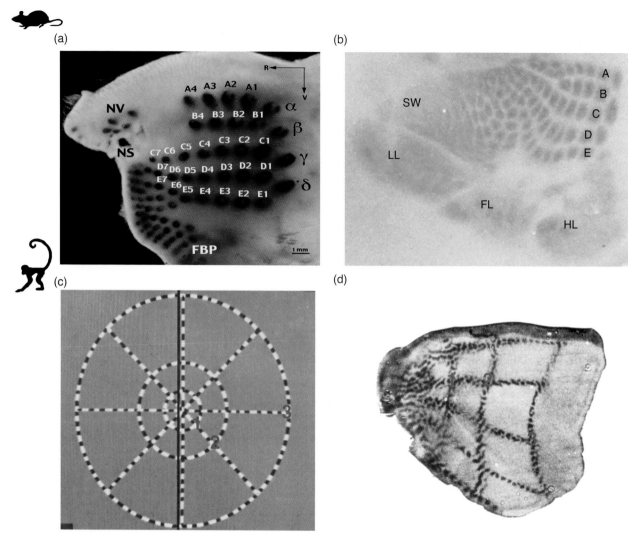

Fig. 9.3 Topographic maps in the mammalian neocortex. (a) The whisker organs (follicles) on the facepad are organized into five rows (A–E) with a group of smaller follicles on the anterior region of the snout (From Haidarliu, S., Simony, E., Golomb, D. and Ahissar, E. (2010) Muscle architecture in the mystacial pad of the rat. *The Anatomical Record*, **293**, 1192–1206, with permission from John Wiley and Sons Inc.; NV = Nasal Vibrissae, NS = Nostril, FBP = Furry Buccal Pad, α – δ = Straddlers, A–D rows of mystacial vibrissae) (b) Picture of a brain slice showing that this pattern of whisker follicles is recapitulated in the layer 4 of the somatosensory cortex of the mouse (a somatotopic map). Each of the whisker-related patches in neocortex is referred to as a 'barrel'. The representation of other body regions is also visible (SW = small whiskers; LL = lower lip; FL = forelimb; HL = hindlimb) (c–d) Visuotopic map in the visual cortex of a monkey. In this experiment the visual stimulus (a wagon wheel) was shown to the monkey. The cells that became electrically active as a result of being shown the wagon wheel (c) were revealed using a method that labels cells showing high levels of activity (d). The pattern of active cells in the cortex closely mirrored the outline of the wheel indicating that adjacent points in visual space project to adjacent points in the cortex. This precise connectivity underlies the construction of the visuotopic map in a similar manner to the somatotopic map shown in (b). Reproduced from Tootell, R. B., Switkes, E., Silverman, M. S. and Hamilton, S. L. (1988) Functional anatomy of macaque striate cortex. II. Retinotopic organization. *J. Neurosci.*, **8**, 1531–1568, with permission from the Society for Neuroscience.

by which they form are likely to be highly conserved. The map of cortical areas is an example of a coarse map. As detailed below, coarse maps
form early on in development.

9.2.2 Fine maps

There are two main types of fine maps: **topographic** and **feature
maps.** Each can be seen in sensory and motor systems throughout
the animal kingdom. Topographic maps often represent the spatial
position of stimuli on a **sensory surface**. They can be formally defined as a neural representation in which the spatial position of the
activity patterns from a sensory surface (or motor representation) is
maintained in a structure in the central nervous system. Examples
of topographic maps from the visual and whisker systems are
shown in Fig. 9.3. Inputs carrying information from adjacent sensory receptors (e.g. **retinal ganglion cells** in the eye, or **whisker
follicles** on the facepad) maintain their spatial relationship in
the brain.

Feature maps are neural representations of a particular physical
feature of a stimulus (e.g. an object's colour, texture, etc.). In general they arise as a result of higher-order connectivity between
brain structures, rather than just spatial position on a sensory surface (but see Box 9.1). Like topographic maps, there are numerous
examples of feature maps in all sensory systems. Examples of feature maps and how they develop will be explained in detail later in
Section 9.7.

> **sensory surface** the region of a
> sense organ that contains the sensory
> receptors, for example the retina in the
> eye.

Box 9.1   The tonotopic map: feature or topographic?

In the auditory system, cells that respond to similar frequencies are found in the same region of auditory
cortex and form a map of sound frequency. In Section 9.2.2 we defined a feature map as a neural representation of a particular physical feature of a stimulus. Since frequency is a particular feature of an auditory stimulus, these frequency maps would appear, at first glance, to be an example of a feature map.
However, in the inner ear unbold and make black sound frequencies are separated along a long thin
structure called the basilar membrane. Different sound frequencies cause the basilar membrane to vibrate
at different locations, such that high frequencies cause vibration at the narrow, stiff basal end and low
frequencies cause vibrations at the more pliable, thick apical end. Hence the frequency of a given auditory stimulus is encoded topographically on the auditory sensory organ and is referred to as the tonotopic
map. The generation of a tonotopic map in the cortex, therefore, arises from the point-to-point projection
of axons between brain structures (i.e. it is topographic) rather than by a more complex, higher-order
connectivity that is typical of feature maps.

This apparent discrepancy highlights the difference between thinking about maps as a representation of a
given area or physical feature of an object (or region) and understanding mapping, which is the connectivity
between two brain structures. As a map, the frequency maps are feature maps, but in terms of the mechanisms
by which maps form (i.e. 'the mapping problem', Section 9.3) the tonotopic map is a topographic map.

9.3 Principles of map formation

Maps result from the ordered connectivity between distinct brain regions. How this ordered connectivity arises is often referred to as 'the **mapping problem**' and it has occupied developmental neurobiologists for some time. In the previous chapter we examined the mechanisms by which axons navigate over distances – in some cases relatively long distances – to reach their target structure. In this chapter we examine the mechanisms by which axons establish precise connectivity *within* target structures and how this connectivity creates maps. We will see that both the **electrical activity** of neurons and molecular cues regulate map formation. We will also see that **computational modelling** (see Chapter 1) is used to help understand the mechanisms of map formation.

For an example of orderly connectivity that generates maps in brain structures we return to the mouse whisker system where spatial patterning of whiskers is relayed through nuclei in the **brainstem** and **thalamus** before reaching the cerebral cortex. At all levels of the pathway, the spatial relationship of the connectivity from each whisker follicle is maintained (Fig. 9.4). Hence the question of how brain maps develop is synonymous with the question of how ordering in neural connectivity arises.

9.3.1 Axon order during development

Because the formation of maps is intricately linked to the connectivity between brain areas, clues to the mechanisms that regulate map formation in a particular system can often come from examining the axon order as they innervate their target structure. These axons could innervate the target in an ordered fashion, showing **directed growth** to their target with relatively few errors. However, as was mentioned at the end of Chapter 8, in many systems axons send out **exuberant** branches that cover wide areas and subsequently refine their

electrical activity the ability of a cell to regulate electrical current at its cell membrane.

brainstem posterior region of the brain between the diencephalon and the spinal cord. Contains the pons, medulla and midbrain.

thalamus a structure in the centre of the vertebrate brain that transmits sensory input to the cerebral cortex, and receives reciprocal output from the cortex.

Fig. 9.4 Cartoon showing how the whisker-related patterns are recapitulated at all levels of the somatosensory pathway. Pseudounipolar neurons in the trigeminal ganlglia (TG, blue oval) extend an axon (red) that carries information from the whisker follicles to the brainstem (BS). Neurons in the brainstem then send axons (grey dashed arrow) to the thalamus (Th, grey dashed oval). Finally these thalamic neurons pass the information on to the somatosensory cortex (S1). At each stage of the pathway, whisker-related patterns are visible. These patterns were first described by Woolsey and van der Loos in the cortex in the 1970s. Henrik van der Loos coined the term 'barrels' for the cortical pattern based on the similarity in shape between the cortical structures and a beer barrel in an etching and carving by Pieter Bruegel (called *A Fair on St. Georges Day, c.*1559–1560). Whisker patterns were subsequently identified in the brainstem and thalamus and were called 'barrelettes' and 'barreloids', respectively.

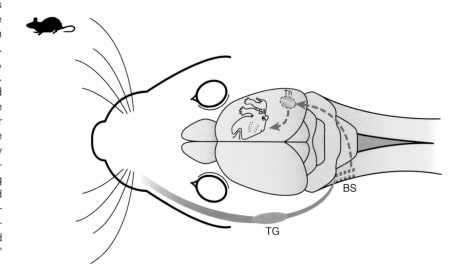

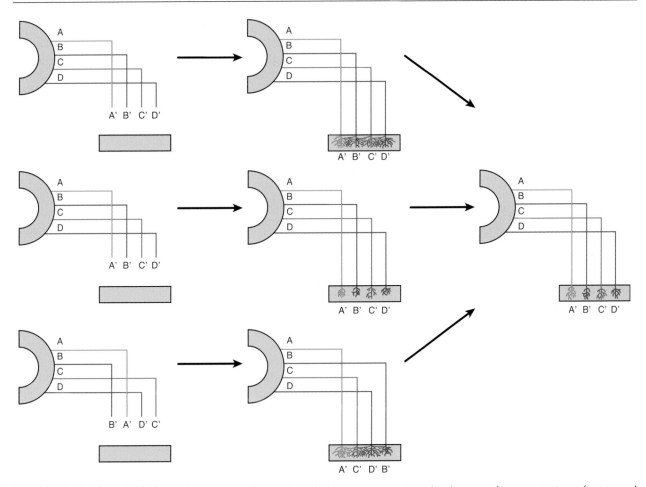

Fig. 9.5 Mechanisms by which ordered connectivity arises during nervous system development. In some systems (upper and middle rows) axons arising from a given tissue maintain their relative spatial order as they innervate their target tissue. For some pathways, axons innervate and elaborate in specific regions of the target tissue with little exuberance, showing directed growth and selective branch elaboration (middle row). Alternatively they may elaborate branches more widely, in some cases over long distances, before retracting inappropriate terminals with branches becoming restricted to correct areas (upper row). Finally, in some cases axons show no signs of relative order before innervating their target and only become refined once they innervate their target tissue (bottom row).

projections to the correct areas (Fig. 9.5). In the case of an exuberant projection, some form of matching of pre- and post-synaptic elements must occur that allows refinement of connectivity into precise maps.

9.3.2 Theories of map formation

In most of this book, discussion of mechanisms of brain development focuses on empirical data from biological systems. For map formation, much of our current thinking is driven not only by experimental evidence but also by another form of analysis, namely computational modelling. The rise of computational modelling owes much to the similarity of the mapping problem in both biology and mathematics. In mathematics, mapping involves associating elements of one set with those of a second set. Therefore, how the precise connectivity between sets of neurons develops readily lends itself to mathematical analysis.

A detailed discussion of the mathematical models devised to gain insight into how biological maps form is beyond the scope of this book (and uses really complicated equations whose inclusion would likely decrease our sales and that we don't understand anyway). However, we have grouped them into two main categories based on the relative role of the projecting axons and the target cells. The second category is further subdivided based on whether the precision of mapping arises as a result of activity or molecular cues.[3]

(1) One set of models hypothesize that the incoming axons have inherent information that specifies their orderly mapping within the target tissue. The target tissue itself is a blank slate, in which the final identity of target cells is induced by information from the incoming axons. Historically, these have been referred to as **induction models**. Induction models often postulate a precise order of axons as they innervate their target structure (i.e. directed ingrowth) but some induction models can form precise maps from a crude ordering of incoming axons.

(2) Another set of models hypothesize that the final connectivity is a product of information initially present in both the incoming axons and target cells. In these models, axons could be either ordered or not but they are instructed, in part, by the target structures to form an ordered connectivity.

> **(a) Cytodifferentiation models** postulate the existence of molecular cues on incoming axons that match them with corresponding cues on target cells.
>
> **(b) Neighbour matching models** postulate that incoming axons contain signals that are more similar between adjacent cells than between distant ones. Neighbouring target cells have the inherent ability to distinguish these signals and selectively establish contact with incoming axons carrying similar signals. Although most neighbour matching models are activity-based, the signals could be in the form of diffusible molecules.

9.4 Development of coarse maps: cortical areas

9.4.1 Protomap vs. protocortex

In the 1980s and 1990s the differentiation of cortical areas (Fig. 9.2) was a very hotly debated topic. The arguments originated from two main hypotheses of cortical area formation that have dominated the literature. The **protomap** hypothesis postulates that the early cortex has an inherent template of the later developing cortical areas that is matched to incoming axons during development (consistent with the cytodifferentiation and neighbour matching models). In contrast,

---

[3] For detailed descriptions see Principles of Computational Modelling in Neuroscience. Sterratt D., Graham B., Gillies A. and Willshaw D. Cambridge University Press. Cambridge, UK (2011) and Mechanisms of Cortical Development. Price D. J. and Willshaw D. J. Oxford University press, Oxford, UK (2002).

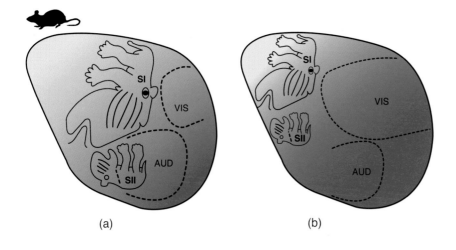

Fig. 9.6 EMX2 regulates areal mapping in the neocortex. (a) The *Emx2* gene is expressed in a high-caudal to low-rostral gradient during cortical development (as shown by the green shading). (b) In mice that overexpress EMX2 protein, the cortical area map is shifted rostrally indicating a role for this transcription factor in patterning of the neocortex. Abbreviations as in Fig. 9.2.

the **protocortex** model hypothesizes that the cortex is a 'tabula rasa' or blank slate and that the identity of individual cortical areas is specified by incoming afferent axons from the thalamus. The protocortex hypothesis, therefore, is an example of the induction model discussed above. Over the last two decades there has been evidence in support of both hypotheses. For example, it is clear that distinct areas of cortex are molecularly pre-specified in the **ventricular zone** of developing cortex suggesting the presence of a protomap prior to axon innervation. However, while certain areas may be pre-specified, it is clear from transplantation studies and studies where sensory axons are rerouted to inappropriate targets, that cortical

ventricular zone the inner side of the neural tube closest to its lumen in the developing vertebrate brain. This transient layer contains neuronal progenitor cells.

Box 9.2   Role of fibroblast growth factor 8 (FGF8) in cortical patterning

Decreasing FGF8 levels in the rostral pole causes an increase in the extent of caudal areas and a decrease in rostral areas. Overproduction of FGF8 in the anterior pole of the cortex has the opposite effect. Finally, creating an ectopic source of FGF8 in caudal cortex creates a double gradient resulting in a partial duplication of the cortical map. These data strongly suggest that FGF8 levels regulate arealization of the neocortex.

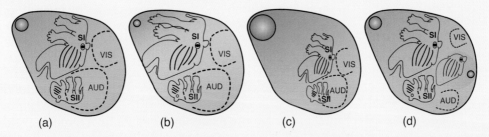

(a)–(d)) Schematics showing the location of primary sensory areas in flattened sections through layer 4 of whole cerebral hemispheres. (a) In a normal animal, FGF8 is generated by cells at the rostral pole (blue circle), and the primary somatosensory cortex (SI, orange ovoid) is located in the middle of the neocortical sheet. (b) When FGF8 signalling is reduced, SI moves more rostrally. (c) When FGF8 is overexpressed rostrally, SI moves more caudally. (d)When an ectopic FGF source is produced in the posterior cortex, SI is partially duplicated. Abbreviations as in Fig. 9.2.

areas can be reprogrammed to process information coming from ectopic sources.[4]

9.4.2 Spatial position of cortical areas

At a molecular level, very little is known about how cortical areas differentiate or what creates the boundaries between them. More is known about the mechanisms that regulate the relative position of cortical areas within the cortical sheet. In previous chapters we have seen how gradients of molecules can regulate numerous aspects of brain development including nervous system patterning (Chapter 4) and axon guidance (Chapter 8). In a similar way, molecular gradients regulate the patterning of arealization in the cerebral cortex.

A key **transcription factor** involved is EMX2 (see Chapter 4, Section 4.3.3). In mice, EMX2 is present in a gradient with high levels of expression in cells located at the **caudal** regions of the cortex and low expression in cells at the **rostral** regions. Ablation of the *Emx2* gene results in the expansion of rostral areas of the cortex and contraction of caudal areas. In contrast when EMX2 is experimentally overexpressed, the caudal areas expand and the rostral areas contract (Fig. 9.6). How transcription factors like EMX2 regulate the position of cortical areas is unclear, but the induction of EMX2 expression is likely to be regulated by diffusible factors such as **fibroblast growth factor** 8 (FGF8), which is expressed in a rostral to caudal gradient and appears to regulate area position within the cortex (Box 9.2).

9.5 Development of fine maps: topographic

The most studied examples of topographic maps in the nervous system are found in sensory systems and can be demonstrated using both physiological and anatomical techniques. Physiologically, the stimulation of adjacent receptors in a sensory array (such as the retina or the skin) leads to the stimulation of adjacent neurons in the brain. In terms of development, the best studied models of topographic map formation are the visual system (Fig. 9.11) and the whisker system of mice (Fig. 9.4).

9.5.1 Retinotectal pathways

In birds and amphibians the primary target of **retinal ganglion cell** (RGC) axons is the **tectum** (see Chapter 2, Fig. 2.4). Neighbouring RGCs project to neighbouring cells in the tectum, so the position of an RGC cell body in the retina is closely correlated with the position of its target cell in the tectum, that is the tectal cells form a map of RGC position. Axons of RGCs located in the **temporal** part of the retina project to the anterior (or rostral) part of the tectum and axons from **nasal** retina project to the posterior (or caudal) tectum (Fig. 9.7). Similarly in the perpendicular axis, axons of RGCs in the **ventral** retina project to the **medial** tectum and **dorsal** RGCs project to **lateral** tectum.

transcription factor proteins that bind to DNA to regulate gene transcription.

fibroblast growth factors (FGFs) a family of growth factors involved in embryonic development as well as other processes such as wound healing.

tectum in non-mammalian vertebrates, a region of the midbrain that receives innervation from retinal ganglion cells. Known as the superior colliculus in mammals.

temporal referring to the position close to the temple (beneath which sits the temporal bone) in a bilaterally symmetric animal (contrast with nasal).

nasal referring to a position close to the nose in a bilaterally symmetric animal (contrast with temporal).

[4] For more information on the evidence for the protomap and protocortex models of cortical arealization see Rakic, P. *et al.* (2009) Decision by division: making cortical maps. *TINS*, **32**, 291; Rakic, P. (1988) Specification of cerebral cortical areas. *Science*, **241**, 170–176; O'Leary, D. D. (1989) Do cortical areas emerge from a protocortex? *TINS*, **12**, 400–406.

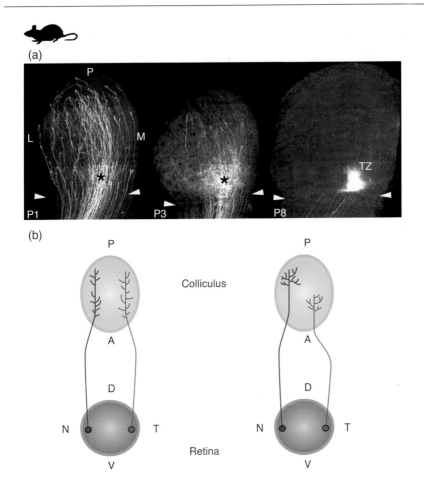

Fig. 9.7 The development of retinotectal projections. (a) Retinal projections from the mouse temporal retina initially invade the entire **superior colliculus** on postnatal day (P) 1. Over the first postnatal week, however, these axons become restricted to the anterior portion of the colliculus (P3 and P8 shown in (a)). (b) Schematic diagram showing that retinal axons are initially exuberant but subsequently refine their termination patterns: axons originating from cells in the nasal (N) retina terminate in the posterior (P) colliculus, while those originating in cells of the temporal (T) retina terminate in the anterior (A) colliculus. (Abbreviations: D = dorsal, V = ventral, M = medial and L = lateral.) Arrowheads indicate the anterior boundary of the colliculus. Asterisks mark the location of the future termination zone. Reprinted from *Neuron*, **35**, Hindges, R., McLaughlin, T., Genoud, N., Henkemeyer, M. and O'Leary, D. EphB forward signaling controls directional branch extension and arborization required for dorsal-ventral retinotopic mapping, 475–87, 2002, with permission from Elsevier.

The precise mapping of retinal position onto the tectum results from an initial exuberant projection and subsequent pruning. Small injections of dyes into the retina early in development result in labelling throughout the tectum. Examination of individual retinotectal axons also shows a clear branching of axons throughout the tectum with neurons in the temporal and nasal retina eventually restricting their axons to the anterior half and posterior portions of the tectum, respectively.

superior colliculus a region of the dorsal midbrain that receives visual input. Generally known as the visual tectum in non-mammalian vertebrates.

9.5.2 Sperry and the chemoaffinity hypothesis

Some classic experiments on map formation were conducted in the 1940s by Roger Sperry and co-workers (Sperry won the Nobel Prize in 1981 for his studies of split brain patients). Using **optic nerve** regeneration in adult amphibians to investigate the development of the **retinotopic map** in the tectum, eyes were removed and rotated by 180° before being replaced. Remarkably, despite this dramatic surgical manipulation, RGCs in the operated eye were able to reform functional connections. These experiments tested the hypothesis that the maps arise as a result of molecular cues. They found that, despite their new orientation, RGCs formed connections with their normal target cells

optic nerve the bundle of axons connecting an eye to the brain.

retinotopic map the map of retinal ganglion cell position in a target brain structure.

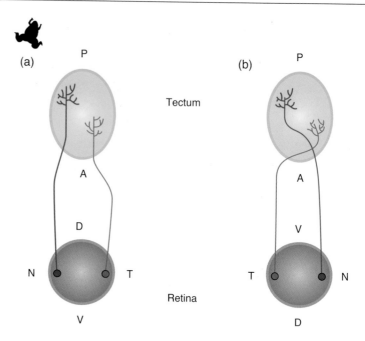

Fig. 9.8 The chemoaffinity hypothesis. (a) Schematic showing the normal pattern of retinal innervation of the tectum. (b) Sperry surgically rotated one eye by 180° and found that the axons still reached their appropriate target region of the tectum, indicating the presence of molecular markers in the tectum acting as postcodes that instruct the targeting of retinal ganglion cell axons. Abbreviations as in Fig. 9.7.

olfactory bulb the brain region that receives input from olfactory neurons.

and as a consequence the animals behaved as if they were seeing the world upside down. When presented with a fly above the rotated eye the animals would consistently strike downwards, indicating that they visualized the fly below rather than above their eye (Fig. 9.8). This indicated that the connections were pre-specified molecularly and could not be adjusted to take into account the changed eye orientation.

The existence of molecular postcodes (or ZIP codes for readers in North America) by which axons find their appropriate targets led Sperry to propose his **chemoaffinity hypothesis**, postulating the existence of 'chemoaffinity labels' on axons and target cells. Sperry reasoned that, given the enormous numbers of cells involved, it is highly improbable that each cell could have a different molecule acting as a chemoaffinity label (although such labels do appear to regulate target selection in the **olfactory bulb**, Box 9.3). Instead, if a molecule were expressed in a gradient, the amount expressed by each cell would vary as a function of the cell's position within the tissue. Sperry hypothesized the existence of perpendicular gradients of signalling molecules that 'stamp each cell with its appropriate latitude and longitude' and complementary gradients of receptors on the axons that interpret this information. In terms of the mathematical models mentioned earlier in this chapter (Section 9.3.2), these findings are consistent with either the cytodifferentiation or neighbour matching models.

9.5.3 Ephrins act as molecular postcodes in the chick tectum

Proteins that are expressed in gradients across the retina and tectum were identified in experiments aimed at isolating the cell surface molecules that could guide retinal ganglion cell (RGC) axons in culture. Using a **stripe assay** (Fig. 9.9), RGCs from the temporal retina were

Box 9.3   Molecular specificity in the formation of olfactory maps

Molecular gradients are not a universal mechanism for the establishment of topographic maps. A quite different mechanism is employed in the olfactory system of a range of species including *Drosophila*, zebrafish, mouse and man. In 1991, Linda Buck and Richard Axel published a landmark study[5] for which they were subsequently awarded a Nobel Prize in Physiology or Medicine in 2004.[6] They showed that there are approximately 1000 genes that encode different **olfactory receptors proteins (ORs)** expressed by **olfactory sensory neurons (OSNs)** in the nasal epithelium, which can be thought of as the olfactory equivalent of the retina. Any one OSN expresses a single OR type and each OR is activated by a single or small number of related odorants in the environment. Each OSN connects to a particular subset of neuronal targets in the olfactory bulb, called **glomeruli**.

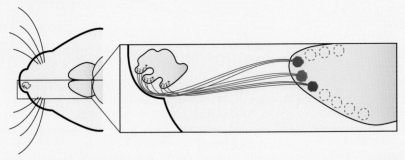

Mapping in the olfactory system. Schematic showing the connection between the olfactory epithelium in the nose of the mouse and the olfactory bulbs in the anterior region of the brain. Different olfactory receptors (coloured in purple, green and blue) are scattered throughout the olfactory epithelium and project to appropriate glomeruli (circles in the olfactory bulb).

As a general rule, each glomerulus receives input from a cohort of OSNs that all express the same OR (although some glomeruli receive input from two cohorts). The complexity of the mapping problem between OSNs in the nasal epithelium and the glomeruli in the olfactory bulb arises when you consider that different OSNs expressing the same OR are distributed throughout the olfactory epithelium, in some species in an apparently random manner. It is now clear that the ORs are not only located in the sensory processes of the OSNs: they are also expressed in axons and growth cones where they play a role in glomerular targeting during map formation. Genetic alteration of individual ORs alters the patterning of the olfactory map. The details of the cellular mechanisms that underlie olfactory map formation remain to be defined completely, but to date it is the only system in which individual axons each express specific molecules that determine their target specificity. Given the heavy genetic cost of such a 1-gene–1-axon system (olfactory receptor genes occupy 3–5% of the mammalian genome) it is unlikely that other such examples exist.

confronted with a choice of cell membranes isolated from either anterior or posterior tectum to grow on. Temporal RGC axons showed a strong preference for anterior over posterior tectal membranes. This repellent activity of the posterior tectum was found to be due to members of a family of surface proteins named **ephrins** (see Chapter 4, Section 4.4.1 and Chapter 8, Section 8.5.3). EphrinA2 and ephrinA5 are both expressed in gradients in the tectum, with low levels in anterior tectum and highest levels posteriorly. The receptors for EphrinAs,

[5] Buck, L. and Axel, R. (1991) A novel multigene family may encode odorant receptors: a molecular basis for odor recognition. *Cell*, **65**, 175–87.
[6] http://nobelprize.org/nobel_prizes/medicine/laureates/2004/ [20 November 2010].

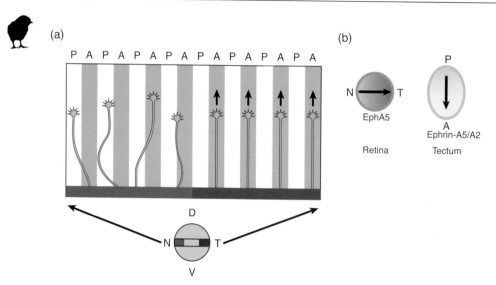

Fig. 9.9 The stripe assay demonstrates the preference of temporal RGC axons for anterior tectum. (a) Membranes were prepared from cells isolated from either the anterior (green stripes) or posterior (white stripes) regions of the optic tectum and applied to glass slides in a pattern of stripes. When confronted with these stripes, RGC axons from temporal retina (blue) showed a strong preference for stripes coated with anterior tectal membranes, while nasal (red) RGC axons showed no preference. (b) Selective outgrowth of temporal retina on anterior tectum is mediated by Eph–ephrin interactions: complementary gradients of Eph expression in the retina (left) and ephrin expression in the tectum (right). Ephrin activity in the posterior tectum repels EphA5-expressing axons preventing stabilization in posterior tectum of axons arising from temporal retina.

growth cones a specialized structure found at the leading edge of migrating axons that detects and responds to guidance cues in the environment.

called EphAs, are expressed in a complementary gradient in the retina: low-nasal, high-temporal. Thus, RGCs in the temporal part of the retina express high levels of EphA on their **growth cones** and are therefore highly sensitive to ephrinA-mediated repulsion. As a result they are repelled by the posterior tectum and establish contacts with the anterior tectum, where ephrinA levels are lowest. Conversely, RGCs in the nasal retina express low levels of EphA, giving their growth cones a low sensitivity to ephrin-mediated repulsion and allowing them to penetrate further into the tectum such that they end up in its posterior domain.

While Eph–ephrin signalling is critically required to set up the pattern of retinotectal mapping, it is not as simple as having a hard-wired molecular postcode; instead there is flexibility built into the system. A series of experiments in goldfish in which parts of the retina or tectum were removed showed that retinotectal maps could expand or retract by removing a portion of the retinal input or tectal tissue, respectively. For example, if the posterior tectum (the natural target for axons coming from the nasal retina) is surgically removed, the retinal projections re-map such that the entire retinal projection maps to the anterior tectum. Similar re-mapping occurs if part of the retina is ablated with the remaining retinal axons expanding their termination zones to fill the tectum while maintaining the retinotopic map (Fig. 9.10).

The plasticity in mapping could be explained by several mechanisms. For example, relative levels, rather than absolute levels, of Eph–ephrins may be crucial for retinotopic mapping. Such a

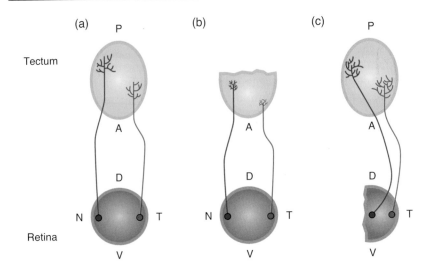

Fig. 9.10 Plasticity of mapping in the retinotectal system. (a) Pattern of retinotectal axon termination in a normal animal. (b) Removal of the posterior tectum results in a remapping of the retinal axons such that the entire retina is represented in the remaining portion of the tectum. (c) Removal of the nasal retina results in the remapping of the temporal retina onto the entire tectum. Abbreviations as in Fig. 9.7.

mechanism could explain the remapping as the gradient of Eph-ephrin expression would still be present on the remaining tectum or axons following ablation. Alternatively, patterns of neural activity (Section 9.6.2) could modify the response of ingrowing axons to molecular cues such as Eph-ephrins to regulate plasticity of neural maps. Finally there are other molecules that regulate retinotopic map formation, which may be key to remapping following lesions.[7]

9.6 Inputs from multiple structures: when maps collide

Up to this point we have examined the pathways and mechanisms by which the axons from a single structure map onto their target. However, in many systems two or more structures need to innervate the same target. For example, both ears must be mapped onto a single auditory structure and both eyes onto a single visual structure in the brain. Importantly, it is the comparison between the information coming from these bilateral sense organs that allows the precise localization of objects. In the visual system, the slight differences in the relative position of objects on the two retinae that is critical for our ability to perceive depth (i.e. stereopsis). Similarly the comparison of auditory input to the two ears allows animals to localize sounds in space. Therefore the maps not only have to come together in a single structure, they must also be in precise registration in order for similar regions of sensory space to be accurately compared. We shall now explore how individual maps from distinct brain regions come together using the mapping of the two eyes in the visual system of mammals as a model system.

---

[7] For more information, see Clandinin, and Feldheim, (2009) *Current Opinions in Neurobiology*, **19**, 174–180.

9.6.1 From retina to cortex in mammals

Perhaps the most salient feature of most sensory systems is the fact that when axons from different brain regions come together in a single target structure, they segregate into specific subregions within that structure. In the adult mammalian visual system, the axon terminals from the two eyes form eye-specific regions or layers in the **dorsal lateral geniculate nucleus (dLGN)** of the thalamus. The dLGN neurons then send axons, known as **thalamocortical afferents** (TCAs), that segregate into eye-specific domains known as **ocular dominance bands** in layer 4 of the primary visual cortex (the primary visual cortex is also known as Brodmann area 17 or V1, Fig. 9.11).

Numerous mammals have been studied to examine segregation of axons carrying information from the two eyes but in recent years the most common models are the ferret and the mouse. Like the retinotectal projections, the **retinogeniculate axons** initially branch throughout the developing dLGN and subsequently retract into eye specific zones or layers. As in the tectum, Eph–ephrin interactions regulate the patterning of eye-specific layers in the dLGN.

We have already discussed the role of Eph–ephrins in map formation. However, it is equally clear that neuronal activity also plays a crucial role in eye-specific segregation in the dLGN. Here, we will focus on the role of activity in regulating eye-specific segregation.

dorsal lateral geniculate nucleus (dLGN) a region of the thalamus that processes visual information; it receives input from the retina and sends information to the visual cortex.

retinogeniculate axons the axons of the retinal ganglion cells that project to the lateral geniculate nucleus of the thalamus.

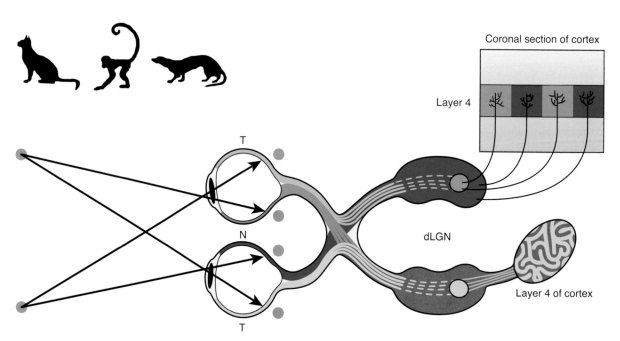

Fig. 9.11 The visual system of mammals. Two points in space represented by blue and pink dots are focused on the retina of the two eyes. The pink dot, located in the right half of the visual field, is imaged on the nasal (N) portion of the right eye (top) and the temporal (T) portion of the left eye. The reverse is true for the blue dot. In mammals with forward facing eyes, such as carnivores and primates, the majority of axons carrying information from the temporal retina project ipsilaterally (light blue and light pink), while those from the nasal retina project contralaterally (dark blue and dark pink). In the dLGN the axons form the two eyes segregate into eye specific zones. The cells in the dLGN then send axons to layer 4 of the cortex where the segregation of eye-specific inputs is maintained in the form of ocular dominance bands. These ocular dominance bands can be seen in both coronal and tangential sections through layer 4.

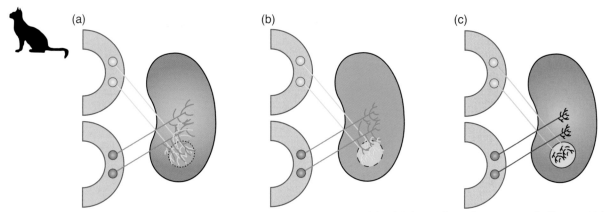

Fig. 9.12 Formation of eye-specific layers in the dLGN is dependent on activity. (a) Axons from the two eyes (yellow and blue axons) project to the dLGN where their branches initially overlap (denoted by green in the dLGN). (b) and (c) The axon terminals slowly segregate into eye-specific zones until distinct eye-specific layers are visible. Blockade of neuronal activity with TTX, a toxin found in pufferfish, results in a loss of eye-specific lamination. In this case the projection pattern would remain as seen in (a).

9.6.2 Activity-dependent eye specific segregation: a role for retinal waves

The first experiments showing a role for neuronal activity in eye-specific segregation in the dLGN came from experiments using injection of **tetrodotoxin (TTX)** into the ventricles of developing cats. Tetrodotoxin is isolated from the puffer fish and blocks the conduction of action potentials by blocking voltage-dependent sodium channels (see Chapter 10, Fig. 10.3). TTX injections into the lateral ventricles of developing cat prevented the segregation of eye inputs (Fig. 9.12).

Lamberto Maffei and colleagues working in Italy in the 1980s provided insight into the mechanism by which neuronal activity regulates dLGN layer formation by showing that cells of the retina show **spontaneous electrical activity** that occurs in bursts and spreads to neighbouring cells. These waves of activity, referred to as **retinal waves,** occur at the same time as RGC axons are segregating (Fig. 9.13).

spontaneous electrical activity electrical activity that arises from the endogenous properties of a neuronal or a neural network.

How could retinal waves instruct segregation of eye inputs? A favoured theory is based on a postulate put forward by Donald Hebb in 1949 (see Chapter 12, Section 12.2.2) that cells active at the same time will connect to the same targets. Retinal waves result from the correlation of the activity of adjacent cells in a single retina. However, such waves will not be synchronized between corresponding positions of the two eyes. The difference in activity patterns between the two eyes could therefore instruct the segregation of eye inputs in the dLGN (Fig. 9.13). This hypothesis has been successfully recapitulated mathematically using neighbour matching models outlined in Section 9.3.2.

Whether or not retinal waves instruct eye-specific segregation in the dLGN is still a matter of debate, the details of which are beyond the scope of this book.[8] However, evidence that patterns of activity can

---

[8] See recent reviews by Chalupa, L. M. (2009) Retinal waves are unlikely to instruct the formation of eye-specific retinogeniculate projections. *Neural Dev.*, **4**, 24; Feller, M. B. (2009) Retinal waves are likely to instruct the formation of eye-specific retinogeniculate projections. *Neural Dev.*, **4**, 24.

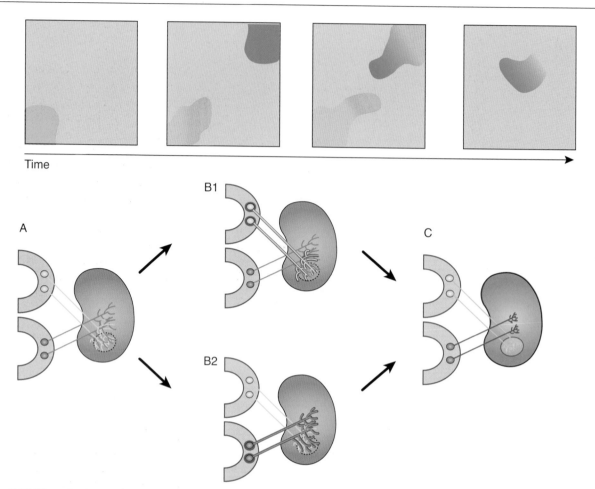

Time

Fig. 9.13 The retinal wave theory of segregation in the dLGN. Top panels: schematics of a region of a developing retina in which waves of activity (orange and green areas) spread across the retinal surface. These waves result from groups of cells becoming simultaneously active and passing on their excitation to the adjacent retinal ganglion cells, thus forming a wave of activity. These retinal waves, therefore, are bursts of correlated activity that spread across small areas of the retina every 1 to 2 seconds. Bottom panels: the retinal waves could instruct the segregation of eye inputs into discrete eye-specific layers in the dLGN. The segregation would arise because waves would correlate the activity of neighbouring cells within an eye (B1 and B2), but not between the two eyes. According to Hebb's postulate, 'cells that fire together, wire together' (see Chapter 12, Section 12.2.2). Retinal waves would cause cells in each eye to fire together, ultimately leading to segregation of eye inputs in the dLGN.

contralateral on the opposite side.

instruct retinal axon segregation comes from work done in the frog (*Xenopus*) tectum. Unlike in mammals, normally all frog RGCs project to the **contralateral** tectum and hence there is only one map and no segregation. However, using surgical grafts, the input from two eyes, or from two half eyes (i.e. two nasal or temporal retinae) can be forced to innervate the same tectum. In both of these cases, the inputs segregate into input-specific bands (Box 9.4) strongly indicating that there is a general underlying mechanism that can drive the segregation of inputs present even in brain structures in which segregation is not normally present. There is no *a priori* reason to assume that the two eyes or two hemi-retinae would contain different chemoaffinity markers, as proposed by Sperry in his

---

Box 9.4   Ectopic segregation in *Xenopus* tectum

Innervation of the tectum by multiple eyes can be achieved by grafting an eye **primordium** into a frog embryo to generate a **three-eyed frog**. One tectum of these animals then receives input from two eyes. The result is striking: the inputs from the two eyes segregate into alternating stripes of eye input similar to the ocular dominance bands seen in layer 4 of the visual cortex of carnivores and primates. Similar findings were seen in frogs in which **compound eyes** were generated by surgically placing two nasal retinae or two temporal retinae together in the same eye-cup. In these experiments, pieces of rudimentary retinae were dissected from developing frog eyes prior to axons exiting the eye; therefore these experiments examined the actual *initial* innervation of the tectum, rather than the innervation of the tectum by newly transplanted eye *after* the normal eye had already innervated the tectum (as is the case with three-eyed frogs). In frogs with compound eyes, hemi-retina specific bands appear indicating the mechanism for creating segregation is present at a developmental stage when the retina normally innervates the tectum. For the three-eyed frog, the formation of eye-specific stripes involves the retraction of initially exuberant retinotectal projections and does not occur if neural activity is blocked. It is difficult to imagine how molecular markers such as those proposed by Sperry's chemoaffinity hypothesis could drive RGC segregation in the three-eyed frog since the eyes innervating the tectum will be expressing the same chemoaffinity molecules. This strongly suggests that patterns of neuronal activity may drive eye segregation.

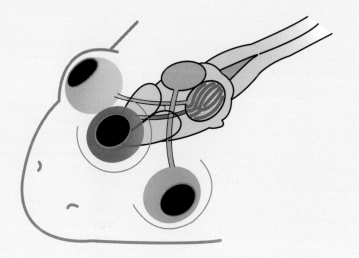

Segregation of eye-specific inputs in the three-eyed frog. Connections to the right tectum (solid orange) come only from the left eye and show no segregation as they have no competing input form the third eye. In contrast connections from the implanted *third eye* (red) compete with axons from the right eye (orange) in the left tectum. The result is eye specific bands similar to the ocular dominance bands seen in layer 4 of the visual cortex (Chapter 12).

primordium an embryological term for a region that will subsequently give rise to a particular organ or tissue.

chemoaffinity hypothesis. Therefore the suggestion is that activity plays a key role in regulating input specific segregation.

9.6.3 Formation of ocular dominance bands

In both the tectum and the dLGN the formation of either retinotopic or eye-specific maps arises from an initial exuberance of retinal axon determination and subsequent retraction of axons from inappropriate target regions. This was also thought to be the case for the segregation of thalamocortical axons that carry information from the two eyes to layer 4 of the cerebral cortex. Furthermore, the start of ocular dominance band formation in the cat correlated well with the time of eye opening, leading to the belief that the formation of ocular dominance

visual experience a visual stimulus or group of stimuli that changes neuronal excitation in neurons of the visual system.

anterograde forward, used to describe the direction between the cell body of a neuron and its axon terminal.

bands in layer 4 was dependent on **visual experience**. However, several experiments suggest a different story.

9.6.4 Ocular dominance bands form by directed ingrowth of thalamocortical axons

Larry Katz and colleagues working in the USA in the 1990s found that thalamocortical axons from a single eye grew directly into layer 4 exhibiting little overlap with terminals carrying information from the other eye. They used small injections of **anterograde** tracer into one layer of the dLGN to label small groups of thalamocortical axons (the same principle shown in Box 8.2 of Chapter 8). They found that axons did not show the pruning that would be expected if axon retraction were responsible for the emergence of ocular dominance bands, indicating that thalamocortical axons appeared to grow directly to their targets (Fig. 9.14).

9.6.5 Activity and the formation of ocular dominance bands

Two further lines of evidence suggest that neuronal activity – and visual experience in particular – was not necessary for the formation of ocular dominance bands. First, newborn monkeys that have had no visual experience have near adult-like ocular dominance bands. Secondly, removal of the eyes prior to ocular dominance band formation in the ferret does not prevent ocular dominance band formation. However, the findings do not rule out a role for action-potential driven activity. As with the retinal waves, patterns of spontaneous activity have been demonstrated in the developing dLGN suggesting correlated spontaneous activity could mediate the segregation of thalamocortical axons into ocular dominance bands. Furthermore, while thalamocortical axons from the dLGN appear to grow directly to their *ultimate* target regions in layer 4, this does not rule out exuberance and retraction and a role for activity *earlier* in the thalamocortical axon pathway. When thalamocortical axons first approach the cortical plate they enter a waiting phase during which they form transient synapses with **subplate** cells. It is possible that at this stage, the axons carrying information from the two eyes are initially intermingled but become sorted prior to entering the cortex. In support of this notion, thalamocortical axons make synapses with subplate cells prior to entering the cortical plate and ablation of subplate prevents ocular dominance band formation. The findings do not directly address the possibility of a role for axon retraction in the formation of ocular dominance bands, but they indicate that numerous mechanisms may be regulating ocular dominance band formation even prior to the formation of synapses in layer 4.

It is important to point out that while ocular dominance band formation is not dependent on visual experience, it is equally clear that the relative size of ocular dominance bands for each eye can be dramatically altered by visual experience. The maintenance of ocular dominance band size is discussed in Chapter 12.

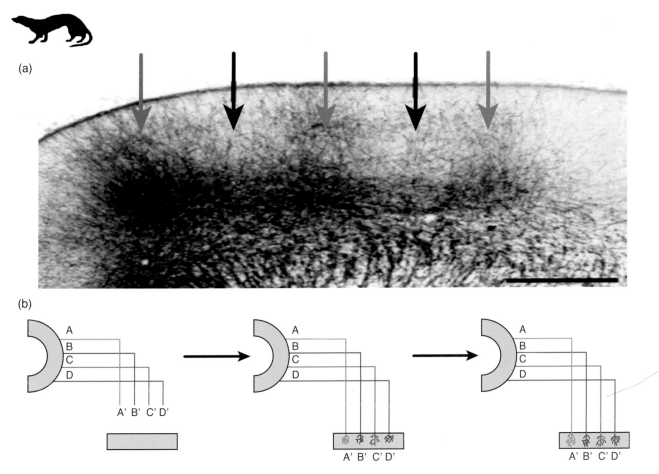

Fig. 9.14 Thalamocortical axons innervating the cortex show directed growth to their appropriate zones. (a) Injections of tracer into one layer of the dLGN as thalamocortical axons are first entering the cortex results in *patches* of label in layer 4 in the visual cortex indicating that axons grow directly to their target cells in eye-specific zones rather than growing into layer 4 diffusely and segregating into patches later. (From Crowley, J. C. and Katz, L. C., (2000) Early development of ocular dominance columns. *Science*, **290**, 1321–4). Reprinted with Permission from AAAS. (b) Schematic from Fig. 9.5 showing directed ingrowth as a mechanism of creating ordered connectivity between structures.

9.7 Development of feature maps

9.7.1 Feature maps in the visual system

The fundamental mechanism by which the brain processes complex information is to extract specific components or features (physical and spatial properties) and process them in parallel before reconstructing them into a complete perception. For example, in the visual cortex, subsets of neurons respond to particular features of objects including their orientation, direction of movement, colour and depth. The two feature maps that will be discussed further are those for **orientation-** and **direction-selectivity** since they illustrate the mechanisms by which feature maps form. The discovery of feature maps followed on from the seminal findings of David Hubel and Torsten Wiesel (who, together with Roger Sperry, won the Nobel Prize in 1981 for their work on how the

Box 9.5   Hubel and Wiesel and feature maps

David Hubel and Torsten Wiesel won the Nobel Prize for Medicine in 1981 for their discovery that neurons in the primary visual cortex are feature detectors and the physiological and anatomical properties of neurons can be altered by an animal's early experience. They placed microelectrodes into the primary visual cortex of anaesthetized cats and set out to determine the visual stimuli that would make cortical neurons fire action potentials. Rather than being stimulated by circles of light or dark or by natural scenes involving other cats or mice for example, neurons in the visual cortex respond to bars of light (or dark) of a particular orientation (i.e. they are **orientation-selective**). With the knowledge that different neurons encoded different features of an object, how these groups of neurons were arranged or mapped in the brain and how these maps develop could then be addressed. The physiological set-up used by Hubel and Wiesel would not have been unlike the one depicted below, without the computer of course.

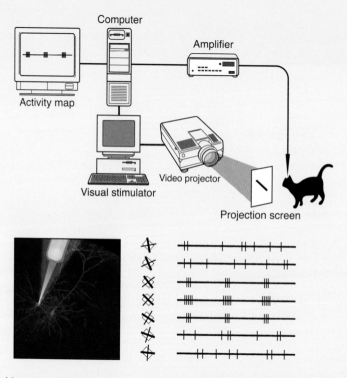

Top: a visual stimulus (in this case a black bar on a white background) is shown to a cat using a video projector or a computer screen. An electrode inserted into the visual cortex of the cat monitors the electrical activity of neurons that results from the visual stimulus. The electrical signal is amplified and recorded on a computer that can generate graphs of activity patterns. The computer can be used to synchronize the recording of electrical activity from the cortical neurons with the timing of the appearance of a visual stimulus. Bottom: a stylized recording electrode monitoring the electrical activity of a layer 3 cortical pyramidal neuron (labelled with **DiI**). The pattern of electrical activity can be monitored as bars of different orientation are shown to the animal. Bursts of activity are only visible in response to a narrow range of orientations around 45° indicating that this cell is highly orientation-selective.

brain processes visual information using experiments such as those outlined in Box 9.5).[9]

The formation of feature maps in the developing nervous system poses some interesting mechanistic questions. Unlike the unique

---

[9] http://nobelprize.org/nobel_prizes/medicine/laureates/1981/ [20 November 2010].

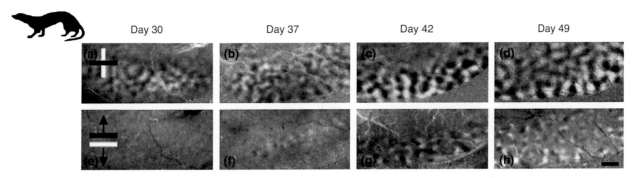

Fig. 9.15 Development of orientation- and direction-selective cells in the ferret visual cortex. (a)–(d) Orientation-selective maps in the ferret visual cortex. Optical imaging shows clear patterns of activation in the cortex (black and white patches) that result from horizontal and vertical stimuli (shown by black and white bars respectively) are first seen just prior to eye opening. (e)–(h) Direction-selective maps for a horizontal bar of light moving upward (black) or downward (white). Direction-selective maps appear approximately 4 weeks after the appearance of direction-selective maps. The finding that eye opening and the appearance of these feature maps occur at similar ages led to the hypothesis that their development is dependent on visual experience. (a) Reprinted from *Neuron*, **56**, White L. E. and Fitzpatrick D. Vision and cortical map development, 327–338, 2007 with permission form Elsevier.

spatial coordinates of a cell that are encoded by a complex interplay between gradients of Eph–ephrins and neuronal activity, there is no reason to believe that any molecular determinants could underlie the precise higher-order connectivity necessary for the formation of feature maps. Furthermore, while ocular dominance and topographic maps develop before visual experience is received (i.e. before birth or eye-opening), the development of orientation and direction maps coincides with the onset of visual experience. Perhaps for these reasons, most research on the development of feature maps has focused on the role of experience-dependent rather than spontaneous activity.

There is no clear anatomical correlate of **orientation** and **direction maps**. Instead they are detected solely by electrophysiological or metabolic techniques. A physiological technique known as **optical imaging** has been used to reveal these maps in both ferrets and cats.[10] Orientation maps can be visualized by presenting moving bars of light of a particular orientation to an anaesthetized animal (generally cats, ferrets or monkeys are used for these types of studies).

Direction selective maps can be considered sub-maps of the orientation maps since they reveal the regions of cortex responding to a stimulus of a particular orientation only if the stimulus is moving in a particular direction. Current evidence suggests that development of orientation and direction maps occurs later than the development of topographic and ocular dominance maps (Fig. 9.15).

optical imaging an imaging technique that measures local changes in oxygen metabolism. Commonly used to visualize topographic and feature maps in the cerebral cortex.

9.7.2 Role of experience in orientation and direction map formation

By rearing ferrets from birth in complete darkness (**dark-rearing**), researchers have been able to address how feature maps develop in

---

[10] For more on optical imaging, see Zepeda, A., Arias, C. and Sengpiel, F. (2004) Optical imaging of intrinsic signals: recent developments in the methodology and its applications. *J. Neurosci. Meth.*, **136**, 1–21.

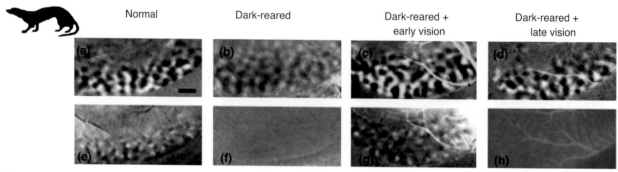

Fig. 9.16 Development of orientation- and direction-selective maps in dark-reared ferrets. The orientation-selective (upper row) and direction-selective (lower row) maps in normal animals (a) and (e), dark-reared animals (b) and (f) and animals that had been dark-reared until about 3 days after normal eye opening (early vision, (c) and (g)) or until 2–3 weeks after eye opening (late vision, (d) and (h)). Dark-rearing does not prevent the formation of orientation maps (b) although the pattern of the maps is blurred relative to normal animals. In contrast, direction-selective maps are absent in dark-reared animals (f). Orientation maps return to normal following restoration of binocular vision either days (c) or weeks after eye opening (d). Direction selective maps can be partially rescued provided visual experience is restored soon after eye opening (g), but not if vision is restored 2–3 weeks later (h). Reprinted from *Neuron*, **56**, White L. E. and Fitzpatrick D. Vision and cortical map development, 327–338, 2007 with permission form Elsevier.

sensitive period distinct time-windows during development when the functional properties of neurons can be altered by experience.

the absence of any input to the two eyes. Unlike the ocular dominance bands and eye-specific segregation in the dLGN, visually-driven activity (i.e. experience) does regulate the initial appearance of orientation and direction selectivity (Fig. 9.16). For orientation maps, dark-rearing does not prevent the formation of the maps *per se*, but the maps are less well defined. On the other hand, direction-selective maps are not present at all in dark-reared ferrets indicating that the development of this attribute is absolutely dependent on visual experience. Importantly, when animals are returned to the light early in their development, direction maps appear to develop normally. If the return to light-rearing is delayed until the animals are several months old, the direction maps never form. These findings indicate the existence of a critical time window (a **sensitive period**) during which visual experience is crucial for the normal development of direction selectivity. Sensitive periods during development are discussed in much greater detail in Chapter 12.

9.8 Summary

- Maps are two-dimensional representations of spatial or physical characteristics of an object.
- Neural maps can be found throughout the animal kingdom and can be divided into coarse and fine maps with the latter being subdivided into topographic and feature maps.
- Map development is underpinned by the precise connectivity between brain areas that can arise through a number of different mechanisms.
- Computer modelling has played a large role in our understanding of map formation.

- Both molecular cues and patterns of neuronal activity regulate map formation.
- Molecules, such as Eph–ephrins, form gradients that guide axons to their correct destination in the target tissue.
- Patterns of activity allow neighbouring cells in the projecting tissue to connect to neighbouring cells in the target tissue.
- Visual experience regulates feature map formation.

Maturation of Functional Properties

10

In previous chapters we have examined how nerve cells acquire their complex shapes, their correct identity and how their axons find the appropriate target. However, the brain is not simply an electronic circuit board and knowledge of the anatomy of neuronal connectivity is insufficient for understanding brain function. Instead we need to view functioning neurons as dynamic integrators of complex information whose integrative properties, and hence their response to a given stimulus, can be altered. In this chapter we will examine how neurons acquire their **functional** or **physiological properties** as well as examining what role **electrical excitability** may play in regulating development. In Chapter 12 we will see how neurons are able to change their properties as a consequence of an animal's experience.

To help understand the complexity of neuronal function and how it underlies what appears to be even the simplest of behaviours, imagine a student sitting in a class listening to their lecturer, taking notes and hopefully storing novel information that can be synthesized with existing knowledge and recalled at a later date. This simple task involves information processing and motor skills that are mediated by a large number of cells in the brain, spinal cord and musculature. Sensory cells in the ear initiate the processing of the lecturer's voice and the information is relayed to the auditory cortex through a series of intermediate brain centres. After further processing in the cortex, the information reaches neurons in the motor cortex that communicate with motor neurons in the spinal cord. These cells then activate muscle fibres that control the movement of the arm and fingers to allow the writing of words. Finally, cells in a variety of brain regions alter their physiological properties to act as a repository for the new information being stored. Each of these processes takes place in millions of neurons and it all relies on their ability to integrate information from a variety of sources, conduct electrical signals with high fidelity and communicate efficiently.

functional properties a general term used to describe the physiological properties of a neuron, especially those that alter the behaviour of a neuronal network or animal.

electrical activity/excitability the ability of a cell to regulate electrical current at its cell membrane.

Building Brains: An Introduction to Neural Development, First Edition.
David Price, Andrew Jarman, John Mason and Peter Kind.
© 2011 John Wiley & Sons, Ltd. Published 2011 by John Wiley & Sons, Ltd.

10.1 Neurons are excitable cells

An **excitable cell** is traditionally defined as one that can propagate **action potentials** along its membrane following mechanical, chemical or electrical stimulation (see Section 10.2.2). Several cell types are excitable including neurons and muscle cells. Excitability is a more general term, defined as the ability to regulate ion movement across the cell membrane without necessitating the propagation of action potentials. Very little is known about the cellular mechanisms that control the development of cellular excitability. More is known about how different forms of cellular excitability regulate development. Prior to reviewing what is known about excitability during development, it is first necessary to discuss the electrical properties of membranes and the proteins that control them.

10.1.1 What makes a cell excitable?

The ability of cells to conduct electrical signals results from unique properties of the cell membranes and the presence of highly salty, ion-rich fluids on either side. Membranes are lipid bilayers that act as barriers to ions, restricting their movement in and out of the cell. Embedded in the lipid bilayer are large numbers of transmembrane proteins known as **ion pumps** and **ion channels** that regulate the distribution and movement of ions across membranes. Ion pumps selectively move ions, thereby establishing and maintaining an uneven distribution across membranes, known as **ionic gradients**. The result is an imbalance of electrical charge across a membrane referred to as the **membrane potential** (measured in volts). The difference in electrical charge and the imbalance in ion concentrations establish an **electrochemical gradient**. The main ions that establish the electrochemical gradient for neuronal membranes are the positively charged cations, sodium (Na^+), potassium (K^+), calcium (Ca^{2+}), and the negatively charged anion, chloride (Cl^-). For most neurons the **resting potential** – the membrane potential when the cell is not conducting an impulse – is about -70 mV inside (Fig. 10.1).

10.1.2 Electrical properties of neurons

Ion channels and ion pumps lie at the heart of neuronal excitability including nerve conduction and cell communication. For example, some neurotransmitter receptors are also ion channels; binding of their cognate neurotransmitter causes channel opening, which allows the flow of ions and thereby changes the membrane potential. The flow of ions across a membrane is referred to as the **electrical current** and is measured in amperes (amps). There are two main forces that drive ionic current: the concentration gradient for that particular ion across the membrane (ions will diffuse from high to low concentrations) and the electrical charge or voltage across the membrane (ions will be attracted towards their opposite charge). For example, if an ion channel that is permeable for sodium ions opens, Na^+ would flow into the cell down its concentration gradient (chemical gradient, see Fig. 10.1). Furthermore, at resting potential, the inside of a cell is

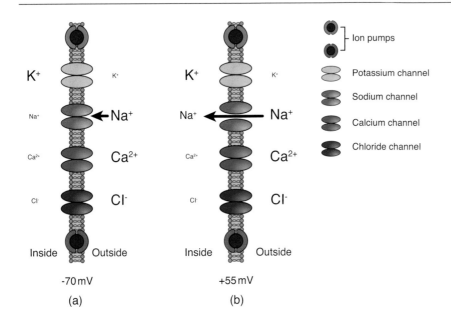

Fig. 10.1 Membrane proteins regulate the concentration of ions across membranes. Schematics showing prototypical neuronal membranes that contain transmembrane proteins, including ion channels and ion pumps, which regulate the flow of ions across the membrane. (a) For most neurons, Ca^{2+}, Na^+ and Cl^- concentrations are much higher outside the cell than inside. In contrast, K^+ concentration is much higher inside the cell than outside. The voltage at which the flow of ions across a neuronal membrane is in equilibrium is called the resting potential (approximately -70 mV). (b) When ion channels open (such as the Na^+ channel here), ions flow down their electrochemical gradient changing the membrane potential. The membrane potential at which there is no net flow of an ion is referred to as the reversal potential. For Na^+ the reversal potential is $+55$ mV. Ion pumps or transporters reset the concentration gradients to restore resting potential.

negatively charged relative to the outside. Therefore, there is also a force exerted to generate a net flow of Na^+ ions from outside to inside the cell (electrical gradient). Na^+ will flow into the cell until equilibrium between these two forces is reached. However, once the electrical gradient is depleted, Na^+ ions will continue to flow inwards, causing a positive membrane potential. This flow of Na^+ continues until the inward force exerted by the chemical gradient is opposed by an equal outward force from the electrical gradient. The membrane potential at which this equilibrium is reached when the membrane is selectively permeable for a particular ion is referred to as the **reversal potential**. For Na^+ the reversal potential is $+55$ mV.[1]

10.1.3 Types of ion channels

There are thousands of different ion channels but they can be broadly subdivided into four groups defined by their mode of activation: **ligand-gated**, **voltage-gated**, **G-protein-gated and second messenger-gated** (Fig. 10.2). Ligand-gated channels include many neurotransmitter receptors and are activated by the binding of a ligand in the extracellular space. Voltage-gated ion channels are activated when the membrane voltage changes following the opening of other ion channels in the cell membrane or in the membrane of intracellular organelles that store calcium (e.g. endoplasmic reticulum). As their name implies, second-messenger gated channels are activated when second messenger molecules such as cAMP and Ca^{2+} activate the intracellular portion of the channel. Similarly, G-protein-gated ion channels are activated when specific subunits of **heterotrimeric** G proteins bind to the intracellular domain of the channels. In many cases an ion channel is made up of several protein subunits, usually encoded by

ligand a molecule or ion that binds to a receptor molecule, for example on the cell surface, to generate a biological response.

G-proteins (guanine nucleotide binding protein) a large family of membrane-associated and soluble proteins involved in intracellular signalling.

second messengers intracellular molecules that act as relays for extracellular signals bound to cell surface receptors; they include cyclic AMP, PIP3 and Ca^{2+}.

---

[1] To see how the reversal potential is determined, see Nicholls, J. G., Martin, A. R., Wallace, B. G. and Fuchs, P. A, (2001) *From Neuron to Brain: A Cellular and Molecular Approach to the Function of the Nervous System*, 4th edn, Sinauer Associates, Inc.

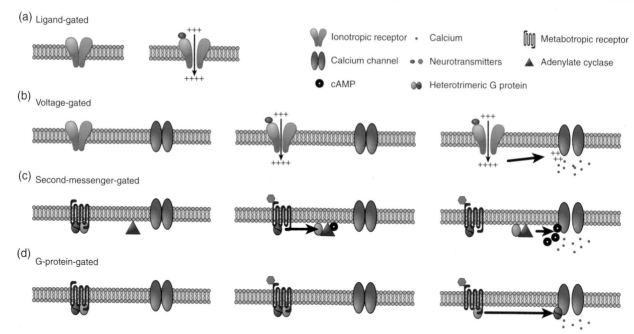

Fig. 10.2 Four different types of ion channels classified by their mode of activation. (a) Ligand-gated ion channels, such as ionotropic neurotransmitter receptors, open as a direct result of ligand binding to the extracellular portion of the protein. (b) Voltage-gated ion channels open (the Ca^{2+} channel here) as a result of a change in the electrical potential near the channel. In the case shown here, an increase in membrane potential results from the activation of a ligand-gated ion channel. (c) Second-messenger gated ion channels are regulated by second messengers such as Ca^{2+} or cAMP, the latter being depicted here. cAMP is generated from the activity of adenylate cyclase, which is activated either by increases in intracellular Ca^{2+} or via **heterotrimeric** G proteins (shown here). (d) In some cases, heterotrimeric G-proteins can directly regulate ion channel opening after activation by the stimulation of **metabotropic** neurotransmitter receptors.

heterotrimeric consisting of three different subunits.

metabotropic receptor a receptor that does not form an ion channel and instead transduces signals to the inside of the cell through the activation of intracellular signalling cascades often using heterotrimeric G proteins.

different genes and it is the ability of these subunits to come together in unique combinations that greatly increases the complexity of ion channels. In other cases an ion channel is formed by a single protein. In all cases, however, the channels open as a result of a conformational change in the protein that opens a pore and allows ions to flow in a direction determined by the nature of the electrochemical gradient.

10.2 Neuronal excitability during development

The vast majority of studies examining the role of neuronal excitability in development have focused on late developmental stages (when it is more commonly known as **neuronal activity**; see Chapters 9 and 12). It is at these later stages when action potentials and synaptic transmission, initiated by either spontaneous activity or sensory and motor stimulation, regulate neuronal maturation. However, there is a growing body of evidence that neuronal excitability also regulates aspects of early brain development including proliferation of neural progenitors (Chapter 5), migration (Chapter 6) and axon pathfinding (Chapter 8).

As we have seen in the preceding section, the electrical properties of neurons are dependent, in large part, on the protein composition of their membranes. In terms of development, there are several key questions that need to be addressed:

- When do the cells in the developing nervous system first become excitable?
- What proteins regulate excitability during development?
- What developmental events are regulated by neuronal excitability?

10.2.1 Neuronal excitability changes dramatically during development

The complexity and shear number of ion channels, and the fact that different neuronal subtypes express different complements of ion channels, has rendered comprehensive studies examining ion channel expression through development impractical. For example, there are more that 70 genes encoding potassium channel subunits that between them can generate more than 1000 different functional channels. Despite the paucity of studies concerning the precise developmental time course of ion channel expression, some dramatic examples of changes in ion channel expression – and hence excitability of neurons – have emerged that make it clear that the development of neuronal excitability is a highly dynamic process.

10.2.2 Early action potentials are driven by Ca^{2+}, not Na^+

An example of changes in ion channel expression and hence changes in electrical excitability with neuronal maturation can be seen in the development of action potentials (Fig. 10.3). In adult animals, action potentials are fast and short in duration. The initial **depolarization** results from the opening of voltage-dependent Na^+ channels and is rapidly followed by a **repolarization** phase that results from an efflux of K^+ through voltage-gated potassium channels. In contrast, the first action potentials that appear during embryonic development are infrequent and have a long duration. They result from the activation of Ca^{2+} channels (as opposed to Na^+ channels). Their long duration results from the delayed expression of the **hyperpolarizing** potassium current (i.e. the outward flow of positive K^+ ions that makes the inside of the cell relatively more negative) and the fact that calcium channels open and close more slowly than sodium channels. It is not known if all neurons go through a phase of Ca^{2+}-based action potentials during development, but for those that do, the phase is brief and rapidly replaced by Na^+-based action potentials. The precise timing of action potential development differs by cell type and brain region, but the first action potentials can be seen in the cortex during embryonic stages, prior to the development of synapses, and in many types of neurons can be measured soon after the neuron becomes post-mitotic.

depolarization an increase in positive charge inside a neuron relative to the outside; a response to a depolarizing stimulus.

repolarization the restoration of the membrane resting potential following the generation of an action potential.

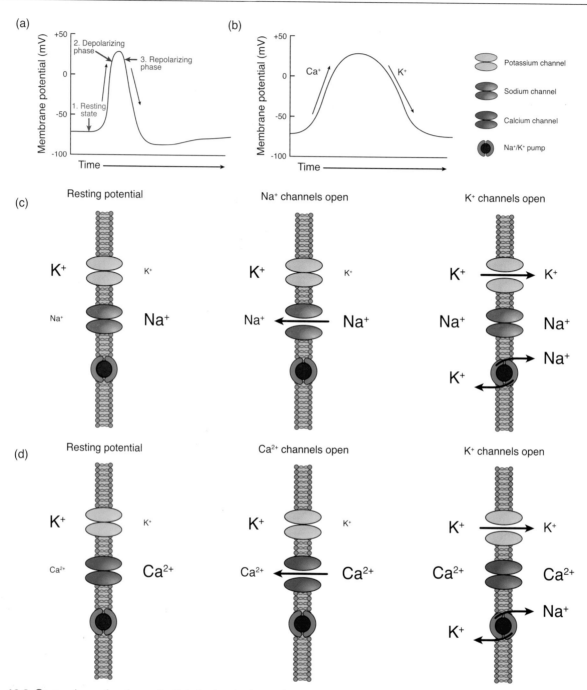

Fig. 10.3 Comparison of action potentials in developing and mature neurons. The action potential can be divided into three phases: the resting state, the depolarizing phase and the repolarizing phase. (a) and (c) For a mature neuron, the depolarizing phase results from the opening of voltage-dependent Na$^+$ channels. This depolarization subsequently activates voltage-dependent K$^+$ channels. Because K$^+$ is present in much higher concentration inside relative to outside the cell, K$^+$ ions flow out of the cell, repolarizing the membrane to its resting potential. (b) and (d) In developing neurons the depolarization phase results from the opening of voltage-gated Ca^{2+} channels, but like mature neurons the repolarization phase results from the activation of K$^+$ channels. In each case, the ionic flux that occurs during the action potential results in a change in the ionic gradient across the cell membrane. This has to be corrected in order for the cell to be ready to conduct another action potential. The establishment and ongoing maintenance of the ionic concentration gradients is achieved by a range of membrane proteins, such as the sodium-potassium pump (shown here) and intracellular storage orgnalles.

10.2.3 Neurotransmitter receptors regulate excitability prior to synapse formation

Neuronal excitability resulting from activation of neurotransmitter-gated receptors is also regulated through development. In particular, the neurotransmitters **γ-aminobutyric acid (GABA)** and **glutamate**, and their receptors are expressed before synaptogenesis; neurotransmitter receptors are among the earliest expressed ion channels. **Neuronal progenitors** in the **ventricular** and **subventricular zones** of mammalian cerebral cortex (Chapter 5, Fig. 5.16) express GABA and glutamate receptors that regulate a range of processes outlined in the sections below. Furthermore, the neuronal activity that results from activating these receptors is also regulated through development. As we will see, activating certain GABA receptors has a very different effect on membrane potential for cortical progenitor cells than it does for mature neurons. Neurotransmitter receptor activity can be modulated in several ways including altering receptor subunit composition, altering ionic pump expression and even altering local ion concentrations. For example, the development of **astrocytes** that secrete potassium changes the external concentration of K^+ and hence the resting potential of neurons.

ventricular zone the inner side of the neural tube closest to its lumen in the developing vertebrate brain. This transient layer contains neuronal progenitor cells.

subventricular zone the transient layer of the forebrain neural tube that contains the basal progenitor cells.

astrocyte a type of glial cell; they are star-shaped with many processes that enwrap neuronal synapses.

10.2.4 GABAergic receptor activation switches from being excitatory to inhibitory

GABA is the dominant inhibitory neurotransmitter in the mature brain. One subtype of GABA receptors ($GABA_A$ receptor) is permeable to Cl^-. In mature neurons the presence of the potassium-chloride cotransporter (KCC2) keeps concentrations of Cl^- 20 times higher *outside* the cell (Fig. 10.4). Activation of a $GABA_A$ receptor leads to an influx of Cl^- ions,

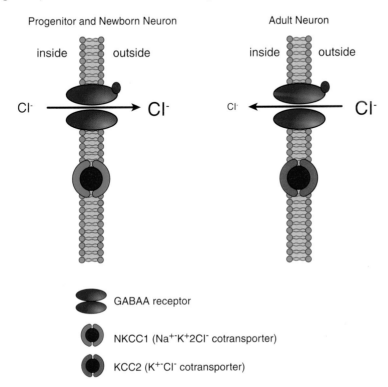

Progenitor and Newborn Neuron

Adult Neuron

inside   outside

inside   outside

GABAA receptor

NKCC1 (Na⁺-K⁺2Cl⁻ cotransporter)

KCC2 (K⁺-Cl⁻ cotransporter)

Fig. 10.4 A developmental switch in chloride ion transporter expression mediates the switch from excitatory to inhibitory effects of GABA (purple oval) during development. Early in development cells express the NKCC1 cotransporter, which keeps the concentration of Cl^- relatively high inside the cell and the reversal potential for Cl^- relatively positive. When $GABA_A$ receptors open, Cl^- flows out of the cell due to the electrical gradient. The net flow of negative ions out of the cell depolarizes the membrane. In adult neurons, the KCC2 cotransporter replaces NKCC1 expression. KCC2 keeps Cl^- concentration relatively low intracellularly making the reversal potential more hyperpolarized. The result is that $GABA_A$ receptor activation causes Cl^- to flow into the cell due to its chemical gradient, hyperpolarizing the membrane.

Box 10.1 Imaging calcium levels

Using dyes that fluoresce when Ca^{2+} concentration in a cell's cytoplasm is increased, several researchers have demonstrated short-lived local increases in intracellular Ca^{2+}, known as **calcium transients**, in neuronal progenitors in the ventricular and subventricular zones of the developing neocortex. Similar Ca^{2+} transients have been seen in almost all developing systems examined throughout development. Furthermore, these transient increases in Ca^{2+} are not restricted to cell bodies, but have also been seen in developing growth cones during axon growth and pathfinding. These spontaneous Ca^{2+} transients could arise from either the activation of calcium channels in the cell membrane or through second-messenger activation of Ca^{2+} channels in the membrane of intracellular organelles that store calcium such as the endoplasmic reticulum and mitochondria.

The first Ca^{2+} dye was discovered in 1985 by Roger Tsien (who also shared the Nobel prize for his discovery of green fluorescent protein – Box 1.4). Tsien and colleagues identified a fluorescent molecule (that they named fura-2), which changes its fluorescent properties (namely the wavelength of light it absorbs) when it binds to Ca^{2+}. By exciting fura-2 with the correct wavelength of light using a laser, a researcher could then distinguish between bound and unbound fura-2. Importantly, cell membranes are permeable to a derivative of fura-2 (fura-2AM), so cells can be easily filled with fura-2AM and any change in free Ca^{2+} inside the cell can be measured following electrophysiological or pharmacological stimulation. Fura-2 and many other similar Ca^{2+}-sensitive dyes are commonly used in neuroscience research.[2]

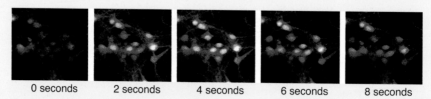

| 0 seconds | 2 seconds | 4 seconds | 6 seconds | 8 seconds |

Individual frames of a time-lapse video showing the transient increase in intracellular Ca^{2+} in response to synaptic stimulation. Cultured cortical neurons were stimulated with a $GABA_A$ receptor blocker (bicuculline) to increase synaptic activity. Individual frames are spaced 2 seconds apart (courtesy of G. Hardingham, University of Edinburgh, UK).

hyperpolarizing the cell (i.e. the inside of the cell becomes more negative and so less likely to generate an action potential).

However, things are very different during early neuronal development. At this stage, the KCC2 pump is not expressed. Instead the sodium-potassium-chloride cotransporter (NKCC1) is expressed, which increases the relative concentration of Cl^- *inside* the cell, thereby making the reversal potential for Cl^- more positive. The result of the altered reversal potential is that when $GABA_A$ receptors open, Cl^- flows out of the cell and the inside of the cell becomes depolarized. The depolarization caused by the efflux of Cl^- then activates other voltage-gated Ca^{2+} channels. In this way, GABA activation of $GABA_A$ receptors can induce an increase in intracellular Ca^{2+} concentration (as measured with calcium indicator dyes, see Box 10.1) in neuronal progenitors and early born neurons. Importantly, $GABA_A$ receptor stimulation results in large, long-lasting depolarizations which are very different in size and duration from typical synaptic currents, and are reminiscent of the early Ca^{2+}-dependent action potentials.

---

[2] A movie of a Ca^{2+} sensitive dye in action can be found at http://www.tsienlab.ucsd.edu/Movies.htm [20 November 2010].

10.3 Developmental processes regulated by neuronal excitability

10.3.1 Electrical excitability regulates neuronal proliferation and migration

In Chapter 5 we described the mechanisms that regulate the proliferation of neuronal progenitor cells in the ventricular and subventricular zones in the vertebrate brain. These mechanisms largely focused on transcription factors as master regulators of neurogenesis and secreted signals that regulate cell–cell interactions. Here we briefly discuss the role of electrical excitability in inhibiting neuronal progenitor proliferation. As mentioned above, GABA receptors are expressed very early in development, well before the formation of synapses. GABA is released from the first GABAergic neurons that migrate from the **ganglionic eminences** into the cerebral cortex (see Chapter 6), where it acts in a non-synaptic, **paracrine** manner (i.e. it acts on nearby cells) to inhibit progenitor cell proliferation. The intracellular pathway by which GABA receptor stimulation leads to altered proliferation is not clear. What is known is that opening of $GABA_A$ receptors leads to the activation of voltage-dependent calcium channels and the resulting increase in intracellular Ca^{2+} inhibits DNA synthesis and hence proliferation (Fig. 10.5).

ganglionic eminences ventral regions of the embryonic telencephalon.

paracrine signalling between adjacent cells either by contact or diffusible factors.

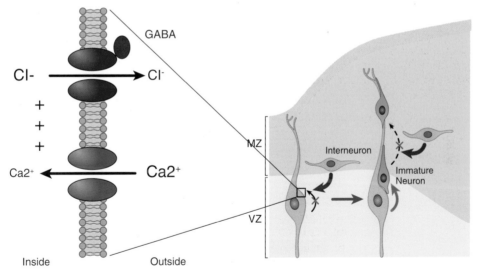

Fig. 10.5 Activation of GABA receptors expressed by neuronal progenitor cells inhibits proliferation and migration. This figure depicts the GABA-containing neurons (orange with red nucleus) that have migrated from the ganglionic eminences. These neurons secrete GABA that activates $GABA_A$ receptors on **radial glia**, which are neuronal progenitors (orange, brown nucleus) in the ventricular zone (VZ), causing an efflux of Cl^- and their depolarization. The high magnification of the progenitor cell membrane (inset) shows how the increase in net positive charge near a voltage-gated Ca^{2+} channel activates the channel resulting in the influx of Ca^{2+}. This Cl^- efflux and membrane depolarisation initiates a cascade of intracellular events to inhibit proliferation (indicated by the black arrow with red cross). The precise nature of these events is not known but it could be through either its role as a second-messenger molecule or the change in membrane excitability. GABA has also been shown to inhibit neuronal migration (dashed black arrow with red cross) of immature neurons (green) in the VZ and subventricular zone (SVZ) into the cortical plate (CP). (Adapted from Wang, D. W. and Kriegstein, A. R. (2009) Defining the role of GABA in cortical development. *Journal of Physiology*, **587**, 1873–1879, with permission from Wiley-Blackwell).

radial glia the neuronal progenitor cells of the vertebrate CNS.

hippocampus a structure of the vertebrate forebrain particularly associated with learning and memory formation.

In the developing **hippocampus,** GABA released from cells that have migrated from the ganglionic eminence acts in a paracrine manner on GABA$_A$ receptors to regulate neuronal migration. Inhibitors of GABA$_A$ receptors dramatically reduce the migration of hippocampal neurons. Numerous cellular events control cell migration (Chapter 6), but it is not known how they are regulated following GABA receptor activation to cause altered migration.

10.3.2 Neuronal activity and axon guidance

As a final example of how neuronal excitability regulates early cellular development and differentiation, we will examine how local alteration in membrane excitability can alter the pathfinding of developing axons (Fig. 10.6). In this case the stimulus is not a neurotransmitter, but the classic axon guidance molecules, the netrins. In Chapter 8 we saw that diffusible factors such as netrins can affect the turning behaviour of growing axons by binding to their receptors on growth cones. The turning of axons as they enter a netrin gradient is mediated by Ca^{2+} entering the growth cone through TRP (transient receptor potential) channels located in the growth cone membranes. Reduction of TRP channel expression blocks the ability of axons to turn towards a netrin source, strongly suggesting that netrins exert their axon guidance effects via the activation of calcium channels in the cell membrane. An increase in the Ca^{2+} concentration inside the cell not only depolarizes the membrane but also alters Ca^{2+}-dependent signal transduction pathways. It is not yet clear which of these two functions of Ca^{2+} is more important in regulating netrin-dependent growth cone turning.

In summary, it is clear that early neuronal excitability arises as a result of the regulated expression of genes and itself regulates numerous aspects of neuronal maturation that are not traditionally associated with activity-dependent development. That said, the complement of proteins that mediate early neuronal and precursor excitability are very different from those that mediate classical neuronal excitation. This is not surprising given the vastly different surroundings of young neurons compared with fully differentiated

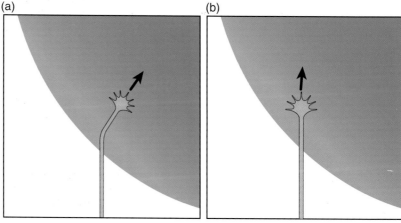

(a)   (b)

Fig. 10.6 Transient receptor potential (TRP) channels regulate axon turning to netrins. (a) Schematic showing the turning of a growth cone of a *Xenopus* spinal cord neuron in response to a netrin gradient (red). (b) This turning response is absent if TRP channel expression is reduced.

neurons. For example, early neurons have no synapses and express a different cohort of ion channels.[3]

10.4 Synaptogenesis

The principal job of a neuron is to integrate information coming from up to thousands of cells and then pass on the relevant information to target cells. This information flow happens at highly specialized structures known as synapses and the process by which these connections are initially formed is termed **synaptogenesis**.

10.4.1 The synapse

A mature synapse has three major parts: (i) a **presynaptic terminal** (also known as a 'synaptic bouton'), a specialization of the axon that is characterized by the presence of large numbers of **synaptic vesicles** and an **active zone**; (ii) the **postsynaptic terminal** located on dendritic spines, dendritic shafts and cell bodies that comes in a range of shapes and sizes and is characterized by a distinctive **electron-dense** structure called the **postsynaptic density** (**PSD**); (iii) the **synaptic cleft**, the 20–25 nm space located between the pre- and postsynaptic terminals (Fig. 10.7). The axon and dendrites of an individual neuron can have hundreds to thousands of both presynaptic boutons and postsynaptic terminals.

The highly characteristic, asymmetric structure of synapses closely reflects their function. An action potential invades the presynaptic terminal but is unable to cross the synaptic cleft between the pre- and postsynaptic terminals. Instead, it must first be converted into a chemical signal mediated by neurotransmitters found within small membranous organelles known as synaptic vesicles (Fig. 10.8). Many different types of neurotransmitter are used, including two that we encountered earlier in this chapter, glutamate and GABA. Neurotransmitters are released from the presynaptic cell in response to an action potential and diffuse across the synaptic cleft and bind to neurotransmitter receptors in the postsynaptic density. This binding activates ion channels in the cell membrane resulting in a change in membrane potential and the conversion of the chemical signal back into an electrical signal. The postsynaptic density is a large multi-protein complex that determines how the postsynaptic cell responds to incoming signals. Pre- and postsynaptic cell membranes are held in close apposition by, for example, cell adhesion molecules.

10.4.2 Stages of synaptogenesis

How are synapses assembled during CNS development? This relatively simple question is proving very difficult to answer. Our understanding of the molecular mechanisms of synaptogenesis is far from complete.

synaptic vesicles membrane-bound organelles in the presynaptic terminal that contain neurotransmitter.

active zone the region of the presynaptic terminal where synaptic vesicles containing neurotransmitter fuse with the membrane to release neurotransmitter.

electron-dense describes a structure that is unable to pass electrons, therefore appearing dark on an electron micrograph.

---

[3] For more on the role of excitability in early development, see Spitzer, N. C. (2006) Electrical activity in early neuronal development. *Nature*, **444**, 707–12; Wang, D. D. and Kriegstein, A. R. (2009) Defining the role of GABA in cortical development. *J Physiol.*, **587**,1873–9.

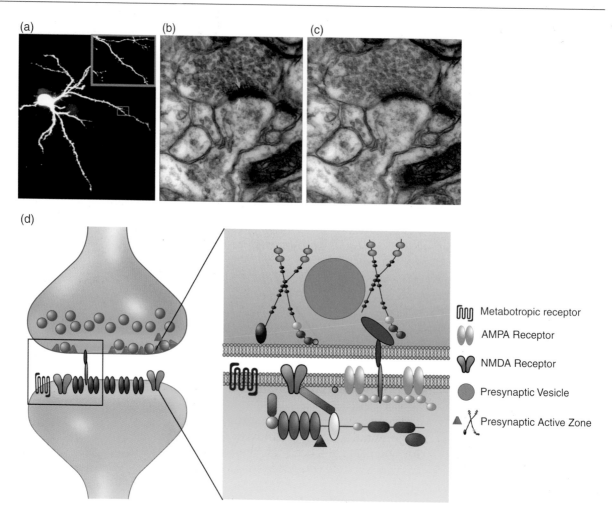

Fig. 10.7 The synapse. (a) A layer 4 excitatory neuron in the somatosensory cortex of the mouse showing the elaborate dendritic morphology of neurons. Inset shows a section of dendrite with numerous protrusions called **dendritic spines** (also see Figs. 10.16 and 10.17). The spines are the sites of excitatory inputs onto the cell. (b) and (c) Electron micrographs of a dendritic spine (orange in (c)) forming synapses with a single presynaptic terminal (blue in (c)). The presynaptic terminal is easily identifiable by the presence of vesicles (red arrows) that contain glutamate, the principal excitatory neurotransmitter of cortical synapses. Where the presynaptic terminal contacts the dendritic spines there is an electron dense darker region on both the presynaptic (blue arrow) and postsynaptic side (yellow arrow) of the synaptic cleft. These are large protein complexes that on the presynaptic side form the active zone and on the postsynaptic side form the postsynaptic density. (d) Schematic of a synapse showing the presynaptic terminal with synaptic vesicles (blue circles) and the active zone (red triangles) and the postsynaptic mushroom spine with its postsynaptic density (PSD, orange). The enlargement shows the molecular complexity of the PSD and the presynaptic active zone. The identities of some of these proteins are shown in the legend and discussed in this chapter and Chapter 12.

There are enormous technical challenges to studying the process of synaptogenesis in the intact brain. For example, most synapses are too small to visualize in detail using light microscopy (the area of contact between the two cells is typically less than 1 micrometre across) so they must be visualized using electron microscopy or, more recently, high-resolution confocal microscopy (see Box 5.3).

In the following sections we will examine the general principles that are emerging with regards to the mechanisms by which synapses form. We will focus mainly on the development of synapses in the CNS

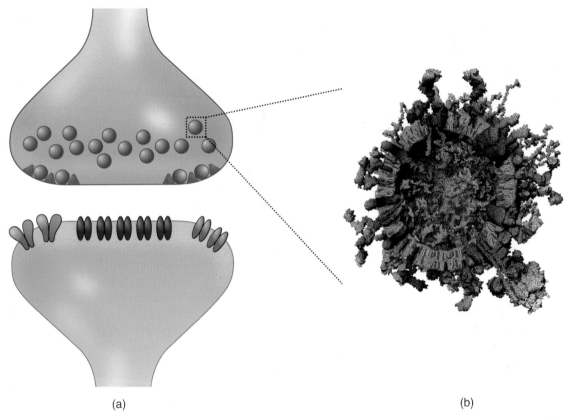

(a)   (b)

Fig. 10.8 The presynaptic vesicle. (a) Schematic showing a synapse and the location of the presynaptic vesicles. (b) Enlargement of a prototypical presynaptic vesicle that has been reconstructed from a detailed protein characterization of its associated proteins. Synaptic vesicles are far from being simple lipid bilayers containing neurotransmitter. Instead they are highly complex organelles whose molecular structure is key to their essential role in neuronal communication. (Reprinted from Cell, **127**, Takamori S. *et al.*, Molecular Anatomy of a Trafficking Organelle, 831–46, 2006, with permission from Elsevier).

although many parallels can be drawn with the development of a highly specialized synapse between neurons and muscle (i.e. the **neuromuscular junction**, see Box 10.2). The predominant viewpoint of synaptogenesis that we will consider here, entails **filopodial** outgrowth from the postsynaptic dendrites (Fig. 10.9) and hence is often referred to as the filopodial model (but see other models in Section 10.5.2). In the filopodial model there are three main stages to synapse construction: (i) synapse specification and induction, (ii) synapse formation and (iii) synapse stabilization (Fig. 10.9). During each of these stages, there is crosstalk between the presynaptic axon and the postsynaptic dendrite, but the relative importance of each component in regulating the differentiation of its counterpart structure varies depending on the type of synapse being examined.

filopodia a finger like cellular outgrowth associated with cell shape changes. They are important for migrating cells, growth cones, and dendritic spine formation.

10.4.3 Synaptic specification and induction

The first step in synapse formation involves the choice of a correct target tissue (specification) and the initiation of synapse formation between the presynaptic axon and postsynaptic dendrite or soma (induction). As we saw in Chapter 8, a variety of soluble and membrane

Box 10.2 The vertebrate neuromuscular junction

The synapse that forms between a motor axon and the muscle fibre that it innervates is known as the **neuromuscular junction (NMJ)**. The NMJ has been widely studied for many years, in part because it is much more accessible than synapses in the CNS. Those parts of each cell that contribute to the NMJ synapse are highly functionally specialized. In the presynaptic cell, the motor neuron terminal contains a large number of synaptic vesicles filled with acetylcholine, the neurotransmitter employed at the NMJ, reflecting its key function in neurotransmitter release. The postsynaptic membrane on the muscle fibre contains a high density of acetylcholine receptor molecules, more than $10\,000/\mu m^2$, compared to just $10/\mu m^2$ in the non-synaptic parts of the muscle cell plasma membrane. This highly localized concentration of receptors allows the muscle cell to respond rapidly and reliably to neurotransmitter released from the motor axon terminal.

How is the massive localized increase in acetylcholine receptor density at the NMJ brought about? Experiments in the 1970s demonstrated that incoming axons are able to organize clusters of AChRs when they come into contact with muscle cells. Attempts to identify the factor(s) responsible for this activity led to the discovery of **agrin**, a secreted **proteoglycan** produced by motor axons and released from motor terminals. Agrin is thought to induce clustering of acetylcholine receptors on the surface of muscles that underlie the incoming motor axon terminal.

In addition to clustering of pre-existing acetylcholine receptors, newly synthesised acetylcholine receptor molecules also become incorporated into the postsynaptic domain of the NMJ. During synaptogenesis, the expression of genes that encode acetylcholine receptor subunits is increased in those parts of the muscle that directly underlie the NMJ. At the same time, expression of these genes is repressed in the remainder of the muscle. These localized differences in transcription are controlled by acetylcholine released from the motor axon terminal. The consequent localized increase in acetylcholine receptor synthesis contributes to the greatly increased density of acetylcholine receptors in the postsynaptic membrane of the NMJ.

Factors released from the presynaptic motor neuron, including agrin and acetylcholine, regulate aspects of differentiation of the postsynaptic cell during synaptogenesis. However, the incoming motor axon is not the only factor regulating postsynaptic differentiation. For example, acetylcholine receptors form localized clusters in muscle membranes before the innervating motor axon arrives. These early-forming clusters are thought to be able to become incorporated into functional synapses, but the mechanism(s) that promote this early clustering are as yet unknown.[4]

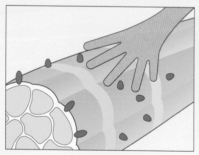 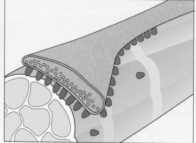

(a) Before innervation, most acetylcholine receptors (green) are distributed widely across the surface of a muscle fibre. (b) During formation of the neuromuscular junction, acetylcholine receptors become clustered at high density at the synapse, while remaining much more sparsely distributed in the rest of the muscle.

proteoglycans extracellular matrix proteins that are heavily modified by the covalent attachment of polysaccharide groups.

associated molecules control axon pathfinding and target selection (such as Slits and ROBO). In many cases, these same molecules also appear to prime neurons for the ability to make synapses but these

[4] More information about development of the neuromuscular junction can be found in: Kummer, T. T., Misgeld, T. and Sanes, J. R. (2006) Assembly of the postsynaptic membrane at the neuromuscular junction: paradigm lost. *Curr Opin. Neurobiol.*, **16**, 74–8.

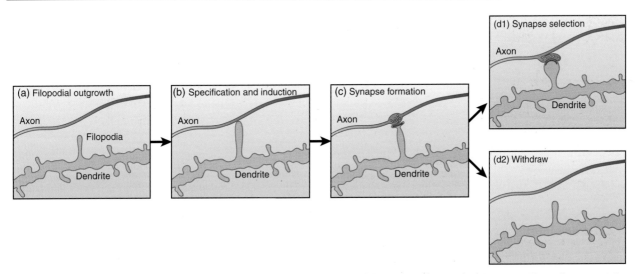

Fig. 10.9 The main steps of synapse formation. (a) Shows the developing dendrite (orange) extending a filopodium towards a passing axon (but see Fig. 10.15 for other modes of spinogenesis). (b) The filopodium makes contact with a passing axon to initiate the specification and induction phase during which a series of molecular interactions determines whether a synapse is formed. (c) During synapse formation the active zone and presynaptic vesicles (yellow) are recruited to the presynaptic membrane as are postsynaptic proteins transported to the tip of the filopodium (red). (d) Once formed, synapses remain plastic and during the final phase of synapse selection, neuronal activity regulates whether a synapse become stable (d1) or is removed (d2).

processes are distinct from the initial specification and induction of synapses within the target tissue. A new set of proteins including cell **adhesion molecules** (e.g. neuroligin, SynCAM), and membrane bound or secreted signalling molecules (e.g. **ephrins**, **Wnts** and **neurotrophins**) play a more direct role in synapse formation. For example, ephrinB has been shown to play a role in the clustering of glutamate receptors at putative synaptic sites, a key first step in the formation of a postsynaptic density. However, perhaps the most studied of the synaptogenesis molecules in the CNS are the neuroligins and their receptors, the neurexins, which have roles in both synaptic specification and induction.

Neuroligins and neurexins are families of transmembrane proteins that are expressed in the dendrites or soma of the postsynaptic neuron and the growth cone of the presynaptic axon, respectively. Neuroligins bind to neurexins to form a bridge between the pre- and postsynaptic membrane. Because both proteins have large intracellular portions capable of binding to other proteins they are perfectly placed to organize the active zone and the postsynaptic density. In fact this is believed to be the principal function of neuroligins and neurexins, to initiate the protein specializations that characterize the synapse (Fig. 10.10).

A key question in synaptogenesis is how presynaptic partners selectively bind to their appropriate postsynaptic partner. For example, while excitatory cells make synapses with axons from both GABAergic (inhibitory) and glutamatergic (excitatory) cells, each synapse type forms on specific parts of the dendrites or soma. For pyramidal cells in the neocortex, GABAergic inputs from a particular type of neuron,

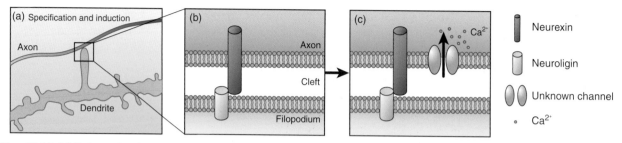

Fig. 10.10 (a) Schematic of synapse specification and induction. (b) High magnification showing that the binding of β-neurexin in the axon with the neuroligin in the dendritic filopodium causes the local influx of calcium into the presynaptic terminal via an as yet unidentified Ca²⁺ channel (c). If this contact is successful, a spine begins to form; if not, the filopodium is quickly retracted.

proximal dendrites regions of the dendrites that are close to the cell soma.

called a basket cell, form on the cell soma and **proximal dendrites**. Inputs from excitatory neurons form further out on the dendritic tree. Furthermore, GABAergic inputs form **symmetric synapses** with relatively small postsynaptic densities, whereas excitatory inputs form **asymmetric synapses** mainly onto dendritic spines with larger postsynaptic densities (Fig. 10.11). The different family members of the

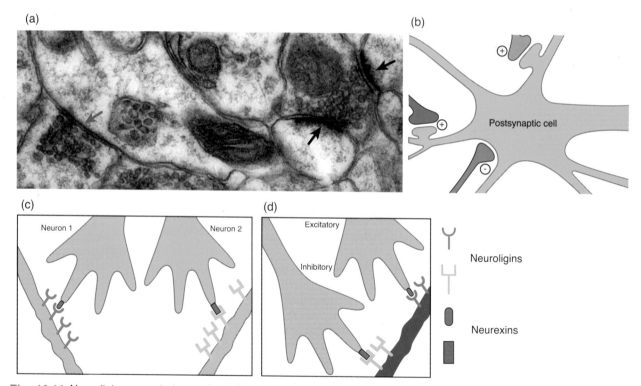

Fig. 10.11 Neuroligin–neurexin interactions determine synapse specificity. Neurons receive excitatory and inhibitory connections often from presynaptic axons from different cell types or different projection neurons. (a) Example electron micrograph showing excitatory (black arrows) and inhibitory synapses (red arrow). Excitatory inputs form asymmetric synapses mainly with dendritic spines that possess a clear postsynaptic density. In contrast, inhibitory synapses mainly form on cell bodies and dendritic shafts, and are distinguishable by the lack of a clear postsynaptic density causing the protein thickening in the presynaptic terminal (i.e. the active zone) to look similar or symmetric to the postsynaptic density. ((b)–(d)) Schematics showing that neurons receive both inhibitory and excitatory synapses (b). During development, specific neurexins expressed on the presynaptic growth cones interact with neuroligin isoforms on the postsynaptic cell (see key) to determine not only the specificity of neuronal connections with their correct partners (c) but also specify GABAergic and glutamatergic synapses (d).

neuroligins and neurexins are important for determining synapse type. For example, neuroligin 1 expression is enhanced in excitatory synapses and neuroligin 2 is present at GABAergic synapses. Over expression of neuroligin 1 or neuroligin 2 in culture increases excitatory or inhibitory synaptic transmission, respectively, indicating that these proteins play a key role in regulating the specification of synapse type (Fig. 10.11).

It is not clear how appropriate contacts form synapses while inappropriate contacts are retracted, but it appears that upon first contact of an axon and dendrite in the hippocampus, Ca^{2+} channels are activated and brief bursts of Ca^{2+} can be observed presynaptically. In some cases these contacts are very short lived, ranging from seconds to a few minutes. In other cases these contacts become stabilized and remain for as long as they can be visualized (more than 1 hour). For those contacts that become stabilized, the Ca^{2+} bursts increase in frequency and synapse formation begins, suggesting a critical role for Ca^{2+}-based excitability in the earliest forms of synaptogenesis. In support of this hypothesis, Ca^{2+} bursts are small and never stabilized at contacts with GABAergic axons, which are inappropriate for this region of the hippocampus.

10.4.4 Synapse formation

This second phase of synaptogenesis occurs, for an individual synapse, over a period of hours to days and is characterized by the molecular elaboration of the presynaptic active zone and postsynaptic density as well as by the recruitment of presynaptic vesicles (Fig. 10.12). The initial stabilization of transient axo-dendritic contacts is mediated by a range of cell adhesion molecules (CAMs) including cadherins, nectins and SynCAM (also discussed in Chapter 6). The cadherins are a family of calcium-dependent cell adhesion molecules found at many CNS synapses. The cytoplasmic domains of cadherins interact with intracellular proteins and the actin cytoskeleton to help stabilize the synapse. The cadherins play a key role in synaptic specification and induction.[5]

Another group of proteins, known as **scaffolding proteins**, are then recruited to the site of membrane contact. As their name implies, the main function of these proteins is to act as bridges between proteins to create protein complexes, such as the presynaptic active zone and the postsynaptic density. A major class of scaffolding proteins are the membrane-associated guanylate kinases (MAGUKs – although the name is misleading since they do not have kinase activity). MAGUKs regulate the formation of both the presynaptic active zone and the postsynaptic density (PSD). Presynaptically, a protein called CASK binds to neurexins to recruit other presynaptic molecules including more scaffolding proteins (such as the homologous multidomain proteins, bassoon and piccolo) as well as presynaptic vesicles. The postsynaptic density protein, PSD-95, and some related MAGUKs bind the neuroligins to recruit neurotransmitter receptors and downstream signalling enzymes. A mature PSD may contain hundreds of proteins. However, it is important to note that neither the PSD nor the

---

[5] For a review of the role of cadherins in synaptogenesis see Arikkath, J. and Reichardt, L. F. (2008) Cadherins and catenins at synapses: roles in synaptogenesis and synaptic plasticity. *Trends Neurosci.*, **31**, 487–94.

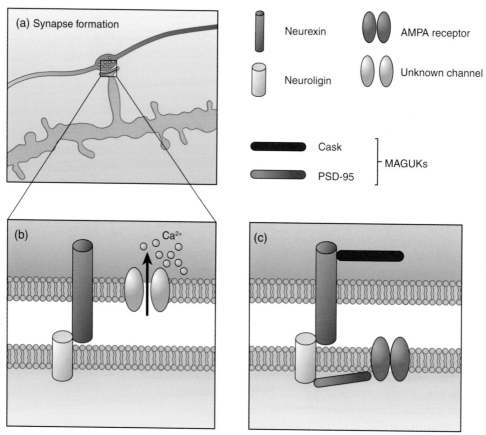

Fig. 10.12 Synapse stabilization. (a) Following the initial contact, and synapse specification and induction (b), the neuroligins and neurexins bind to scaffolding molecules that recruit active zone and PSD proteins (including AMPA receptors, see section 12.2.4), respectively (c). Cadherins also play a key role in linking the PSD to the actin cytoskeleton to help stabilize the synapse (not shown).

presynaptic active zone is a static structure. Instead they are highly dynamic with individual proteins or modules of proteins binding and releasing as activity patterns or developmental stages change. It is the dynamic nature of the PSD that allows activity patterns to alter synaptic development and is believed to be at the heart of learning and memory in mature **neural networks**.

Interestingly there may be a key difference in the way presynaptic and postsynaptic elements form. Postsynaptically it appears that proteins are gradually added singly or in small complexes until an adult, dynamic structure is formed. In contrast, the presynaptic active zone appears to be added en masse by the fusion with the plasma membrane of **transport vesicles** that already contain the protein complexes of the active zone.[6]

neural networks a group of neurons that form a circuit.

transport vesicles membrane-bound organelles that transport proteins to their correct location within a cell.

10.4.5 Synapse selection: stabilization and withdrawal

During the early phase of synaptogenesis, synapses accrue rapidly such that, in rodent cortex, thousands of synapses and dendritic spines per

[6] For further reading on presynaptic construction see Owald, D. and Sigrist, S. J. (2009) Assembling the presynaptic active zone. *Curr. Opin. Neurobiol.*, **19**, 311–8.

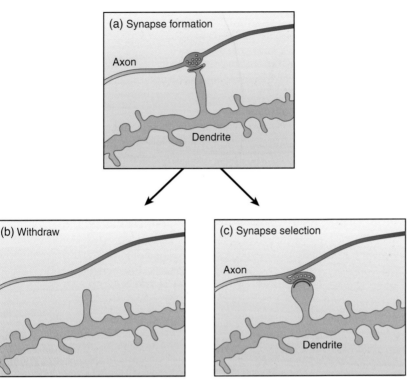

Fig. 10.13 Synapse selection. Once formed (a) synapses remain plastic during development and can be strengthened and stabilized or weakened or withdrawn ((b) and (c)). Synaptic activity and molecular cues play a key role in synapse selection and are covered in Chapters 9 and 12.

neuron are added in a period of one to two weeks. In fact, in many neural systems, there is an overproduction of synapses followed by period of removal or withdrawal (Fig. 10.13). Neuronal activity plays a key role in the stabilization and withdrawal of developing synapses. It is not surprising, therefore, that many of the molecules that affect synapse selection are known to regulate activity patterns at developing synapses. In fact many proteins located in the developing PSD have been shown to regulate synapse number and size. How neuronal activity regulates synaptogenesis will be covered in Chapter 12. However, it is important to note that some synapses in some regions of the brain remain plastic well into adulthood. It is this plasticity of synapses that underlies childhood behavioural development as well as learning and memory in both children and adults.

10.5 Spinogenesis

A key step in the maturation of glutamatergic neurons is the formation of dendritic spines, the anatomical postsynaptic structures that are the site of most excitatory, glutamatergic input. Not all synapses form on spines. Inhibitory, GABAergic synapses onto excitatory neurons occur directly on the cell soma or dendritic shaft rather than on spines. Moreover, in contrast to excitatory neurons, GABAergic cells themselves have few spines, so both excitatory and inhibitory synapses are made on the dendritic shaft and soma.

Box 10.3 Fragile X Syndrome (FXS) and related synaptopathies

Synaptopathies are a group of conditions whose main symptoms are believed to result from altered synaptogenesis that include certain forms of autism, severe learning disability and schizophrenia. Since the sequencing of the human genome, a large number of neurodevelopmental psychiatric conditions have been linked with mutations in particular genes. In some cases mutations that result in the silencing or deletion of a single gene were discovered to be the cause of numerous forms of autism or learning disability, making them particularly amenable to research because of the relative ease with which they can be examined in animal models.

Fragile X Syndrome (FXS) is the most common form of inherited mental retardation. It is caused by the genetic silencing of the fragile X mental retardation gene (*FMR1*), which leads to the absence of the fragile X mental retardation protein (FMRP). FXS is also the most common genetic cause of autism with approximately one third of FXS individuals meeting the clinical diagnosis for autism and almost all FXS individuals meeting the criteria for **autism spectrum disorder (ASD)**. FMRP is an mRNA binding protein that regulates several aspect of mRNA function including mRNA stability, mRNA trafficking to dendrites and local mRNA translation. The most prevalent morphological change in cortical neurons resulting from the loss of FMRP is the increased density of immature spines and filopodia. Many neurons also show altered synaptic plasticity including exaggerated **long-term depression (LTD)** or reduced **long-term potentiation (LTP)** (see Box 12.3). These and other findings have led to the hypothesis that the loss of FMRP results in altered synaptogenesis and these alterations cause the developmental delay in cognitive development observed in FXS individuals.

Drosophila and mouse models have been created that accurately recapitulate many of the anatomical and behavioural phenotypes seen in human patients. Neurons in *Fmr1* knock-out mice show an increase in the density of immature spines as well as alterations in spine plasticity and physiology (see Chapter 12). Furthermore, potential pharmacological treatments have been developed for FXS that, in both mice and flies, prevent and in some cases reverse, abnormal synaptic function and behaviour. Some of these are now in clinical trials. For this reason, many believe that FXS will be a success story of modern day molecular medicine, whereby silencing of a single gene was discovered to be the cause, animal models were generated to model the disease, theories were devised and tested based on the findings from animals models, pharmaceutical compounds were generated based on these theories and are now in clinical trials.

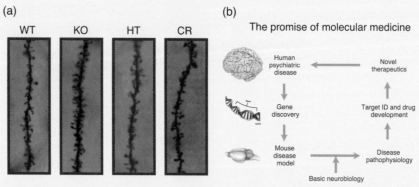

(a) Dendrites of layer 3 pyramidal neurons from wild-type (WT), *Fmr1* knock-out (KO), *Mglur5* heterozygous (HT) and *Fmr1* knock-out/*Mglur5* heterozygous (CR) animals showing that the increase in dendritic spine density on cortical neurons in *Fmr1* knock-out mouse is prevented by genetically reducing mGluR5. (b) Shows the cycle of research that is proving to be the cornerstone for modern day molecular medicine. (b) Reproduced from *Neuron*, **56**, Dölen, G., Osterweil, E., Rao, B. S., Smith, G. B., Auerbach, B. D., Chattarji, S. and Bear, M. F. Correction of fragile X syndrome in mice, 955–62, 2007, with permission from Elsevier. b) Kindly provided by and reproduced with the permission of Mark Bear.

autistic spectrum disorder (ASD) a term used to describe psychological conditions that share abnormalities in social interactions and communication as well as repetitive behaviours.

long-term depression (LTD) a long-term decrease in synaptic strength resulting from uncorrelated activity between pre- and postsynaptic elements.

long-term potentiation (LTP) a long-term increase in synaptic strength resulting from coordinated activity between pre- and postsynaptic elements.

Much more is known about spine development during the formation of glutamatergic synapses on glutamatergic neurons than about the development of GABAergic synapses or the presynaptic development of either type of synapse for several reasons. First, spines can be labelled relatively easily *in vivo* and *in vitro*, and hence are more amenable for study. Secondly, altered spine morphologies have been linked to numerous developmental neurological diseases (see Box 10.3). Finally, spine morphology correlates with the number of **AMPA receptors** in the postsynaptic density (PSD) and hence is believed to be an effective read-out of synaptic function.

10.5.1 Spine shape and dynamics

Dendritic spines have been subdivided into up to 16 distinct categories based on their shape. However, there are three main types: mushroom, long-thin and stubby (Fig. 10.14). **Mushroom** spines are mature spines, with a spine head that can be clearly defined from the shaft or spine neck. In contrast, immature spines are classifed as **long-thin** spines with small heads and **stubby** spines with short bulbous protrusions on a dendritic shaft that show no evidence of a spine neck. Spine head size is closely linked to the size of the PSD, and hence the number of neurotransmitter receptors and strength of the synapse. The likely precursors to spines are dendritic **filopodia** (as mentioned in Chapter 7). They are generally referred to as dendritic processes rather than spines since it is not known whether they contain PSD proteins.

Not surprisingly the rapid phases of synaptogenesis and spinogenesis are closely correlated and both processes are highly dynamic. Recent advances in confocal microscopy (Box 10.4) have demonstrated that during development, dendritic spines show rapid formation and withdrawal that is regulated, in part, by changing activity patterns of the developing neural circuit. Therefore, like synaptogenesis, the various stages of spine formation (outlined below) are seen throughout development as appropriate synapses are stabilized and inappropriate ones are removed.

In vivo pertaining to the context of the intact organism.

In vitro pertaining to experiments conducted outside the organism.

AMPA receptor a type of glutamate receptor that is responsible for the majority of the initial depolarization of the excitatory postsynaptic potential following activation of an excitatory synapse.

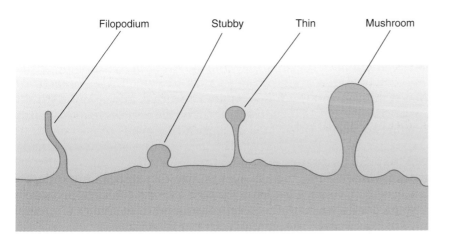

Filopodium   Stubby   Thin   Mushroom

Fig. 10.14 Morphology of filopodia and dendritic spines are closely linked to their function. Filopodia are immature protrusions that sample incoming axons and can be thought of as precursors of dendritic spines. Long-thin spines are immature or weakened forms of spines that have fewer neurotransmitter receptors in their PSD. Mushroom-shaped spines are characterized by a long-thin spine neck and a larger spine head. The shape is believed to be crucial to spine function with the thin spine neck isolating the physiological identity of individual spines.

Box 10.4 Confocal microscopy and spine dynamics

Arguably the single biggest technical advance to influence our knowledge of spinogenesis was the development of two-photon confocal microscopy. This form of fluorescent microscopy was pioneered by Winfried Denk in the 1990s and has allowed the high-resolution imaging of individual spines over time in the cerebral cortex of living animals and in cultured or **acute slices** from brain tissue. Until this time, spines could only be analysed post-mortem, giving a freeze-frame of spine density and shape at the moment of death. Scientists are now able to image spines on cortical cells in the somatosensory cortex of mice while individual whiskers are being stimulated. These types of studies have demonstrated that developing spines are incredibly motile, being able to change shape, appear or disappear over tens of minutes. Although there is still much to learn, there is emerging evidence that altered spine motility may be a principal problem in many development brain disorders, such as FXS (see Box 10.3), that involve alterations in spine density and shape.

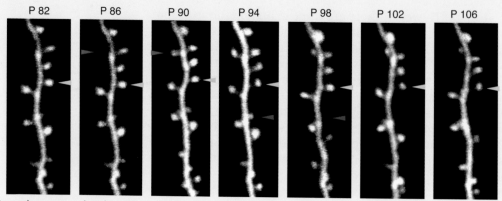

Two-photon microscopy showing the dynamics of spine morphology *in vivo*. Individual frames from time-lapse imaging of spine dynamics from layer 3 pyramidal neurons in the visual cortex of the mouse. Some spines remain stable (yellow arrowheads) throughout the imaging period (P = postnatal day) while others are added and remain (red) and some are added and subsequently withdrawn (blue). Reprinted by permission from Macmillan Publishers Ltd: *Nature*. Hofer, S. B., Mrsic-Flogel, T. D., Bonhoeffer, T. and Hübener, M. Experience leaves a lasting structural trace in cortical circuits. **457**, 313–7, copyright, 2009.

acute slices thin sections taken from a brain (or brain region) immediately after sacrificing an animal in order to keep the cells alive, generally for physiological recording or live cell imaging.

10.5.2 Theories of spinogenesis

There have been numerous theories about how spines develop. These differ notably in the role of the dendritic filopodia and presynaptic terminals in regulating spine formation (Fig. 10.15). As we have seen above, one model suggests that filopodia on postsynaptic dendrites contact axons that are growing past (*en passant*). These contacts are then stabilized and the filopodia are converted into spines with the tips of the filopodia expanding to form heads as postsynaptic density proteins are added. Other models suggest that axons contact dendritic shafts directly and these contacts *initiate* spine formation. Such a model could explain the presence of stubby spines. Stubby spines are also immature. Finally, some models hypothesize that spines form independently of axon contact. Evidence for such a model comes from analysis of spine development in the **cerebellum** and from studies of mutant mice such as *weaver, shaker* and *reeler* (see Chapter 6).

cerebellum meaning 'little brain' is a discrete structure at the base of the brain that lies above the brain-stem. It regulates a range of functions including motor control, attention and cognition.

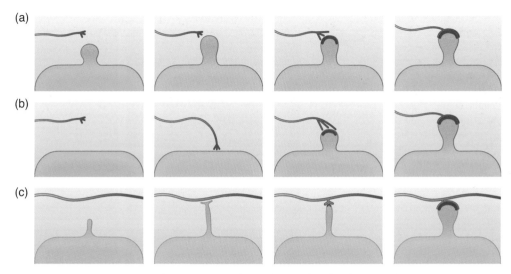

Fig. 10.15 Models of spine development. There are several models of spine development that focus on the relative involvement of the pre- and postsynaptic terminals. (a) One model supposes that dendritic spines develop and elaborate independent of presynaptic terminals. This model appears to explain spine development in the cerebellum (see below). (b) Another model hypothesizes that axons contact dendritic shafts and spines mature gradually from these sites of contact. (c) Finally, the filopodial model, which appears to be the principal mode of spinogenesis in the forebrain, hypothesizes that the dendrites elaborate filopodia that contact axons to initiate synapse formation. This filopodial model is the most prevalent model (see Fig. 10.9). Adapted by permission from Macmillan Publisher Ltd: Nature Reviews: Neuroscience. Yuste, R. and Bonhoeffer, T. Genesis of dendritic spines: insights form ultrastructural and imaging studies. **5**, 24–34; 2004.

10.5.3 Mouse models of spinogenesis: the weaver mutant

In the **weaver** mouse the gene encoding a potassium channel (*Girk2*) has been mutated. Studies of this mouse found that cerebellar **granule neurons** fail to migrate properly and make synapses with their targets, the **Purkinje neurons**. In *weaver* mutants the dendritic tree of Purkinje neurons is reduced in size and complexity, but the remaining dendrites are covered in spines, despite the fact that they have lost their major input. A similar result was found for the **reeler** mouse in which part of the cerebellum develops with ectopic Purkinje neurons and many fewer granule cells (see Fig. 6.17). Again, these Purkinje neurons develop a large number of spines on their dendritic trees despite the lack of synapse formation. Hence, for cerebellar Purkinje neurons, spines can develop in the absence of presynaptic partners (Fig. 10.16) providing evidence for the model shown in Fig. 10.15(a). It is important to note that these models are not mutually exclusive. While it appears that different cell types may use different mechanisms as the main mode of spinogenesis, the use of multiple mechanisms by a single cell type cannot be ruled out.

granule cells small neurons, with a diameter of around 10um found in large numbers in the granule layer of the cerebellum.

10.5.4 Molecular regulators of spine development

At a molecular level, numerous proteins have been shown to regulate the development of dendritic spines. These include diffusible factors, cell-adhesion molecules and proteins that regulate neuronal activity – most notably neurotransmitter receptors and their downstream signalling complexes. Overall these regulators of

Fig. 10.16 Spine development in the *weaver* mouse. In *weaver* mice a K⁺ channel is mutated resulting in the complete loss of **parallel fibres**, the main presynaptic partner for Purkinje neuron dendrites. (a) and (b) Despite the loss of their main synaptic target, Purkinje neurons elaborate a dendritic tree although the overall size is reduced. More surprising is the fact that spine density in the *weaver* mouse (d) appears very similar to that found in Wild-type mice (c). Therefore, spinogenesis in the cerebellum can occur in the absence of presynaptic partners, indicating a minor role for the presynaptic terminal in regulating spine density (Fig. 10.15a). Images kindly provided by John O'Brien and Nigel Unwin (some of which appeared in O'Brien, J. and Unwin, N. (2005) Organization of spines on the dendrites of Purkinje cells. *PNAS*, **103**, 1575–1580). Information on the diolistics technique used here to label these cells can be found at www.genegunbarrels.com [22 November 2010].

parallel fibres axons from the granule cells in the cerebellum that run parallel to the pial surface in the molecular layer where they form synapses with Purkinje cell dendrites.

knock-out an organism that has been engineered to carry genes that have been made inoperative.

knock-down to reduce the levels of an mRNA or protein.

Wild-type   Weaver

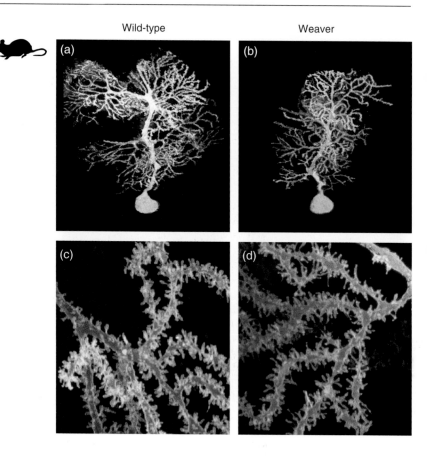

spinogenesis can be subdivided into two main categories: those that promote spine maturation and those that inhibit spine maturation. The role of particular proteins in spinogenesis has largely been elucidated by studying genetic **knock-out** (or **knock-down**) mice (See Chapter 1, Section 1.5.4 and Fig. 1.7) or overexpression of particular proteins followed by examination of spine morphology. For example, knock-out of an inhibitor of spinogenesis may lead to the premature appearance of large, mushroom spines. This is precisely what is seen in mice lacking SynGAP (synaptic GTPase activating protein), a key signalling protein in the PSD. In contrast, genetically removing a promoter of spine development may result in the overproduction of immature spines or filopodia as is seen in mice lacking **FMRP** (Fragile X mental retardation protein – see Fig. 10.17 and Box 10.3). Interestingly, genetic disruption of either promoters or inhibitors of spine maturation often results in severe learning difficulties or other developmental neurological disorders in humans, suggesting the rate at which spine development proceeds is critical for normal neuronal communication.[7]

---

[7] Boda, B., Dubos, A. and Muller, D. (2010) Signalling mechanisms regulating synapse formation and function in mental retardation. *Curr. Opin. Neurobiol.*, **20**, 519–27.

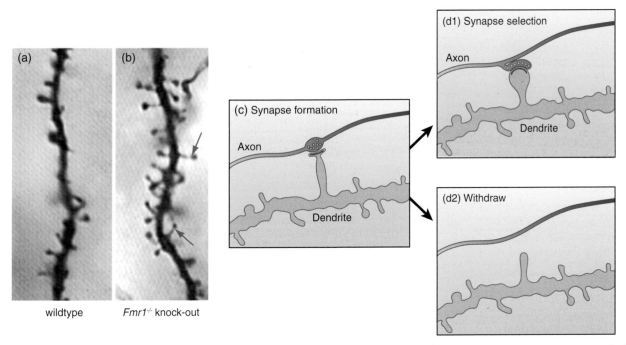

Fig. 10.17 Mice lacking the Fragile X mental retardation protein (FMRP, see Box 10.3). A segment of dendrite from a cortical neuron from a wild-type (a) and an *Fmr1* knock-out (b) animal. *Fmr1* knock-out neurons exhibit a preponderance of immature filopodia and long-thin spines (red arrows) indicating that FMRP normally acts to regulate spine maturation. Recently, mutations in several synaptic genes, including *Fmr1*, have been shown to result in severe learning disability and autism spectrum disorder. These genes all appear to share a role in spine formation (c) and selection (d1) (d2).

10.6 Summary

- The development of neuronal function is a complex process that involves the development of intrinsic neuronal properties such as the acquisition of ion channels and pumps as well as the development of appropriate connectivity.
- Early neuronal excitability plays a key role in CNS development, even before the formation of synapses.
- Synaptogenesis can be subdivided into discrete stages of specification and induction, synapse formation and synapse selection.
- Numerous postsynaptic and presynaptic processes and molecules work together to regulate the timing of synaptogenesis. Mutations in these proteins lead to a range of clinical syndromes, including severe learning disability, autism and schizophrenia.
- Dendritic spines are the main sites of excitatory synapses onto excitatory cells. There are several models of spine formation, but the filopodial model is the most prevalent for CNS neurons. Altered spine density and morphology is a prevalent phenotype in many forms of developmental disorders.

Life and Death in the Developing Nervous System

11

11.1 The frequency and function of cell death during normal development

Most people might associate cell death with pathological processes resulting from injuries or diseases that kill cells by depriving them of oxygen or exposing them to toxins that inhibit metabolism. It might seem odd, therefore, to find a discussion of cell death in a book about the physiological mechanisms controlling normal neural development. In fact, we have known for many decades that cell death is widespread during normal development of both neural and non-neural tissues.

An astonishing amount of cell death occurs in normal developing animal tissues: in the developing vertebrate nervous system, as many as 50% of nerve cells normally die soon after they are formed. What is the function of this naturally-occurring cell death? In some non-neural tissues its functions are particularly obvious. In some cases, cell death is essential for generating the shapes of tissues. For example, digits are sculpted through the action of localized cell death at precise moments during normal limb formation: mouse paws begin as spade-like structures within which individual digits separate because the cells between them die. In other cases, cells die when the structure they form is no longer needed. Spectacular examples of this are found during metamorphosis of insect larvae and tadpoles. For example, when a tadpole changes into a frog cells in the tail die and the tail disappears.

Similarly, in the developing nervous system, cell death is important for sculpting tissues during morphogenesis, for removing sets of cells that carry out transient functions that are no longer needed and for ensuring that each region has an appropriate number of neurons. For example, the shape of the normal mammalian brain is formed by processes that include the death of many of its cells; the development of persistent neuronal circuitry is often guided by transient circuitry acting as a scaffold that is later removed; cell death adjusts the numbers of nerve cells in neural tissues to match the numbers of cells in the target regions that they innervate. The importance of cell death for normal neural development is illustrated by the fact that severe defects

Building Brains: An Introduction to Neural Development, First Edition.
David Price, Andrew Jarman, John Mason and Peter Kind.
© 2011 John Wiley & Sons, Ltd. Published 2011 by John Wiley & Sons, Ltd.

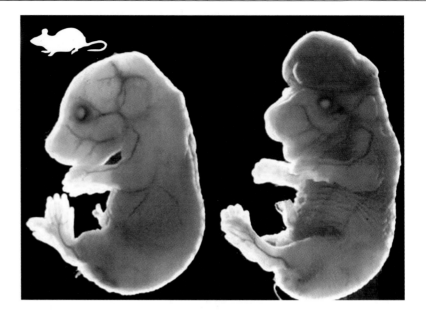

Fig. 11.1 Photographs of two mouse embryos: the embryo on the left is normal whereas the embryo on the right lacks the enzyme caspase 9, which is needed for normal cell death. The mutant embryo is highly abnormal with an expanded brain protruding from the head, known as exencephaly, showing that normal cell death is vital for correct development. (Reprinted from Kuida, K., Haydar, T. F., Kuan, C. Y., Gu, Y., Taya, C., Karasuyama, H., Su, M. S., Rakic, P. and Flavell, R. A. (1998) Reduced apoptosis and cytochrome c-mediated caspase activation in mice lacking caspase 9. *Cell*, **94** 325–337 with permission from Elsevier.)

of neural development occur if cell death is blocked, for example by making transgenic mice carrying mutations in genes required for cell death (Fig. 11.1: these genes will be discussed later in this chapter). These defects include failure of neural tube closure, overgrowth of the brain's proliferative zones and disordered differentiation.

Where cells are no longer needed, they effectively commit suicide by activating an intracellular death program, a process known as **programmed cell death**. Clearly, control over such a potently lethal intracellular program is essential for an organism's normal development, survival and well-being. Many diseases are associated with breakdown in the normal regulation of programmed cell death (Box 11.1).

Box 11.1 Diseases associated with defective programmed cell death

Understanding the mechanisms of programmed cell death is likely to help explain and treat some human diseases. Abnormalities in programmed cell death are associated with a broad range of human diseases, including cancers and neurodegenerative disorders. For example, genes that prevent programmed cell death from occurring are often overactive in cancer and this is likely to contribute to uncontrolled growth. In neurodegenerative diseases, the progressive loss of neurons is often due to the occurrence of deregulated programmed cell death. In a neurogenetic degenerative disease called Huntington's chorea, for example, neurons which seem to function normally for decades in the **basal ganglia** and cerebral cortex suddenly start to die, often in middle age. Why neurons die is unknown and the disease is currently incurable. Similarly, pathological programmed cell death can affect neurons that have functioned normally for many years in the cerebral cortex (causing Alzheimer's disease), in the **substantia nigra** (causing Parkinson's disease) and in the motor neuron pool of the spinal cord (causing amyotrophic lateral sclerosis, sometimes known as Lou Gehrig's disease). Why do certain neurons suddenly start dying? If we can understand the molecular events that activate and mediate programmed cell death it might be possible to interrupt them, offering the remarkable therapeutic possibility of rescuing the dying brain and spinal cord in these types of disorder.

To understand the mechanisms of naturally-occurring programmed cell death we need to know when and where it occurs, how cells recognize that they are not needed and the nature of their intracellular death program. In general, we know more about when and where cell death occurs during development and about the molecular pathways by which cells kill themselves than we do about the mechanisms that determine whether a cell lives or dies. However, before discussing these issues we shall describe the distinguishing cellular features of programmed cell death and how they differ from the features of pathological cell death.

11.2 Cells die in one of two main ways: apoptosis or necrosis

Seminal work by John Kerr, Andrew Wyllie and Alastair Currie in Aberdeen in the early 1970s distinguished between two types of cell death, called **apoptosis** and **necrosis** (Fig. 11.2).[1] In the context of this book, apoptosis is by far the most important. The term apoptosis was derived from a Greek word meaning dropping off of leaves from a tree and is often used synonymously with programmed cell death. Necrosis is a pathological process resulting from overwhelming cellular injury. Other types of cell death have been described but to what extent they are variations of these two major types is not yet clear.

The early features of apoptosis include the disintegration of intercellular junctions and condensations of the cytoplasm. Cells undergoing apoptosis shrivel up and lumps of condensed **chromatin** aggregate in the nucleus (Fig. 11.2 and photograph in Box 11.2), which later splits into a number of membrane-bound fragments. These are cleared away by specialized scavenger cells in the vicinity (in the nervous system these are called **microglia**). These nuclear changes are energy-dependent, reflecting the fact that they are caused by changes in the expression of specific genes that dismantle the cell, for example those encoding endonucleases that disrupt nuclear DNA. It is the DNA cleavage that allows detection of apoptotic cells by the TUNEL method described in Box 11.2.

Necrosis (Fig. 11.2) is characterized at early stages by swelling of the cytoplasm and of cytoplasmic organelles, including mitochondria. This is followed by disintegration of these organelles and the breaking of intercellular junctions, separating affected cells from their neighbours. Later, the nucleus swells and ruptures at around the same time as the cell membrane, releasing cytotoxic cellular components that induce tissue damage and inflammation. These events are thought to be precipitated by injury or disease causing changes in the permeability of the cell membrane, leading to a loss of control over cell volume. The process becomes irreversible once there is significant damage to mitochondrial structure and function and the

chromatin DNA wrapped up with histone proteins in the nucleus.

[1] Kerr, J.F., Wyllie, A.H. and Currie, A.R. (1972) Apoptosis: a basic biological phenomenon with wide-ranging implications in tissue kinetics. *British Journal of Cancer*, **26**, 239–57.

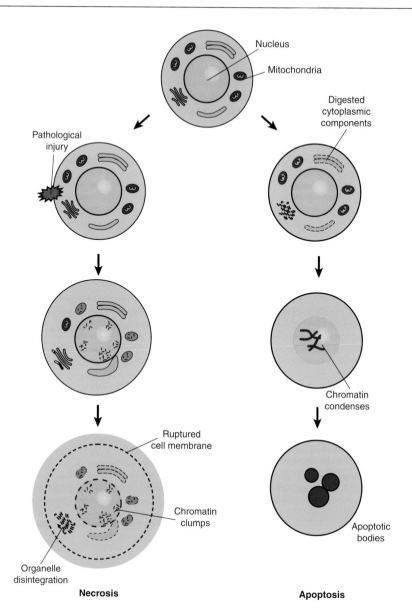

Fig. 11.2 Major distinguishing features of necrosis and apoptosis. Necrosis (on the left) is caused by disruption to the cell as a result of injury or disease: organelles swell and disintegrate, chromatin clumps and the cell membrane ruptures. In apoptosis (on the right), a well-controlled chain of catabolic reactions controlled by specialized enzymes digests cytoplasmic components and fragments nuclear DNA, the cell shrinks and chromatin condenses, resulting in the formation of small membrane-bound apoptotic bodies (see also Box 11.2).

lysosome a membrane-bound organelle containing enzymes found in the cytoplasm of most cells.

lysosomes rupture, releasing their enzymes into the cytoplasm of the cell where they catalyse its destruction.

Apoptosis and necrosis are probably not completely distinct. For example, the breakdown of proteins and cellular organelles by enzymes of the lysosome, referred to as autophagy, is intimately associated with naturally-occurring programmed cell death in invertebrates such as *C. elegans* and *Drosophila*. In these species autophagy is thought to be a mechanism precipitating programmed cell death during normal development. In mammals, on the other hand, autophagy is thought to be primarily an important way in which cells recycle their constituents rather than a mechanism of cell death. Autophagy is essential for normal development in all species, probably because it allows the large-scale turnover of cellular constituents required for processes like proliferation, migration and differentiation. Defects of

Box 11.2   The TUNEL method

The TUNEL method detects breaks in the cell's DNA made at an early stage in programmed cell death; in normal cells there are very few such breaks and they are repaired rapidly. (a) TUNEL stands for Terminal deoxynucleotidyl transferase dUTP Nick End Labelling and it identifies apoptotic cells in tissues or in cultures by using the enzyme terminal deoxynucleotidyl transferase to transfer labelled dUTP to breaks in the DNA strands. The label on the dUTP is then detected in a second reaction that, for example, generates a coloured or fluorescent signal. (b) Here, TUNEL has been applied to mammalian neurons in culture resulting in yellow fluorescence from those that are undergoing programmed cell death (a non-specific stain has been used to colour all cells orange); (c) a DNA stain for the nuclei of the same cells as in (b) showing that the nuclei of the TUNEL-positive cells (the dying cells) are small and bright, an appearance that is characteristic of chromatin condensation, whereas the other cells have larger less brightly stained nuclei.

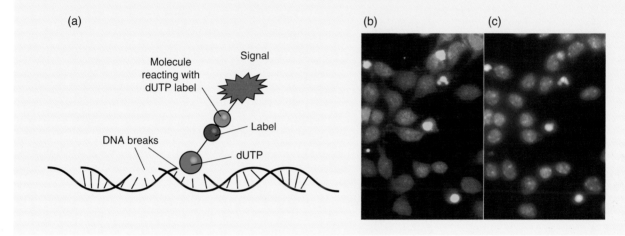

autophagy in humans are likely to cause degenerative disease by precipitating abnormal cell death.[2]

11.3 Studies in invertebrates have taught us much about how cells kill themselves

We now know a great deal about the molecular genetic pathway that results in the dismantling of those cells that are triggered to die for whatever reason. Our knowledge extends from invertebrates to humans and has arisen largely as a result of work on *C. elegans* (Section 1.4.2 in Chapter 1). The field was pioneered by work in this species because it has two key advantages.

First, it is relatively easy to observe cells undergoing programmed cell death in normal living *C. elegans*, since changes in the appearance of dying cells allow their detection using standard microscopy (Fig. 11.3). The **lineages** of all the cells in *C. elegans* have been worked

lineage the sequence of divisions that generated a cell, in other words its cellular ancestry.

[2] For a more detailed description of autophagy in development, see Cecconi, F. and Levine, B. (2008) The role of autophagy in mammalian development: cell makeover rather than cell death. *Developmental Cell*, **15**, 344–357.

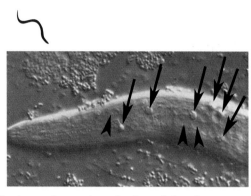
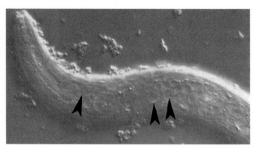

Fig. 11.3 *C. elegans* larvae viewed using a light microscope; the one on the left contains several dead cells (called corpses), which are round and appear raised (indicated by arrows). Arrowheads point to some examples of living cells, which can be seen faintly in both. The animal on the right lacks a normal apoptosis-promoting gene *ced-3*, which is why dead cells are not seen. Reprinted from Ellis, H. M. and Horvitz, H. R. (1986) Genetic control of programmed cell death in the nematode *C. elegans*. *Cell*, **44**, 817–29 with permission from Elsevier.

signal transduction a process in which intercellular signalling, involving the binding of a ligand to its specific receptor, activates a set of intracellular reactions.

adaptor proteins usually lack any enzymatic activity but mediate specific interactions between other proteins in intracellular signalling cascades by promoting the formation of protein complexes.

out and we now know that precisely 131 of its 1090 cells undergo programmed cell death; we know which cells die and when and where they die.

Secondly, unlike in many other animals, genetic manipulations designed to test the molecular basis of programmed cell death in *C. elegans* can modulate cell death without compromising the viability of the whole animal, allowing greater scope for analysing the results of the manipulations. Interestingly, if cells normally fated to die are prevented from dying, the majority become neurons, suggesting that cell death might act to limit the numbers of neurons produced.

The process by which cells go through programmed cell death in *C. elegans* has been divided into three stages: (1) in the specification phase, cells are instructed to undergo programmed cell death; (2) in the killing phase, the apoptotic program is activated; (3) during the engulfment phase, cells are dismantled and engulfed by neighbouring cells. Early work showed that mutations in two genes, called *ced-1* and *ced-2* (standing for *cell-death abnormal-1* and *-2*[3]), result in the accumulation of dead cells by disrupting the engulfment phase. The *ced-1* and *ced-2* genes encode different types of molecule involved in the interaction of the engulfing cell with the apoptotic cell: CED-1 is a membrane protein while CED-2 is an intracellular protein essential for **signal transduction** (it is an example of an **adaptor protein**). Thus, *ced* genes (of which there are other examples given below) are defined on the basis of the abnormal phenotypes produced by their mutation rather than by their normal molecular functions. Identification of *ced-1* and *ced-2* was a first step in identifying many other genes involved in apoptosis and unravelling molecular mechanisms underlying all three phases of programmed cell death in this and other species.

---

[3] The names of these genes reflect the nature of the abnormalities seen in mutant *C. elegans* lines from which the genes were originally identified in forward genetic screens (see Chapter 1, Section 1.4).

11.3.1 The specification phase

It appears that most of the cells that die in *C. elegans* are programmed to this fate from the time of their birth. This contrasts with higher animals in which the triggering of much cell death is attributed to extracellular signals (discussed further below). Current evidence indicates that in cells destined to survive, expression of the death-promoting gene *egl-1* (standing for *egg-laying defective-1*) is low while in the cells destined to die, *egl-1* expression is high. Control of *egl-1* expression is exerted by networks of **transcription factors** whose expression varies from cell to cell and is determined in each specific cell by its lineage. EGL-1 protein acts within the cell by interacting directly with, and inhibiting, the mitochondrial protein CED-9 (which itself promotes survival, discussed below). Thus, cells expressing high levels of *egl-1* die because of changes in the activities of members of the *ced* family, as outlined in the next section.

transcription factors proteins that bind to DNA to regulate gene transcription.

11.3.2 The killing phase

The genes *egl-1*, *ced-3*, *ced-4* and *ced-9* control the activation of programmed cell death in *C. elegans*. Activation of *egl-1*, *ced-3* and *ced-4* promotes apoptosis, whereas activation of *ced-9* protects against apoptosis. These genes act in a genetic pathway shown in Fig. 11.4: *egl-1* inhibits the action of *ced-9* by binding to CED-9 protein, relieving CED-9's

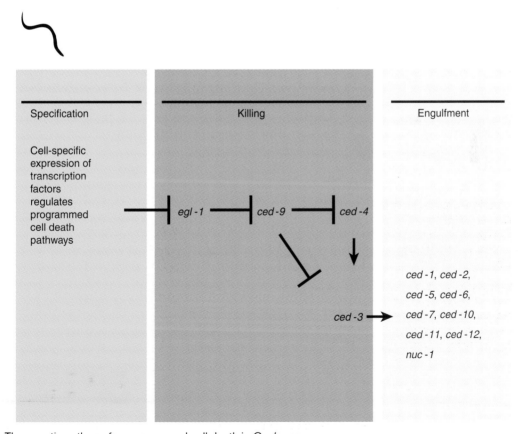

Fig. 11.4 The genetic pathway for programmed cell death in *C. elegans*.

protease an enzyme that breaks down proteins.

inhibition of the apoptosis-promoting genes *ced-4* and *ced-3*. CED-3 is a **protease** whereas CED-4's mechanism of action is still unclear.

11.3.3 The engulfment phase

During the engulfment phase, dying cells undergo morphological changes, their DNA is degraded, and they are recognized by neighbours that engulf them. The morphological changes that occur in the dying cell and the degradation of its DNA are regulated by genes including *ced-11* and *nuc-1* respectively (*ced-11* is thought to encode an ion channel; *nuc-1* encodes a <u>**nuclease**</u>). Dying cells express *ced-7*, which encodes a molecule that marks them as dying cells and allows engulfing cells to recognize them. This recognition is possible because engulfing cells express CED-1, as mentioned above, which is a receptor for the CED-7 protein. During engulfment, the engulfing cell changes its shape and this is achieved by the actions of *ced-2*, *ced-5*, *ced-10* and *ced-12*, which encode proteins involved in **intracellular signalling**.

nuclease a type of enzyme that breaks down nucleic acids such as DNA.

intracellular signalling the process (and molecules) that mediate a cell's response to an extracellular signal.

11.4 Most of the genes that regulate programmed cell death in *C. elegans* are conserved in vertebrates

Most of the genes involved in the killing and engulfment phases of programmed cell death in *C. elegans* have counterparts in vertebrates, all the way through to humans (Fig. 11.5). The killer gene *ced-3* encodes an enzyme called a **caspase** and was the first enzyme of its type shown to have a function in programmed cell death. Caspases are <u>cysteine-aspartic</u> acid <u>proteases</u> that exist in cells as inactive forms that are cleaved proteolytically to generate active enzymes following the

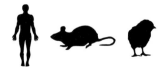

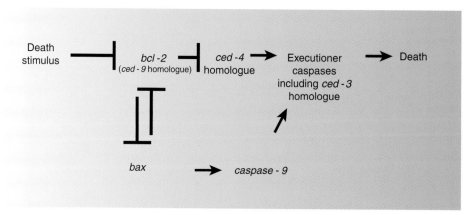

Fig. 11.5 Simplified versions of the vertebrate cell death pathways. Many more molecules are involved than are included here. By stripping away the complexity, the diagram stresses the similarity of this pathway with that of *C. elegans* (Fig. 11.4).

induction of apoptosis. The discovery of the protease *ced-3* in *C. elegans* led to the identification of many caspases that act in apoptosis in invertebrates and vertebrates. The protein encoded by *ced-3* was discovered to have properties similar to mammalian interleukin-1-beta converting enzyme (or ICE), which is now known as caspase 1. Subsequently, other mammalian caspases were identified and numbered in the order in which they were found. About a dozen caspases have been identified in humans and some are involved primarily in apoptosis while others are involved primarily in other processes such as inflammation. Those involved in apoptosis fall into two functional types: initiator caspases and executioner caspases. These caspases act in a molecular cascade: initiator caspases activate executioner caspases by cleaving them and executioner caspases then cleave other cellular proteins. The cascade is regulated by caspase inhibitors. An example of what happens to brain development if caspases are not produced was shown earlier, in Fig. 11.1.

Activation of executioner caspases results in the cleavage of key cellular proteins, causing the cytoplasmic and nuclear changes typical of apoptosis. A characteristic feature of apoptosis is the cleavage of chromosomal DNA into **nucleosomal** units (see Box 3.2 in Chapter 3): caspases contribute to this process by regulating caspase-activated DNase (or CAD), by inhibiting DNA repair enzymes and by breaking down structural proteins in the nucleus. The enzyme poly(ADP-ribose) polymerase (or PARP), which was one of the first molecules to be identified as a substrate for caspases, is normally involved in the repair of damaged DNA and its actions are prevented following cleavage by caspase-3. Proteins that maintain the structure of the nucleus, such as lamins, are degraded by caspase-6, resulting in the chromatin condensation and nuclear fragmentation that is observed in apoptotic cells (Fig. 11.2).

The *C. elegans* gene *ced-9*, which protects against apoptosis, encodes a protein similar to that encoded by the **proto-oncogene** *bcl-2*, which prevents apoptosis in mammals and whose product is a protein integral to the membranes of the endoplasmic reticulum, nuclear envelope and mitochondria. The mammalian gene's name derives from its association with B-cell lymphoma. Since its discovery, 25 other genes have been found in the same family. Their products govern the permeability of the outer mitochondrial membrane. Only some family members protect against apoptosis whereas others, such as Bax (Bcl-2-associated X protein), promote apoptosis. Much research is still going on to understand how this family of proteins suppresses or promotes apoptosis, particularly in view of its importance for human disease; current hypotheses focus on the possibility that through actions on the membranes of mitochondria and possibly other organelles they control cytoplasmic pH and levels of cytochrome c and calcium, which regulate the activities of caspases. How the expression of these molecules is regulated remains enigmatic.[4]

proto-oncogene a normal gene, commonly involved in controlling cell proliferation, that has the potential to promote the formation of a tumour when disregulated by mutation, overexpression or misexpression.

---

[4] For further reading on this topic, see De Zio, D., Giunta, L., Corvaro, M., Ferraro, E. and Cecconi, F. (2005) Expanding roles of programmed cell death in mammalian neurodevelopment. *Semin. Cell Dev. Biol.*, **16**, 281–94.

11.5 Examples of neurodevelopmental processes in which programmed cell death plays a prominent role

Many good examples could be used to illustrate where and when programmed cell death plays a prominent role during neural development and it is not possible to cover them all here. Indeed, it is likely that programmed cell death plays at least some role in almost all aspects of neural development. The examples in this section cover major phases of neural development in vertebrates.

Some of the examples give insights into ways in which programmed cell death might be *triggered* in vertebrates. This is an important issue about which we still know relatively little. In vertebrates it is likely that many triggers originate external to the cell rather than from the cell's own lineage. This contrasts with many (but certainly not all) cases of cell death in invertebrates such as *C. elegans*, where the cell's lineage is often very important in determining whether it survives or dies, as mentioned above.

11.5.1 Programmed cell death in early progenitor cell populations

neural progenitor defined in this book as a cell that divides to give daughter cells, some of which will differentiate as neural cells. Progenitor cells are often multipotent. Cf precursor.

Programmed cell death has been observed even during the early stages of neural development within populations of proliferating **neural progenitors** in a range of organisms from *C. elegans* to mouse. Why this occurs and how it is regulated is not understood. The dying cells have not migrated, elaborated axons, or formed synapses before they die. Perhaps they die because they make errors during their cell division and/or perhaps there are as yet unknown ways in which the developing nervous system cuts back on initially overproduced progenitor cells to achieve the correct numbers. There might be advantages for a system that first produces too many progenitors: if errors do occur in some cells their removal might be possible without reducing the numbers of remaining healthy cells below what is needed.

An interesting example of cell death affecting progenitor cells is found in the proliferative zones of the developing rodent cerebral cortex. This example illustrates some of the practical problems involved in working out how many cells die in a developing tissue. Early estimates based on counting cells that were very obviously apoptotic suggested that only a few percent of cortical progenitors die. The development of very sensitive methods for the detection of cells that might be in the earliest stages of programmed cell death led to a dramatic upwards revision of these early estimates. The new estimates suggested that astonishingly large proportions of progenitors undergo programmed cell death – about 50–70% on some gestational days. The new estimates were based on techniques for detecting breaks in the DNA of cells (Box 11.2). Such breaks occur in cells in the very early stages of programmed cell death. What is not clear, however, is whether all cells with DNA breaks eventually die, or whether only some die, and how much time elapses after DNA breaks appear before cells die and their debris is cleared away. While it is widely accepted that many cells in the proliferative zones of the rodent cerebral cortex die during normal development, the issue of how many die remains controversial.

11.5.2 Programmed cell death contributes to sexual differences in the nervous system

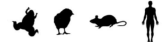

The sexes of many animals, including humans and other vertebrates, have important differences in the structure of their nervous systems as well as their behaviour. In other words, the nervous system exhibits **sexual dimorphism**. In vertebrates, these differences are generated during development through the influence of the circulating steroid hormone testosterone. Testosterone masculinizes the developing nervous system and establishes male behaviour, suppressing female behaviour. One of the ways in which this is achieved is by the regulation of programmed cell death in some areas of the nervous system. These areas comprise groups of cells, called **nuclei**. These nuclei are of different sizes and organization in males and females (i.e. they are sexually dimorphic).

One example of a sexually dimorphic nucleus is located in the **hypothalamus** and is known as the 'sexually dimorphic nucleus of the preoptic area'. It has been studied mostly in rats. It influences copulatory behaviour and becomes much larger in males than in females due to sex differences in the amounts of programmed cell death. In this nucleus, there are more dying cells in newborn females than in newborn males because the presence of testosterone in males prevents programmed cell death. If testosterone is given to newborn females, programmed cell death in this nucleus is reduced and it ends up larger than normal. Giving testosterone to adult females has no such effect. If newborn males are castrated, depriving the nucleus of testosterone, it loses extra cells through programmed cell death and ends up abnormally small.

Testosterone works by entering cells and being converted by the enzyme aromatase into estrogens that bind the intracellular estrogen receptor. This complex then translocates to the nucleus where it binds DNA to regulate gene expression (Fig. 11.6). The nature of the eventual cellular response to testosterone is, however, variable. While in the case of the sexually dimorphic nucleus of the preoptic area described above testosterone inhibits programmed cell death, in other sexually dimorphic nuclei, such as the anteroventral periventricular nucleus of the hypothalamus, testosterone induces programmed cell death. Consequently, this nucleus is larger in females than in males, and it controls ovulation. Whether testosterone promotes or inhibits programmed cell death depends on other factors in the cell's molecular make-up, which ultimately depend on the cell's previous developmental history. These other factors are likely to include the levels of expression of members of the programmed cell death pathways within the cell. These pathways will be discussed later in this chapter; as yet, we know very little about the link between the trigger, testosterone, and the effector pathways leading to programmed cell death in the development of sexually dimorphic nuclei in mammals.

hypothalamus a ventral neural region at the base of the forebrain that regulates hormone secretion and controls many autonomic functions.

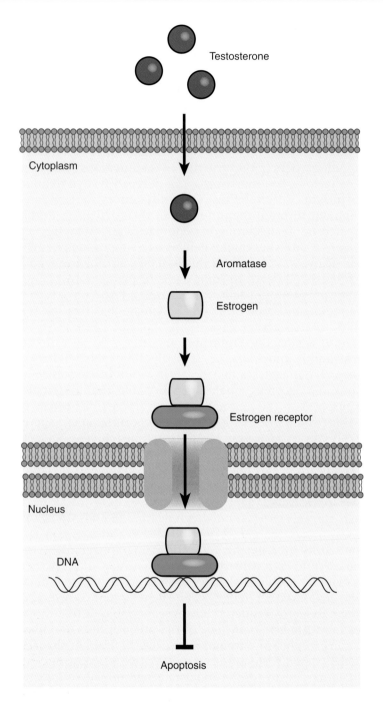

Fig. 11.6 Testosterone crosses the cell membrane into the cytoplasm where it is converted by the aromatase enzyme to estrogen, which binds to its receptor. The receptor–ligand complex enters the nucleus and regulates gene expression. This pathway can lead to the inhibition of apoptosis, as in the sexually dimorphic nucleus of the pre-optic area of the hypothalamus. In other cell types, however, this pathway can activate apoptosis.

hermaphrodite an organism with both male and female sexual characteristics and organs.

Sexually dimorphic neurons are also found in invertebrate species. Individual *C. elegans* are either **hermaphrodite** or male. Whereas hermaphrodites have two hermaphrodite specific neurons (or HSNs) that innervate the vulval muscles and drive egg-laying, males do not need HSNs. In males, HSNs are generated but undergo programmed cell death. Conversely, male *C. elegans* have four sensory cephalic neurons (called CEMs – the name CEM is derived from <u>c</u>ephalic <u>m</u>ale) in their head whereas hermaphrodites do not. CEMs are generated in both sexes but die in hermaphrodites; they probably allow the males to detect chemicals that attract them to hermaphrodites. The sex-specific regulation of programmed cell death in these neurons is regulated at least in part by the actions of transcription factors that they express as a consequence of their cell lineage. These transcription factors regulate the expression of genes of the cell death pathway that were discussed earlier in this chapter.

11.5.3 Programmed cell death removes cells with transient functions once their task is done

Several types of transient function are fulfilled by cells that later die during development in vertebrates and invertebrates. Some transient cells produce axons that provide guidance for the development of subsequent persistent axonal connections, others provide cues on their cell bodies that developing axons use on their journey to their targets and others carry out temporary neural functions while persistent circuitry matures.

As discussed in Chapter 8 (Section 8.5.1), during axon formation many axons follow paths laid down by the axons of **pioneer neurons**. In some cases, these pioneer axons are temporary: they are made by neurons that later die. There are many examples in both invertebrate and vertebrate developing nervous systems of early-generated neurons undergoing programmed cell death after providing a scaffold for the development of later persistent connections. Thus, the development of persistent axonal connections often follows the earlier development of a transient axon scaffold.

pioneer neurons early migrating neurons or navigating axons which act as developmental cues for later developing neurons or axons.

In insect development, some of the first neurons to grow axons in the CNS (which differentiate from midline **neural precursors**) lay out the basic pattern of fascicles and commissures in the segmental ganglia (see Fig. 2.2 in Chapter 2 for a reminder of what these structures are). Subsequent axons use this scaffold for guidance (see Section 8.5.1 in Chapter 8 on the labelled pathway hypothesis). Later in embryonic development, after fulfilling their guidance role, many of these pioneer cells die. Some do not, however, illustrating the important point that programmed cell death is not the only fate for neurons whose functions are no longer required. Some of the cells derived from midline precursors lose their first axon, grow a new one and take on a new function. This recycling of obsolete neurons is not restricted to insect development; it also occurs in later stages of *C. elegans* development, for example.

Populations of pioneer neurons have been identified not only in the CNS but also in the PNS of invertebrates and vertebrates. In grasshopper embryos, for example, pioneer neurons located at the ends of the limb buds grow axons through the limb to the CNS (Fig. 11.7; see also Fig. 8.4 in Chapter 8). The axons of later-generated sensory neurons need these axons for guidance to the CNS but once they have reached their targets the pioneer neurons die.

neural precursor defined in this book as a cell that has committed to become a neural cell, but not yet differentiated; Cf progenitor.

In vertebrates, well-known examples of transient neurons include the **Rohon-Beard cells** in the spinal cord of embryonic fish and amphibians (Fig. 11.8). Rohon-Beard cells are transient sensory

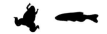

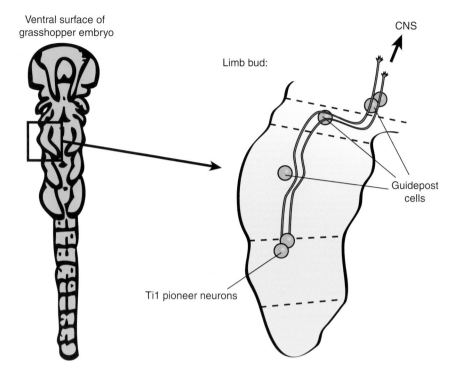

Fig. 11.7 Diagram of the Ti1 pioneer neuron pathway in a grasshopper embryo: a pair of sibling Ti1 pioneer neurons develops and extends axons away from the tip of the limb towards the CNS. The growth cones are oriented by guidepost cells that they encounter along their path. These Ti1 axons provide a pathway along which the axons of later-arising neurons grow to provide a major nerve trunk of the leg. The Ti1 pioneer neurons undergo programmed cell death later in development once their task is done.

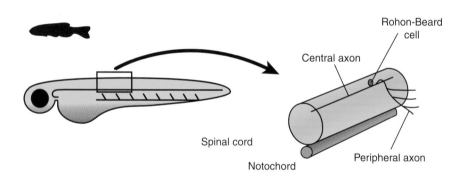

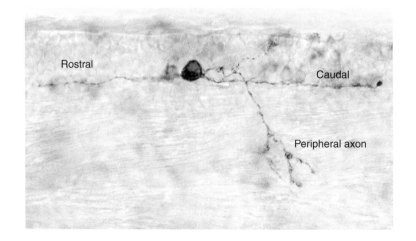

Fig. 11.8 A segment of the spinal cord of a zebrafish embryo showing a single Rohon-Beard cell body (red) and its central and peripheral axons. The photograph shows a single labelled Rohon-Beard neuron in a one day old zebrafish embryo viewed from the side. Rostral and caudal axons in the spinal cord as well as the branched peripheral axon in the epidermis are visible (photograph is courtesy of Thomas Becker, University of Edinburgh, UK).

neurons that extend axonal branches both within the central nervous system – in the spinal cord – and peripherally to the skin. They temporarily provide sensory input for newly born fish or tadpoles, and then die at a particular stage of development when their function is taken over by **dorsal root ganglion** cells. Their gradual – but eventually complete – disappearance begins a few days after the electrical properties of their membranes mature. Blocking their electrical activity reduces the numbers of Rohon-Beard cells undergoing programmed cell death, indicating that electrical activity is required for their normal elimination (this topic is discussed further later in this chapter, Section 11.7).

In mammals, the **subplate** of the developing mammalian cerebral cortex (Fig. 11.9) is a good example of a transient population of differentiated neurons that provides guidance cues. In this case, the transient neurons guide incoming axons from the **thalamus** and possibly other locations. The subplate is located beneath the developing cortex (which is known at this stage as the cortical plate). The functions of the subplate, as currently understood, fall into two categories: first, subplate cells produce long-range pioneer axons used for the guidance of other sets of **afferent** and **efferent** axons; secondly, subplate cell bodies provide incoming axons with a temporary synaptic target until cortical plate neurons (the ultimate targets of incoming axons) have completed their own migration to the overlying layers of the cortex (as was described in Chapter 9, Section 9.6.5). When thalamic axons later grow beyond the subplate into the cortex, subplate neurons lose their temporary thalamic synaptic inputs and undergo programmed cell death. Interestingly, the subplate is very much larger and more highly developed in primates (Fig. 11.9), indicating its importance for the formation of complex cortical circuitry. There is considerable uncertainty as to whether all subplate cells die, especially in rodents. There is evidence that some subplate cells survive and become integrated into the overlying cortical layers, where they might take on new functions, mirroring the examples of neuronal recycling in invertebrates that were mentioned above.[5]

What triggers the death of subplate cells? Experiments have shown that the death of subplate cells can be affected by manipulations that modify either their access to survival-promoting signalling molecules or their receipt of synaptic input. It is possible that subplate cells die when they lose their transient synaptic inputs because these inputs deliver survival-promoting levels of electrical activity and/or signalling molecules. The functions of survival factors and electrical activity in subplate cell death remain speculative; the functions of these regulators of neuronal survival and death are better understood in other systems, as discussed in the following sections.

dorsal root ganglion (DRG) a collection of cell bodies of peripheral sensory neurons whose axons enter the spinal cord. DRGs are located bilaterally along the dorsolateral side of the spinal cord (see Fig. 11.10).

thalamus a structure in the centre of the vertebrate brain that transmits sensory input to the cerebral cortex, and receives reciprocal output from the cortex.

afferent an axon passing impulses *to* a specified region of the nervous system, for example from peripheral receptors *to* central nervous system or from spinal cord *to* brain.

efferent an axon passing impulses *from* a specified region of the nervous system, for example *from* brain to spinal cord or *from* spinal cord to muscle.

---

[5] For an interesting review of the subplate in the context of human development, see Kostović, I. and Judas, M. (2010) The development of the subplate and thalamocortical connections in the human foetal brain. *Acta Paediatr.*, **99**, 1119–27.

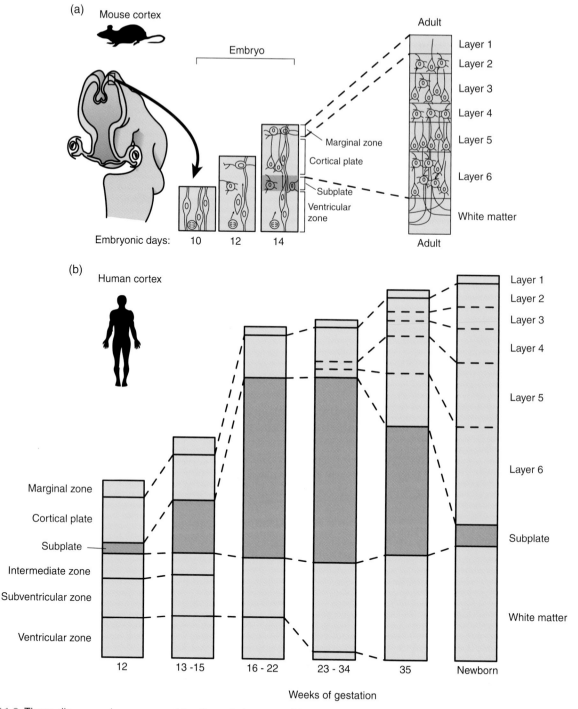

Fig. 11.9 These diagrams show narrow strips through the cortex (drawn as in Fig. 2.8 in Chapter 2) of (a) mouse and (b) human brains of increasing age (from left to right), with the outer surface of the brain at the top of each strip. The subplate is highlighted in a darker shade of orange. (a) In mice, the subplate is a relatively thin layer that forms beneath the cortical plate during embryogenesis and it disappears in postnatal life. (b) In human embryos, the subplate lies in the same relative position as in mouse embryos but it becomes relatively very thick compared with the overlying cortical plate before disappearing as the cortical layers mature.

11.5.4 Programmed cell death matches the numbers of cells in interacting neural tissues

There are many examples of developing neural systems in which more neurons are produced than survive into adulthood. A widely accepted hypothesis is that neurons are initially overproduced, and then normal programmed cell death matches the number of neurons to the size of the target field that they innervate. This might occur through a conceptually rather simple mechanism: innervating neurons might compete for a limited supply of one or more survival-promoting, or **neurotrophic**, molecules whose levels are proportional to the size of the target. Innervating neurons that do not receive enough neurotrophic factor die. This is known as the **neurotrophic hypothesis**.

The neurotrophic hypothesis arose from observations on cell death among developing motor neurons and dorsal root ganglion cells. Early studies on chick embryos by Viktor Hamburger (1900–2001) and his colleagues working in Germany and the USA showed that there is substantial motor neuron and dorsal root ganglion cell death in normal development. An interesting observation was made on the timing of this cell death: it occurs during a specific time-window *after* the neurons have made contact with their targets (i.e. muscles in the case of motor neurons). The amount of cell death is not the same at all positions along the neural axis: in regions innervating larger tissues, such as legs and wings, there is less cell death. One possible interpretation of this observation is that interactions between the motor and dorsal root ganglion neurons and their targets adjust cell survival – the larger targets allow more cells to survive. The outcome is that neuronal numbers are matched to the size of their target tissue. The results of experimental manipulations support this interpretation (Fig. 11.10): (i) experimental reduction of target size by removal of the limb bud increases levels of motor neuron death; (ii) conversely, some of the motor neurons that would have died during normal development are rescued by grafting in an extra limb bud. Similar findings have been reported in other species. The abnormally high rates of cell death induced among motor neurons when their target is removed can be prevented by exposing them to a solution containing molecules extracted from muscle. We now know the explanation for these experimental findings: muscle produces neurotrophic molecules which promote the survival of the neurons that innervate them. Consequently the numbers of motor neurons that survive during normal development is regulated by the amount of neurotrophic support available in the target tissue.

Although many experimental findings support the neurotrophic hypothesis well, others do not; for example, some experiments have indicated that increasing the number of motor neurons innervating a single limb (by diverting axons that would normally grow to other sites) does not increase the proportion of those motor neurons that die, as would be predicted if there were increased competition for a normally sized pool of neurotrophic molecules. Despite these issues, the hypothesis has led to the identification of molecules discussed in

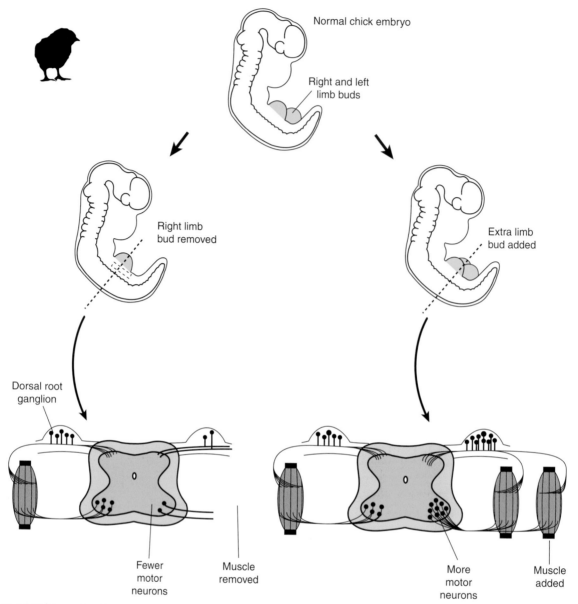

Fig. 11.10 Evidence leading to the formulation of the neurotrophic hypothesis: removing or increasing the size of the limb bud causes a corresponding reduction or increase in the numbers of neurons projecting to it. Removing the limb bud causes a reduction in the numbers of motor neurons and dorsal root ganglion neurons due to an increase in cell death. The neurotrophic hypothesis suggests that this cell death is caused by an absence of trophic support from the target cells in the limb bud. Grafting additional limb buds increases the numbers of motor neurons and dorsal root ganglion neurons due to a reduction in cell death, indicating that bigger targets can support more innervation. The neurotrophic hypothesis suggests that this is caused by an increase in trophic support from the target cells in the limb bud.

the next section that regulate the survival of neurons and for which innervating neurons might compete. Overall, this work has strengthened the general conclusion that in vertebrates programmed cell death is triggered by factors *external* to the cell, rather than being determined autonomously by the lineage of the cell.

11.6 Neurotrophic factors are important regulators of cell survival and death

Neurotrophic factors are extracellular molecules that enhance the survival of neurons. Whilst important for cell survival, in fact the actions of many neurotrophic factors are very broad and many were discovered through their effects on promoting axonal growth (see Chapter 7, Section 7.4.2). In addition, they can affect other developmental processes including neural progenitor proliferation, neuronal differentiation and synaptic plasticity. As well as having functions in the nervous system, they can also act in non-neural tissues. Many neurotrophic factors are relatively small diffusible proteins. They can be classified into two groups – **growth factors** and **cytokines** – based largely on the nature of the receptors through which they operate: growth factors operate through receptors that are **tyrosine kinases** (e.g. Fig.11.11 and Box 11.3) whereas cytokines use distinct multicomponent receptor systems.

tyrosine kinase a type of enzyme that transfers phosphate groups onto (i.e. phosphorylates) tyrosine residues in a protein.

11.6.1 Growth factors

Nerve growth factor (**NGF**) was the first neurotrophic factor to be isolated. Its discovery was due largely to the research of a remarkable Italian scientist called Rita Levi-Montalcini. Working in Viktor Hamburger's laboratory in the USA, she found that when mouse tumour cells were transplanted to chick embryos they stimulated

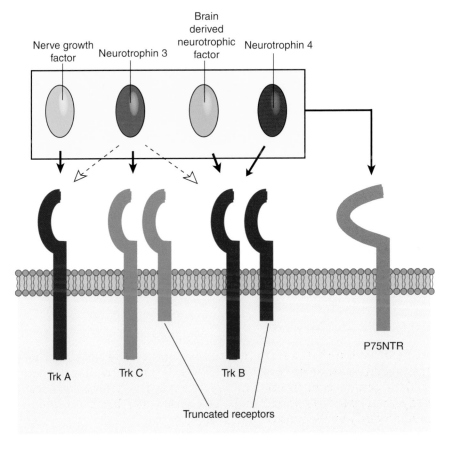

Fig. 11.11 Trk receptors comprise an extracellular domain containing the neurotrophin binding site, a transmembrane segment and an intracellular domain that has tyrosine kinase activity. There are three members of the Trk receptor family: TrkA, which is the receptor for nerve growth factor (NGF), TrkB, which is the receptor for brain derived neurotrophic factor (BDNF) and neurotrophin 4 (NT-4), and TrkC, which is the receptor for neurotrophin 3 (NT-3). There is evidence that the binding between these ligands and their receptors is not entirely specific. There are truncated forms of TrkB and TrkC receptors which lack the intracellular tyrosine kinase domains. Their functions are poorly understood; they might, for example, inhibit the actions of the full-length receptors by dimerizing with them. The neurotrophins also bind with relatively low affinity to a receptor known as p75NTR.

Box 11.3   A simplified example of some well-known intracellular pathways involved in transducing signals from neurotrophins

On binding to neurotrophin, Trk receptors form homodimers and **autophosphorylate**, triggering their intracellular signalling cascades (phosphorylation is indicated by small green circles). The initial steps involve the formation of a protein complex between the Trk receptor and Shc, which becomes phosphorylated and associates with Grb2 (growth factor receptor-bound protein 2). Grb2 couples with other proteins to activate the Akt and MAP kinase (MAPK) pathways (Fig. 3.5 in Chapter 3), which result in the phosphorylation of the transcription factor CREB (cAMP response element binding protein), thereby regulating gene expression. (PI3K = phosphoinositide 3-kinase.)

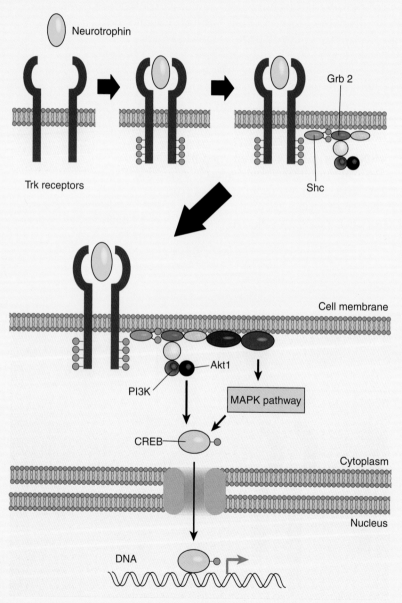

autophosphorylation the phosphorylation of a kinase protein by its own enzymatic activity.

the growth of axons in the chick and that this happened even when there was no direct contact between the tumour and the embryo. Rita Levi-Montalcini concluded that the tumour released a diffusible substance which promoted nerve growth. She and her collaborator, the American biochemist Stanley Cohen, isolated NGF and showed that it was the diffusible molecule responsible for the effect. They were awarded the Nobel Prize in Medicine in 1986 for their work.[6]

We now know that NGF is a member of a small family of growth factors known as the **neurotrophins**. Members of this family have numerous effects throughout the developing and adult nervous system and beyond, not just on axon growth but also on neuronal survival and many other developmental processes. The other members of the family include brain-derived neurotrophic factor (BDNF), neurotrophin-3 (NT-3) and neurotrophin-4 (NT-4). The neurotrophins act on one of two types of receptors on the cell surface. Many of their effects are mediated by high affinity tyrosine receptor kinases, or **Trk receptors** (Fig. 11.11; intracellular pathways from the Trk receptors are illustrated in Box 11.3). The neurotrophins also bind with relatively low affinity to a receptor known as p75NTR which is found in both neuronal and non-neuronal cells. While the Trk receptors signal survival, p75NTR can relay a survival or cell death signal, depending on the cellular context and the ligand, and it might modulate the sensitivity of the Trk receptors to the neurotrophins.[7]

Many growth factors other than the neurotrophins have the ability to promote neuronal survival. For example, members of the multifunctional fibroblast growth factor (FGF) family can promote neuronal survival as well as regulate many other developmental processes (their intracellular signaling pathways have been discussed in the context of early neuronal induction in Fig. 3.5 in Chapter 3).

11.6.2 Cytokines

Cytokines are small proteins that were first discovered in the immune system. They are now known to have much broader roles including important functions in the developing nervous system. Members of this group include ciliary neurotrophic factor (CNTF), leukaemia inhibitory factor (LIF) and interleukins (ILs). LIF is well-known in stem cell biology since it supports the self-renewal of mouse embryonic stem cells (Fig. 1.6 in Chapter 1). Cutting the axons of motor neurons during development, such as by limb bud removal, causes many of them to die (Fig. 11.10). If LIF, CNTF or IL-6 are given to these motor neurons then the number that die is reduced. These and other related findings generated optimism that cytokines might be used therapeutically to treat cases of neurodegenerative disease (Box 11.1), but these hopes have not yet been fulfilled. Information on cytokine receptors and their intracellular signalling pathways can be found in Box 11.4.

---

[6] http://nobelprize.org/nobel_prizes/medicine/laureates/1986/levi-montalcini-lecture.html [20 November 2010].
[7] For more detail on these receptors and their signalling pathways, see Reichardt, L. F. (2006) Neurotrophin-regulated signalling pathways. *Philos. Trans. R. Soc. Lond. B Biol. Sci.*, **361**, 1545–64.

Box 11.4   Cytokine receptors differ from growth factor receptors

Whereas the transduction pathways for cytokine signalling often involve tyrosine kinases, cytokine receptors are not themselves tyrosine kinases, unlike growth factor receptors. For example, the receptor for one well-known cytokine called ciliary neurotrophic factor (CNTF) consists of three subunits, one of which binds CNTF causing the complex to assemble and activate the intracellular Janus tyrosine kinases (Jaks), which phosphorylates molecules called STATs (<u>s</u>ignal <u>t</u>ransduction <u>a</u>nd <u>t</u>ranscription proteins). These phosphorylated proteins translocate to the nucleus where they bind to CNTF response elements in the DNA to initiate gene transcription. This is known as the Jak–STAT pathway. Small green circles indicate phosphorylation.

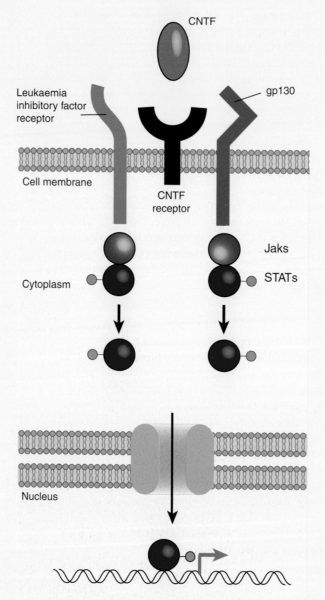

11.7 A role for electrical activity in regulating programmed cell death

Earlier in this chapter we saw that cell death could be regulated by levels of electrical activity (for example, in Rohon-Beard cells and possibly in subplate cells, Figs 11.8 and 11.9). As the nervous system matures, neurons become connected and their electrical properties and neurotransmitter systems develop (see Chapter 10), then the potential for electrical activity to regulate developmental events including cell death is greatly enhanced. Neuronal activity can promote survival or death under different circumstances and depending on the level of activity. We now know that for many neurons survival becomes dependent on electrical activity, but too much stimulation is harmful.

The principal mediator of the regulation of cell death by electrical activity is the **N-methyl-D-aspartate** (**NMDA**) subtype of ionotropic glutamate receptors (see Chapter 12 for more on the importance of this receptor in development). Physiological levels of NMDA receptor activity generally promote neuronal survival as well as playing important roles in synaptic plasticity and transmission. In pathological scenarios such as **ischemia**, however, over-stimulation results in cell death via excessive levels of intracellular calcium, which influxes through the NMDA receptor (and probably other channels). There is a growing understanding of the signalling events that mediate the opposing effects of NMDA-receptor activity and of the factors that determine whether an episode of NMDA-receptor activity will promote survival or death. Whether over-activation of NMDA receptors is a significant factor inducing programmed cell death during normal development remains to be seen.[8]

Ischemia the lack of adequate blood flow to support the normal functioning of a tissue.

11.8 Summary

- Many neural progenitors and nerve cells die during normal development. This is essential for normal development, allowing tissues to develop their correct shapes and sizes, for ensuring that each region has an appropriate number of neurons and removing cells that have only transient functions in development.
- Cells that undergo cell death naturally during development do so by a process called apoptosis which is, in effect, programmed cellular suicide.
- Much of what we know about the molecular genetic pathway that results in the naturally-occurring death through apoptosis of cells during development originated from research on *C. elegans*.
- Most of the genes involved in programmed cell death in *C. elegans* have homologues in vertebrates, including humans.
- Programmed cell death contributes to sexual differences in the nervous system.

[8] To read more on this topic, see Hardingham, G. E. (2009) Coupling of the NMDA receptor to neuroprotective and neurodestructive events. *Biochem. Soc. Trans.*, **37**, 1147–60.

- Programmed cell death removes cells with transient functions once their task is done, for example pioneer neurons in axonal pathway development and subplate neurons in the mammalian cerebral cortex.
- Programmed cell death matches the numbers of cells in interacting neural tissues. The neurotrophic hypothesis proposes that axons that innervate a neural structure compete for a limited supply of one or more survival-promoting – or neurotrophic – molecules whose levels are proportional to the size of the target. Innervating neurons that do not receive enough neurotrophic factor die.

Experience-Dependent Development

12

In Chapters 9 and 10 we considered how **innate** neuronal activity, such as the retinal waves, regulates neuronal development. In this chapter we will examine how **experience-dependent** neuronal activity regulates development of the brain. In this sense, **experience** refers to a stimulus, group of stimuli, or in some cases lack of stimuli that changes neuronal **excitability**. Similarly, experience-dependent neuronal activity can be defined as neuronal activity that results from stimulation of sensory receptors, such as touch of the skin. Experience-dependent activity is essential for young animals to learn sensory and motor skills like seeing and walking as well as for emotional and cognitive development. While much has been learned about experience-dependent development from research in invertebrates and non-mammalian vertebrates, the majority of research has focused on mammals.

The role of experience in development is best demonstrated by examining the effect of cataracts on visual capacity in young infants compared with adults. In the former, unless the cataract is removed and replaced with an artificial lens soon after cataract formation, the child will be left with permanently reduced vision in the affected eye that cannot be corrected with glasses, a condition known as **amblyopia**. In contrast, a cataract that forms in an adult eye can be present for years, but following corrective surgery adults will see as well as they did prior to cataract formation. This simple example highlights two key points about the developing nervous system. First, during development, experience shapes the anatomical and physiological properties of neurons, a process known as **experience-dependent plasticity**. Secondly, there are distinct time-windows during development when experience shapes neural connectivity and hence brain function. These windows are known as **sensitive** or **critical periods**. In this chapter we shall explore the mechanisms by which experience, in combination with innate neuronal activity, refines the physiological and anatomical properties of neurons, essentially teaching neural circuits how to communicate efficiently.

innate arising from the genetic programme of the animal. cf. experience.

Building Brains: An Introduction to Neural Development, First Edition.
David Price, Andrew Jarman, John Mason and Peter Kind.
© 2011 John Wiley & Sons, Ltd. Published 2011 by John Wiley & Sons, Ltd.

12.1 Effects of experience on visual system development

Much of what we know about the mechanisms that underlie experience-dependent development comes from experiments conducted on sensory systems, most notably the visual system. In fact, experience has been shown to alter the physiological and anatomical properties of neurons in the visual system of numerous species, from flies to humans. However, by far the majority of what we know about experience-dependent plasticity has come from experiments on the visual system of mammals.

12.1.1 Seeing one world with two eyes: ocular dominance of cortical cells

Before examining the experimental evidence for experience-dependent plasticity, it is first necessary to review what is known about the anatomical and physiological properties of neurons in the mature visual cortex. A central issue in visual system processing is how images coming through the two eyes merge to create a single perception of the visual world. As we saw in Chapter 9 (Fig. 9.11), axons carrying information from the two eyes segregate in the **dLGN**, and cortical layer 4 where they form **ocular dominance bands**. As a result of this segregation, the majority of the visual input to an individual neuron in layer 4 will be from a single eye, so that neuron will be **monocular**. Layer 4 cells then project axons that synapse with dendrites in layers 2 and 3. It is in layers 2 and 3 that most neurons begin receiving input from both eyes, so that they are **binocular**.

In a typical physiological experiment examining the role of visual experience in development (the experiment would be set up as shown in Box 9.5 of Chapter 9), an electrode that records the activity of a single neuron is placed into the visual cortex and a visual stimulus, such as a bar of light, is shown to each eye separately. In this way the experimenter can determine the level of activity that results from stimulation of each eye. This is referred to as the **ocular dominance** of the neuron. Moving the electrode allows the experimenter to sample the responses of numerous neurons (in some cases several hundred in a single experiment) and plot an **ocular dominance histogram** showing the percentage of neurons with a particular ocular dominance classification that are encountered in the visual cortex of a given animal (Fig. 12.1). If a given cell is monocular, responding to stimulation of either the **contralateral** or **ipsilateral** eye only, it is classified in ocular dominance group 1 or 5, respectively. Cells responding equally to stimulation of either eye are placed in group 3. Cells showing physiological activation to stimulation of either eye, but showing more activity to either contralateral or ipsilateral eye stimulation, are placed in groups 2 and 4, respectively. The vast majority of cells in the visual cortex (outside of layer 4) of most carnivores and primates are binocular (i.e. they fall within groups 2–4).

dLGN a region of the thalamus that processes visual information; it receives input from the retina and sends information to the visual cortex.

ocular dominance bands the overall pattern of synaptic terminals in cortical layer 4 of axons carrying information from the **dLGN**.

contralateral on the opposite side.

ipsilateral on the same side.

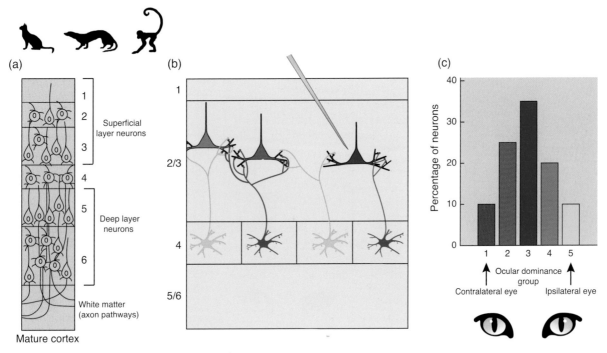

Fig. 12.1 The ocular dominance histogram. (a) Schematic showing the six layers of the cerebral cortex, as shown in Fig. 5.16. (b) A view showing the neuronal connectivity between neurons in layer 4 and those in layer 2/3 that gives rise to a range of cells with differing degrees of input from each eye. The experimental set-up for recording ocular dominance is shown in Box 9.5. Cells in layer 4 are monocular, receiving input from either the eye that is contralateral (ocular dominance category 1, blue) or ipsilateral (ocular dominance category 5, yellow) to the brain hemisphere in which neurons are being sampled with an electrode (grey needle shape). Most layer 2/3 cells are binocular, and may receive approximately equal input from both eyes (ocular dominance category 3, green) or relatively more input from the contralateral eye (ocular dominance category 2, blue-green) or the ipsilateral eye (ocular dominance category 4, yellow-green). (c) An example of an ocular dominance histogram from a cat showing the relative frequency with which neurons of each ocular dominance category are encountered. Tens to hundreds of neurons can be sampled in a single animal.

12.1.2 Visual experience regulates ocular dominance

The first experiments that demonstrated a role of visual experience in nervous system development were part of a series of experiments that eventually earned David Hubel and Torsten Wiesel a Nobel Prize (see Box 9.5). They made extensive use of ocular dominance histograms as measures of the eye preferences of neurons in the visual cortex. Hubel and Wiesel showed that depriving cats or monkeys of input through one eye, a procedure known as **monocular deprivation** (MD), during early postnatal development caused a near-complete loss of **functional connectivity** from the deprived eye to the visual cortex (Fig. 12.2 – note that the deprived eye is reopened immediately prior to the experiment so that the functional connectivity of both eyes can be tested). These changes in ocular dominance in response to altered visual experience are an example of experience-dependent plasticity. Physiological recordings from single cells or small groups of cells in the visual cortex showed that almost all of the neurons responded solely to stimulation of the non-deprived eye. This alteration in the eye preference of neurons is referred to as an **ocular dominance shift**. It is important to note that while dramatic changes in the response

functional connectivity the connections between neurons that, when stimulated, contribute to the generation of action potentials in the postsynaptic neuron.

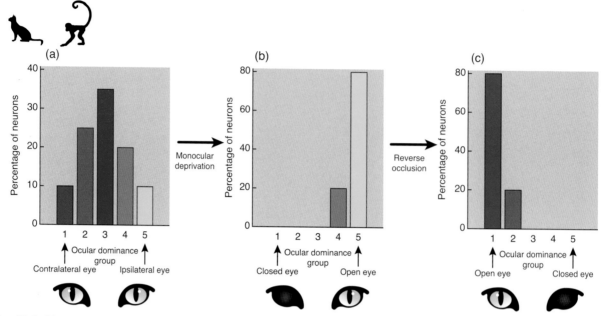

Fig. 12.2 Changes in ocular dominance that result from monocular deprivation and reverse occlusion. (a) An ocular dominance histogram for a normal animal. (b) Monocular deprivation causes a shift in the OD histogram such that cells become dominated by visual stimulation through the non-deprived eye, that is, most cells fall into ocular dominance groups 4 and 5 (yellow-green and yellow bars). (c) Restoring vision to a previously closed eye and closing the previously open eye (known as reverse occlusion) during early postnatal development causes an opposite shift in the ocular dominance pattern, such that cortical neurons become responsive selectively to visual stimulation of the eye that was initially closed (OD groups 1 and 2, blue and blue-green bars).

properties of cortical neurons were visible following monocular deprivation, relatively minor changes were seen in the response properties of cells in the retina and dLGN. As a result the majority of subsequent studies focused on the cerebral cortex as the main site of experience-dependent plasticity.

The shift in ocular dominance that results from monocular deprivation does not reflect an irreparable degeneration of the cells or connections carrying information from the deprived eye. This conclusion came from studies using a procedure known as **reverse occlusion** in which vision is restored to the initially deprived eye and at the same time the initially open eye is deprived of vision. Provided reverse occlusion is initiated sufficiently early in the animal's life, neurons in the visual cortex lose their ability to respond to stimulation of the initially open eye and subsequently increase their excitability to visual stimulation of the initially closed eye (Fig. 12.2).

12.1.3 Competition regulates experience-dependent plasticity: the effects of dark-rearing and strabismus

As we saw in Chapter 10, several key features of neuronal development occur even in animals that have been deprived of all visual experience by rearing them in complete darkness. Physiological recordings from these animals revealed that **dark-rearing** has very little effect on the ocular dominance of cells in visual cortex (although protracted periods of dark-rearing do increase the proportion of cells that do not respond

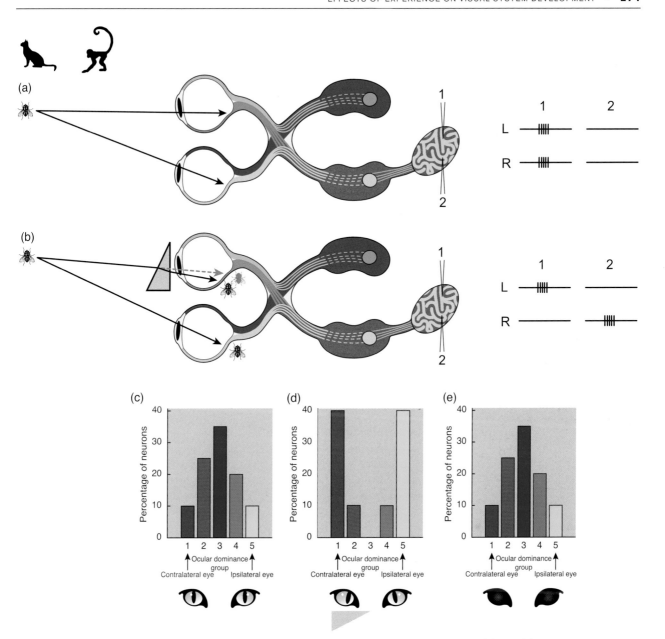

Fig. 12.3 Effects of strabismus and dark-rearing on the ocular dominance of cortical neurons. (a) and (b) Schematics showing how strabismus decorrelates the input from the two retinae to cortical neurons. In a normal animal (a), a fly in the animal's visual field is detected by cells located in corresponding parts of the two retinae that will ultimately send their information to the same cells in the visual cortex. The physiological response of these neurons as monitored with electrodes placed in the visual cortex is shown on the right hand side of the figure. Each vertical line represents an action potential (like that shown in Fig. 10.3 but on a more condensed timescale). The position of the fly leads to activation of neurons present at position 1 in the cortex, but no neuronal activity is seen at position 2. (b) When strabismus is induced by placing a prism in front of one eye the image of the fly is displaced to a different region of the retina. As a result, a different set of retinal ganglion cells is activated that connects to a different group of cortical neurons (located at position 2 in the figure). Therefore in a strabismic animal, the fly generates left-eye activation at position 1, but right-eye activation at position 2 (each eye can be tested alone by covering the other eye). (c)–(e) Ocular dominance histograms for a normal (c), strabismic (d) and dark-reared animal (e). Strabismus imposed during the critical period causes a near-complete breakdown in cortical binocularity with the vast majority of cells being driven solely by stimulation of a single eye (d) while dark-rearing has little effect (e). Although numerous species have been used, most studies examining the physiological effects of strabismus and dark-rearing have been conducted in the cat and monkey.

receptive field region of sensory space that elicits a response in the cell being examined.

to visual stimulation). Since dark-rearing has far less effect on the OD histogram than monocular deprivation, the loss of functional connectivity from the deprived eye that results from monocular deprivation is *not* caused by visual deprivation per se, but instead results from the *imbalance* of activity between the two eyes. A similar conclusion came from experiments in which the integration of the visual information coming through the two eyes was prevented by surgically inducing a misalignment of the two eyes, referred to as **strabismus** or squint (Fig. 12.3). Retinal ganglion cells in the two eyes whose **receptive fields** sample from the same part of the visual world send information to the same binocular neurons in the visual cortex. Therefore action potentials generated in the retinal ganglion cells in the two eyes as a result of stimulation from a particular part of the visual world will arrive at a particular set of cortical neurons at the same time; in other words, the inputs from the two eyes are **correlated**. Inducing strabismus causes a mismatch of the inputs from the two eyes onto cortical cells because retinal cells whose receptive fields should be sampling the same point in the visual world no longer do so. Hence cortical neurons no longer receive coincident stimulation from the two eyes – the inputs from the two eyes become **uncorrelated** (Fig. 12.3). If strabismus is induced early in post-natal development, cells lose their ability to respond to both eyes, becoming activated only by stimulation of the eye that caused the greater response prior to the strabismus being induced.

The near complete dominance of one or the other eye following strabismus and monocular deprivation led to the conclusion that axons carrying information from the two eyes compete for the ability to activate postsynaptic neurons in the visual cortex. In fact, a modification of the neurotrophic hypothesis (introduced in the context of cell death in Chapter 11, Section 11.6) was invoked to explain competition in the visual cortex. The hypothesis was based on the idea that axons carrying information from the two eyes compete for one or more molecule(s) (such as growth factors) that determine the number of synapses they form on cortical neurons. Such a mechanism could explain the changes in thalamic input to layer 4 of the cortex that occur as a result of monocular deprivation.

12.1.4 Physiological changes in ocular dominance prior to anatomical changes

As we saw in Chapter 9, the ocular dominance bands present in layer 4 of carnivores and primates develop independently of visual experience. However, subsequent experiments showed that the *maintenance* of these ocular dominance bands is regulated by visual experience. Hubel and Wiesel showed that a month of monocular deprivation in monkeys caused a large increase in the extent of cortical territory innervated by the non-deprived eye and a corresponding decrease in territory innervated by the deprived eye (Fig. 12.4). These dramatic alterations in neuronal connectivity suggested that the physiological changes in ocular dominance that result from monocular deprivation reflect anatomical changes in the number of synapses representing each eye.

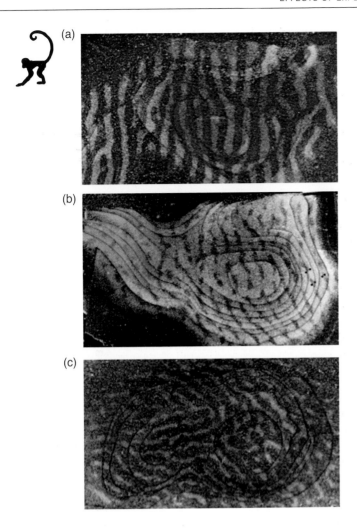

Fig. 12.4 Effect of monocular depri-vation on the pattern of ocular domi-nance bands in layer 4 of the monkey. Experimental results (from Hubel, D. H.,Wiesel, T. N. and LeVay, S. (1977) Plasticity of ocular dominance col-umns in monkey striate cortex. *Phil. Trans. R.Soc.Lond.B,* **278**, 377–409) in which a tracer was placed in one eye. The tracer is picked up by retinal ganglion cells and transported to the dLGN where it is released and picked up by neurons that extend axons to layer 4 of the visual cortex (similar in principle to the method outlined in Box 8.2, but using a different type of tracer that crosses synapses). Panels (a)–(c) show the location of the tracer (white areas) in the synaptic terminals of these thalamocortical axons in layer 4 of a normal (a) and a monocularly deprived (b) and (c) animal. In normal animals, approximately 50% of the to-tal area of visual cortex is innervated by each eye. In contrast, following a month of monocular deprivation, the area of label is increased if the open eye is injected (b) and decreased if the closed eye is injected (c).

We now know that this simple explanation is not correct. The physi-ological changes in ocular dominance of cortical neurons occur very rapidly during early life with a complete shift (i.e. few if any cells responding to the deprived eye) occurring within 48 hours after mo-nocular deprivation has begun. In contrast, even small changes in axon territories or synaptic density in layer 4 are not visible until about a week after the initiation of monocular deprivation. Hence, the physiological effects of monocular deprivation occur too rapidly to be explained by the loss and gain of *anatomically identifiable* syn-apses as proposed by traditional models of competition. Instead, synapses carrying information from each eye lose or gain their *abil-ity to cause a physiological response* in the cortical cells, such that al-though the same number of synapses carrying information from the deprived eye is present, they lose their **functional connectivity** (Fig. 12.5). The changes in functional connectivity of inputs coming through the two eyes are mediated by differences in the timing and patterns of activation of the synapses carrying information from the two eyes. For monocular deprivation and strabismus these interac-tions are competitive (see Section 12.1.3). However, not all interac-tions between the two eyes are competitive.

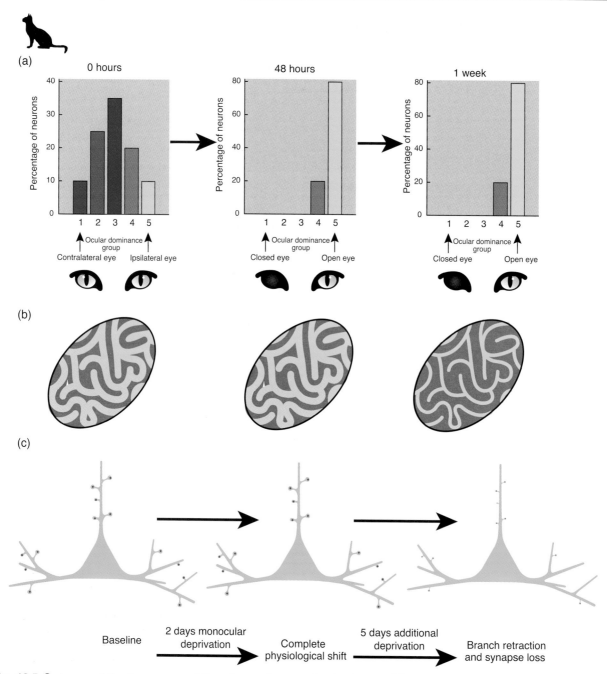

Fig. 12.5 Summary of the time-course of the effects of monocular deprivation. (a) The *physiological* shift in eye dominance that occurs in response to monocular deprivation is observed within 48 hours of the initiation of monocular deprivation (middle graph) and is indistinguishable from that seen after 1 week (right graph). (b) Schematics showing that the change in the pattern of ocular dominance bands in layer 4 is not seen until almost a week of monocular deprivation. Areas that receive input from the deprived eye are shown in light pink; regions that receive input from the non-deprived eye are shown in dark pink. (c) Schematic drawings of layer 2/3 cortical pyramidal neurons showing that the decrease in the number and size of deprived-eye synapses (represented by black dots in the dendritic spines) does not occur until after 1 week of monocular deprivation.

12.1.5 Cooperative binocular interactions and visual cortex plasticity

Although the results from the rearing paradigms mentioned above highlight the importance of competitive interaction between the two eyes during development, the fact is that most neurons receive inputs from both eyes that are *jointly* strengthened during development. This finding suggests that inputs from the two eyes also have the ability to *cooperate* such that they can both be stabilized onto a single neuron. Synaptic changes that result in type of cooperative interaction are referred to as **associative plasticity**. In fact, as long as inputs from the two eyes are correlated, strong input from one eye can help a weaker input from the other eye to gain synaptic strength. In cats, opening an eye after early monocular deprivation results in good re-covery of vision as measured behaviourally using the jumping stand technique (Box 12.1), provided it is done during early postnatal devel-opment. Inducing strabismus when the deprived eye is opened dramat-ically reduces its recovery indicating that correlated activity through the non-deprived and deprived eyes instructs the recovery of vision of the deprived eye, suggesting an associative mechanism (Fig. 12.6).

Interestingly, in monkeys there is little if any recovery of vision fol-lowing monocular deprivation, even if binocular vision is restored early in post-natal development. This evidence seemed initially to sup-port the idea of competition. However, monocular deprivation often induces a strabismus that will decorrelate the input from the two eyes and prevent their cooperation after eye re-opening. Given the results in cats, it is certainly possible that the lack of recovery following mono-cular deprivation in monkeys results from a lack of correlated activity between the two eyes.

12.1.6 The timing of developmental plasticity: sensitive or critical periods

As mentioned previously, a key finding from the initial studies of Hubel and Wiesel was that physiological and anatomical changes in response to monocular deprivation do not occur in adult animals. In-stead there are time-windows during development, referred to as **sen-sitive** or **critical periods**, when the functional properties of neurons can be altered by experience (Fig. 12.7).

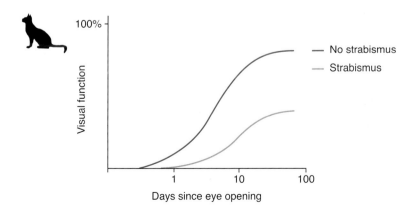

Fig. 12.6 This graph shows that if a deprived eye is re-opened following a period of monocular deprivation in a kitten, correlated activity from the two eyes significantly enhances recovery. Visual function was measured using the jumping stand (Box 12.1). In some cases, animals simply had the de-prived eye re-opened (blue line). In other cases, animals had the deprived eye re-opened but had strabismus in-duced to decorrelate the inputs from the two eyes (orange line). The graphs show recovery of visual function of the deprived eye over time (tested while the non-deprived eye is covered with an opaque contact lens): animals with no strabismus recovered much better vision.

Box 12.1   Behavioural testing of visual function

Testing visual function in laboratory animals employs the same principle as standard eye charts for humans in which the sizes of the letters on the lines on an eye chart are gradually reduced until they are no longer visible. However, instead of getting a verbal response as to whether a given visual stimulus (e.g. letters) are visible, experimenters have to come up with another way that an animal can indicate what it can see. In the case of cats Donald Mitchell, working in Canada in the 1970s, invented the jumping stand (figure below).[1] Cats are trained to jump from a platform a predetermined height above a stage with two distinct sides. On one side of the stage is a picture of a series of black and white vertical lines; on the other side is a picture of horizontal lines. The cats are trained to jump to the side with the vertical lines, which varies randomly with each successive trial. The thickness of both the vertical and horizontal lines are gradually decreased in unison until the cat can no longer distinguish the side with the vertical lines. The experimenter can then extrapolate its **visual acuity**. By placing an opaque contact lens in each eye at a time, the visual acuity of each eye can be determined.

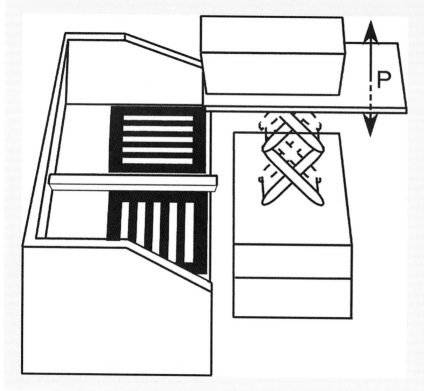

Diagrammatic representation of the jumping-stand apparatus used to test the visual ability of cats. Cats are trained to jump from a moveable raised platform (P) to the side of the stage showing the vertical lines. Cats are encouraged to learn the task using a reward system that involves rewarding correct responses with either their favourite food (such as liver) or petting. During the training period, the stage starts at a low height and large black and white lines are used, making the task relatively easy. Once the animal understands the task, the stage is raised and the width of the black and white lines is decreased gradually until the animal can no longer tell the difference.

visual acuity a functional measure of visual capability.

dendritic spine small outgrowths on the dendrites of excitatory neurons of vertebrates that are sites of excitatory synapses.

A sensitive period in developmental biology can be defined as a time-window during which a particular developmental event has a heightened sensitivity to changes in the animal's environment. The concept of sensitive periods during childhood development has been around for just over a century and has been applied to a range of phenomena from human behaviour to **dendritic spine** development (see Chapter 10).

---

[1] Mitchell, D. E., Giffin, F., Wilkinson, F., Anderson, P. and Smith, M. L. (1976) Visual resolution in young kittens. *Vision Res.*, **16**, 363–6.

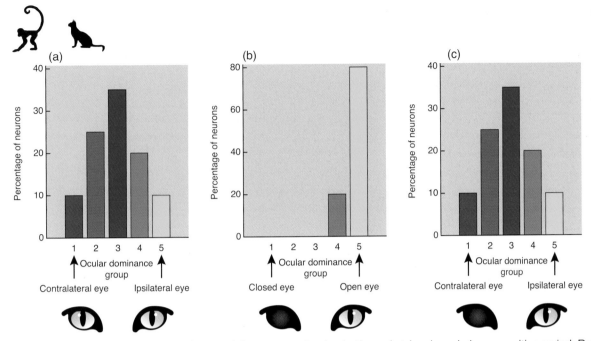

Fig. 12.7 Changes in ocular dominance that result from monocular deprivation only take place during a sensitive period. Representative ocular dominance histograms from (a) normal and (b) and (c) monocularly deprived animals. Monocular deprivation induced at the peak of the sensitive period (4 to 5 weeks of age in the cat) (b) has a dramatic effect on the ocular dominance histogram whereas no effect is seen in adult cats or monkeys (c). Notably, these critical periods do not apply to all species. For example, a shift in ocular dominance as a result of monocular deprivation can still be elicited in adult mice.

12.1.7 Multiple sensitive periods in the developing visual system

The visual system has many different sensitive periods the timing of which vary as a function of brain region, the physiological or anatomical feature being examined and the method being used to alter the environment. For example, in layers 2/3 of the cat visual cortex, a shift in ocular dominance is observed when a one-month period of monocular deprivation is applied at any point up to 10–12 months of age. In contrast, for layer 4 cells ocular dominance cannot be altered by monocular deprivation after three months of age. Similarly, the sensitive period for **orientation selectivity** (see Chapter 9) ends well before the sensitive period for ocular dominance (Fig. 12.8), and the sensitive period for reverse occlusion also ends before the sensitive period for monocular deprivation. As we will see (Section 12.2) there are multiple cellular and molecular mechanisms that regulate the expression of ocular dominance plasticity and there is growing evidence that different critical periods may be linked to different mechanisms.[2] Similarly, many brain regions maintain a high degree of plasticity well into adulthood, which forms the basis of how we learn and remember events throughout life. So some mechanisms discussed below are not necessarily unique to development, but instead show region-specific time courses that can extend well in to adulthood.

orientation selectivity a physiological feature of neurons in the visual cortex by which they only respond to stimuli (e.g. a bar of light) of a particular orientation.

---

[2] For a detailed discussion of this topic see Berardi, N., Pizzorusso, T., Ratto, G. M. and Maffei, L. (2003) Molecular basis of plasticity in the visual cortex. *Trends Neurosci.*, **26**, 369–78.

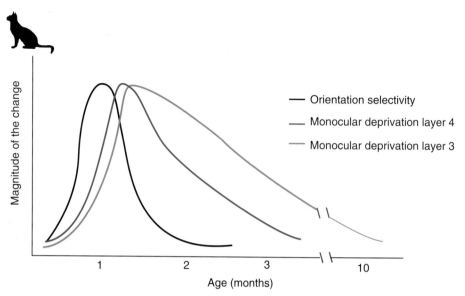

Fig. 12.8 There are numerous sensitive periods during development of the visual cortex. The sensitive period for altering orientation selectivity is the shortest (black line), ending by about 5 weeks of age in a cat. In contrast, sensitive periods for altering ocular dominance end much later and vary by cortical layer being examined. Monocular deprivation after 4 months of age has little effect on the ocular dominance of cortical cells in layer 4 (blue line). In contrast, monocular deprivation can alter ocular dominance of layer 3 cells until approximately 1 year of age (green line). The time-courses of the sensitive periods are not absolute; for example, dark-rearing from birth delays the onset and termination of the sensitive period for monocular deprivation.

Box 12.2 Rett syndrome

Conventional wisdom states that alterations in brain development that occur during sensitive periods are unresponsive to treatments initiated in adulthood. However, a recent paper using a mouse model of Rett syndrome has challenged this viewpoint. Rett syndrome is neurodevelopmental disorder that first presents between the ages of 6 and 18 months and affects 1 in 12 000 females (affected males die *in utero*). The majority of cases of Rett syndrome are caused by mutations in the *MECP2* gene, which is located on the X-chromosome and encodes a protein that binds to methylated DNA and regulates gene expression. Rett syndrome is characterized by numerous physical and mental abnormalities including a decrease head growth, cognitive impairment, anxiety disorder and autism-like behaviours. A mouse model of Rett syndrome, in which the *Mecp2* gene is deleted, exhibits neurological phenotypes very similar to those seen in humans. Adrian Bird and colleagues at the University of Edinburgh re-expressed MECP2 in adult mice lacking MECP2 and found many mice showed a complete reversion of neurological symptoms, including alterations in synaptic plasticity, and a substantial increase in life expectancy. These findings indicate that the neurological symptoms associated with the loss of MECP2 in mice do not result from an irreversible disruption of brain development. Whether such reversal of symptoms would be possible in humans with Rett syndrome and whether scientists will devise effective methods of gene therapy that can be used reliably and safely to treat such conditions is still unknown. However, it is important to remember that while many areas of the adult brain in carnivores and primates seem resistant to experience-dependent plasticity (e.g. primary visual cortex), those responsible for learning and memory and higher cognitive function (e.g. the hippocampus and prefrontal cortex) maintain a high degree of plasticity in adulthood. Therefore, rescue of function in adulthood could become a reality (see Box 10.3 on Fragile X Syndrome), provided appropriate pharmacological and genetic therapies are developed that can reverse the cellular alterations that cause these diseases in the first place.

Another important point concerning sensitive periods is that they are not immutable; their time-course can be altered by an animal's visual experience. For example, dark-rearing an animal from birth delays both the onset and termination of sensitive periods such that monocular deprivation in adult dark-reared animals has a much more dramatic effect than that found in similarly aged normally-reared animals. Furthermore, traditional viewpoints on sensitive periods suggest that once they are missed, function is permanently impaired. This belief has led to the current clinical dogma that developmental disorders, especially those with an obvious genetic basis, cannot be reversed in adulthood. However, recent exciting findings in mouse models of neurodevelopmental disease, most notably Rett syndrome, indicate that the story may not be so simple (Box 12.2).

12.2 How does experience change functional connectivity?

Now that we have seen that experience can change the way neurons communicate in the developing brain, it is time to focus on *how* experience changes brain connectivity. When discussing the cellular mechanisms that underlie developmental plasticity, there are three main questions that need to be addressed: (1) what determines the way in which a neuron or a synapse will change (i.e. what causes one eye's inputs to strengthen and another eye's inputs to weaken); (2) what determines if a neuron or synapse is **plastic**; (3) what determines the timing of the sensitive period? In the remainder of this chapter we shall examine the most prevalent theories that address these three questions (Sections 12.2–12.5), especially as they relate to regulating the effects of monocular deprivation and dark-rearing.[3]

plasticity the ability to change.

12.2.1 Electrical properties of dendrites

To examine the mechanism by which experience regulates neuronal development, it is first necessary to return to and extend some principles examined in Chapter 10. We saw that neurotransmitter released from a **presynaptic** terminal binds to receptors in the **postsynaptic density**. Some of these receptors are **ionotropic** and act as conduits for ions to flow across the membrane when open. These receptors open upon neurotransmitter binding, thereby causing a change in the membrane potential of the cell. At excitatory synapses, ionic flow causes the cell to **depolarize**, that is the inside of the cell becomes more positive relative to the outside. This depolarization is referred to as an **excitatory postsynaptic potential (EPSP)**. The change in membrane potential that results from the activation of a single synapse is called a **miniature excitatory postsynaptic potential (mEPSP)**. At inhibitory synapses, the ionic flow causes

presynaptic the cell generating a signal, generally in the form of a neurotransmitter, at a synapse.

postsynaptic density the **electron dense** protein complex of the postsynaptic terminal that is comprised of the neurotransmitter receptors, scaffolding molecules, signalling enzymes and cytoskeletal elements.

---

[3] For greater depth on the mechanisms of synaptic plasticity see Bliss, T., Collingridge, C. and Morris, R. (eds) (2004) *LTP: Long-term Potentiation, Enhancing Neuroscience for 30 Years.* Oxford University Press, Oxford.

the inside of the cells to become more negative, or **hyperpolarized**, relative to the outside of the cell. This hyperpolarization is called an inhibitory postsynaptic potential, or IPSP. At a single synapse, the hyperpolarization is called a miniature IPSP (mIPSPs). Individual mEPSPs are too small to depolarize a neuron's membrane to the threshold required to initiate an action potential. Instead, several mEPSPs must be combined to trigger an action potential. mEPSPs are short events that decay in size as they spread through a cell and so presynaptic inputs need to generate multiple mEPSPs sufficiently close together in time and cellular location so that they can combine to give an aggregate EPSP. The combination of EPSPs and IPSPs is referred to as **temporal** and **spatial summation**. All mEPSPs and mIPSPs are integrated at the cell soma and if their summed value (the EPSP) is above a certain threshold, an action potential will be initiated at the **axon initial segment** – a specialized region of the cell that is rich in voltage-dependent Na$^+$ channels necessary for initiation of the action potential. A critical point here is that dendritic EPSPs are *not* the same as axonal action potentials. Action potentials are all-or-nothing electrical events that result from the integration of all EPSPs and IPSPs generated at synaptic contacts in the dendrites and soma.

12.2.2 Cellular basis of plasticity: synaptic strengthening and weakening

As mentioned above, the physiological changes in ocular dominance that result from monocular deprivation occur much faster than changes in gross morphology of neurons or synapse number. This finding suggests that the shift in ocular dominance relies on a neuron's ability to modify the relative influence of existing synapses, that is neurons have the ability to change the **synaptic weight** of the synapses that process information from each eye. Synaptic weight (also referred to as **synaptic efficacy)** can be broadly defined as the amplitude of the depolarization or hyperpolarization associated with a certain level of activation of a given synapse. In other words it is the size of the mEPSP or mIPSP for that synapse.

The ability of a synapse (or group of synapses) to change its synaptic weight is referred to as **synaptic plasticity**. As mentioned briefly in Chapter 10, Donald Hebb proposed a theory of synaptic plasticity that has formed the basis of our understanding of activity-dependent development as well as how we store memories as adults. Hebb stated:

> When an axon of cell *A* is near enough to excite a cell *B* and repeatedly or persistently takes part in firing it, some growth process or metabolic change takes place in one or both cells such that *A*'s efficiency, as one of the cells firing *B*, is increased.

Hebb's postulate has now been captured in the common phrase, '*cells that fire together, wire together*'. Strong support for Hebb's postulate came with the discovery of **long-term potentiation (LTP)** by Bliss

(a): LTP

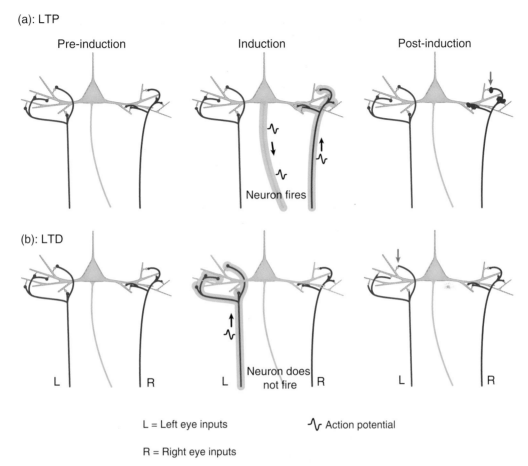

Pre-induction   Induction   Post-induction

Neuron fires

(b): LTD

Neuron does
not fire

L   R   L   R   L   R

L = Left eye inputs   ⏦ Action potential

R = Right eye inputs

Fig. 12.9 Induction of LTP and LTD results from the level of correlation between presynaptic and postsynaptic activity. Schematic of a neuron forming synapses with inputs from two axons (shown in blue and green). Activity is represented by bright yellow highlighting and shown with the schematics of action potentials. (a) LTP: left panel shows the state of the neuron prior to LTP induction (pre-induction). The middle panel shows that strong stimulation of the green axon causes the generation of action potentials in the axon of the postsynaptic cell (as indicated by yellow highlighting and schematic action potential) and induces LTP (depicted in the panel on the right by an increase in synapse size (e.g. red arrow). (b) LTD: in contrast, if a set of synapses (synapses of the blue axon) are active but do not lead to the generation of action potentials (middle panel), they will be weakened (depicted in the right panel by a decrease in size of the synapse, e.g. red arrow).

and Lomo in 1973.[4] LTP is defined as a long-term increase in synaptic weight resulting from coordinated activity between pre- and post-synaptic elements (these elements were discussed in Chapter 10). Key to the induction of LTP is that a sufficient number of synapses are co-activated to generate a summed depolarization that will result in action potentials in the postsynaptic cell (Fig. 12.9).

Neuronal networks and individual synapses also have the ability to weaken in response to a particular stimuli. In this case, when a pre-synaptic terminal is repeatedly active but does not lead to the genera-tion of action potentials in the postsynaptic neuron, the synapses will be weakened. In other words, '*cells that fire out of sync, lose their link*'.

[4] Bliss, T. V. and Lomo, T. (1973) Long-lasting potentiation of synaptic transmission in the dentate area of the anaesthetized rabbit following stimulation of the perforant path. *J Physiol.*, **232**, 331–56; an example experiment is shown in Box 12.3.

Box 12.3   LTP and LTD

Panel (a) shows a schematic of a typical experimental paradigm used to induce LTP/LTD similar to that used by Bliss and Lomo. A group of neurons (here depicted as a single neuron) is activated using an extracellular stimulation electrode (red, by the lower cell). These neurons make synaptic contacts with a group of postsynaptic neurons and the response of the postsynaptic neurons is examined using a recording electrode (blue). Recording electrodes can either monitor the physiological response of a single neuron or a small group of neurons. In either case, the size of the postsynaptic potential or EPSP (black traces in inset panels in (b) and (c)) is recorded every 5 s or so to determine the average baseline response to a given level of stimulation. The magnitude of each EPSP is represented as a percentage of the baseline response and plotted as a blue dot on the graphs below. Once a stable baseline is determined, an LTP or LTD-inducing stimulus is applied through the stimulating electrode. High frequency stimulations (i.e. 50–100 Hz) result in a large depolarization of the postsynaptic cells (and many action potentials) and induce a lasting increase in the magnitude of the EPSP in the postsynaptic cell (blue trace in inset in panel b). This is known as long-term potentiation or LTP. Low frequency (1–2 Hz) stimulations result in weak stimulation of the postsynaptic cell (and few action potentials) and a long-lasting reduction in EPSP amplitude in the postsynaptic cell (blue trace in inset in panel c). This is known as long-term depression or LTD. The precise magnitude of the LTP and LTD varies depending on the precise stimulation frequency employed. Most neurons are capable of undergoing either LTP or LTD depending on the frequency with which they are being stimulated, indicating that they are 'bidirectional'. Thus plotting the magnitude of the synaptic weight change (LTD or LTD) against the stimulation frequency used to induce that change, results in a quasi-continuous line forming a sine wave (see Fig. 12.16).

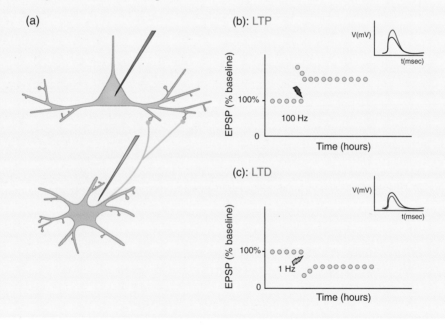

The persistent weakening of synaptic weight following a particular stimulus is called **long-term depression (LTD)**.

12.2.3 The time-course of changes in synaptic weight in response to monocular deprivation

It is widely believed the loss of functional connectivity of the deprived eye and the subsequent gain of functional synapses of the non-deprived eye are mediated, in part, by LTD and LTP, respectively, at

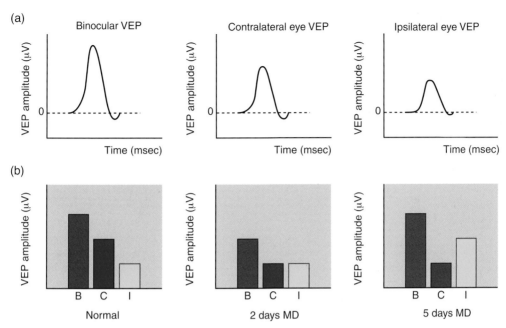

Fig. 12.10 Effects of monocular deprivation on visually-evoked potentials (VEPs). (a) Schematic showing typical waveforms of three VEPs arising from the stimulation of both eyes simultaneously (left panel), only the contralateral eye (middle panel) or only the ipsilateral eye (right panel). The experiments are very similar to those of Hubel and Wiesel outlined in Box 9.5, with the exception that the electrode used is capable of recording from small groups of cells (generally around 30). The VEPs shown here represent the combined activity of neurons in the binocular region of primary visual cortex of the mouse where the contralateral eye has a larger input to cortical cells (compare the middle to the right panel). (b) Bar graphs showing the amplitude of the binocular (B: blue bar), contralateral (C: green bar) or ipsilateral (I, yellow bar) VEPs in a normal mouse immediately before monocular deprivation (left panel) and 2 days (middle panel) or 5 days (right panel) after the start of monocular deprivation. Two days of monocular deprivation induces a decrease in the binocular VEP. This reduction results from a decrease in the deprived eye VEPs (in this case the contralateral eye was deprived). After 2 days of monocular deprivation there is no change in the non-deprived, ipsilateral, eye VEPs. By 5 days, the binocular VEP response has returned to normal levels as a result of an increase in VEP amplitude of the non-deprived, ipsilateral, eye along with a sustained reduction in the contralateral VEP.

cortical synapses. Importantly, LTP and LTD do not occur in unison. Instead, during monocular deprivation, deprived eye synapses are weakened prior to the strengthening of non-deprived eye synapses. This time-course of synaptic plasticity can be demonstrated by conducting experiments very similar to those illustrated in Box 9.5, with the exception that the electrodes used sample the activity levels from of small group of cells rather than single cells. The combined activity of a group of cells to a given visual stimulus is known as a **visually-evoked potential** or **VEP** (Fig. 12.10). By using an opaque contact lens, a stimulus can be shown to one eye only. Alternatively a stimulus can be shown to both eyes simultaneously. In the former scenario, the VEP will represent the activity of either the contralateral or ipsilateral eye; in the latter scenario the VEP will represent the combined activity from both eyes. During monocular deprivation, binocular VEP activity falls over the first 2 days as a result of depression of closed eye synapses (of course the closed eye needs to be reopened or uncovered for the experiment). As the period of monocular deprivation increases, there is a gradual increase in the binocular VEP activity as the connections from the open eye become stronger. After a week of monocular

visually-evoked potential VEP the physiological response of a small group of neurons in the visual cortex to visual stimulation.

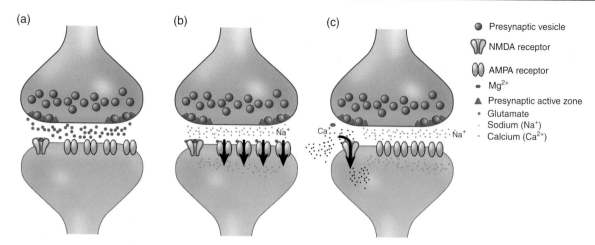

Fig. 12.11 The NMDA receptor is a coincidence detector. (a) Schematic of a synapse containing the NMDA receptors (orange) and AMPA receptors (blue) in the postsynaptic membrane. (b) Glutamate (orange circles) binds to both types of receptors but initially only the AMPA receptors open and Na$^+$ ions pass into the postsynaptic cell. No ions pass through the NMDA receptor because of the presence of a magnesium ion (red hexagon). The Mg^{2+} ion is only removed from the pore of the NMDA receptor if enough positive ions enter the cell through the AMPA receptors, i.e. if the membrane becomes sufficiently depolarized. (c) Once the Mg^{2+} is removed from the pore, the NMDA receptor is open to pass ions, including Ca^{2+}, which enters the cell and activates a range of intracellular signalling pathways that mediate LTP. Because NMDA receptors are only activated if there is sufficient correlated input to depolarize the cell enough to remove the Mg^{2+} block, it acts as a detector of coincident activity.

deprivation, binocular VEP levels are similar to those observed prior to the monocular deprivation.

12.2.4 Cellular and molecular mechanisms of LTP/LTD induction

A necessary feature of any cellular process that induces synaptic plasticity is that it must be able to sense correlated presynaptic and postsynaptic activities, that is, it must be a **coincidence detector**. The first hint at a molecular basis of LTP induction came with the discovery of the **NMDA receptor** (mentioned in Chapter 11 in the context of its role in regulating cell death). NMDA receptors are **glutamatergic** receptors that act as cation channels. A unique feature of NMDA receptors is that they are blocked by a magnesium ion (Mg^{2+}) that sits in the pore of the channel at the resting membrane potential. Therefore, glutamate binding does not by itself cause the opening of the channel (Fig. 12.11). Instead the channel is only free to pass cations when the intracellular membrane depolarizes sufficiently to repel the positive Mg^{2+} (i.e. to unblock the pore). This level of depolarization arises with the activation of sufficient numbers of another type of glutamate receptor, the **AMPA receptor**. When AMPA receptors are open, the resulting influx of Na$^+$ ions depolarizes the cell membrane and expels the Mg^{2+}. Ca^{2+} can now enter the cell through the open NMDA receptor channel. In this way, the NMDA receptor acts as a coincidence detector, only becoming active when there is coincidence between presynaptic activity (glutamate release) and postsynaptic activation (sufficient depolarization) via AMPA receptors.

coincidence detector a cellular mechanism that detects whether presynaptic and postsynaptic activation occur during a defined time-window.

AMPA receptor a type of glutamate receptor that is responsible for the majority of the initial depolarization of the excitatory postsynaptic potential following activation of an excitatory synapse.

A role for NMDA receptors in inducing ocular dominance plasticity was first demonstrated using pharmacological inhibition of NMDA receptor activation. Infusion of NMDA receptor blockers into primary visual cortex of cats prevented the shift in ocular dominance associated with monocular deprivation (Fig. 12.12). Some of the intracellular pathways that mediate NMDA receptor plasticity resulting from monocular deprivation have also been identified using both pharmacological inhibition of particular enzymes or genetic deletion in mouse of particular genes encoding these proteins. Several examples of pathways involved in ocular dominance changes in response to monocular deprivation are shown in Fig. 12.12.

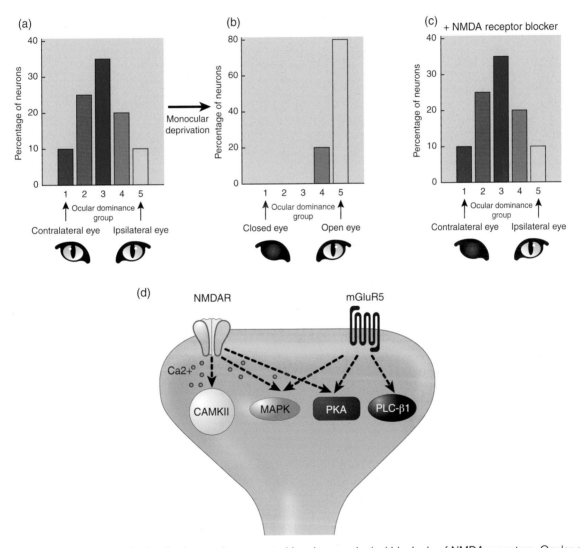

Fig. 12.12 Effects of monocular deprivation can be prevented by pharmacological blockade of NMDA receptors. Ocular dominance histograms from a normal (a) and a monocularly deprived (b) cat (as seen in Fig. 12.2). The shift in ocular dominance in response to monocular deprivation does not occur if an NMDA receptor blocker is infused into the visual cortex during the period of monocular deprivation (c). (d) Schematic summarizing some of the neurotransmitter receptors and their associated intracellular pathways that have been demonstrated to regulate ocular dominance plasticity. Dotted arrows indicate the intracellular pathways that can be activated by NMDA receptors and metabotropic glutamate receptors (mGluR5), although which receptors activate which intracellular pathways, to mediate ocular dominance plasticity, is not known.

12.2.5 Synaptic changes that mediate the expression of LTP/LTD and experience-dependent plasticity

One of the most heated debates in neuroscience through the 1990s concerned the nature of the cellular changes that underlie LTP and LTD. At the heart of the debate was whether the site of cellular changes lay within the presynaptic terminal or in the postsynaptic cell. While this debate is still active for certain cell types, what is now clear is that there are numerous mechanisms, both pre- and postsynaptic, that can underlie synaptic plasticity, including the following examples.

(1) Postsynaptic: changes in the number of AMPA receptors
While NMDA receptors have been shown to regulate the *induction* of certain forms of synaptic plasticity, other proteins mediate the *expression* of synaptic plasticity, that is, the actual change in the amplitude of the EPSP. Perhaps the most studied mechanism underlying the expression of LTP and LTD is the insertion and removal of AMPA receptors in the postsynaptic membrane (Fig. 12.13).

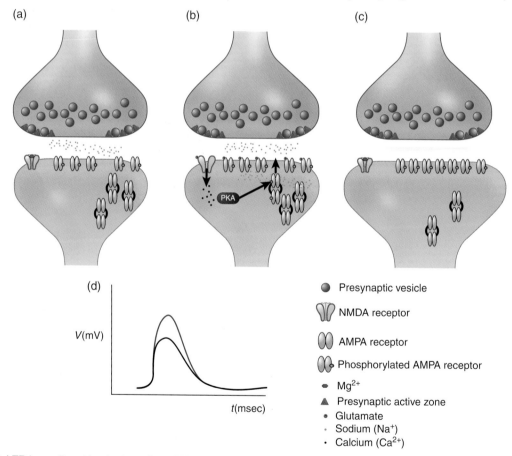

Fig. 12.13 LTP is mediated by the insertion of AMPA receptors. Schematic of prototypical synapse (a) in which an LTP induction protocol results from Ca^{2+} (coming through the NMDA receptor) activating intracellular kinases, such as protein kinase A (PKA) (b). PKA phosphorylates AMPA receptors contained in transport vesicles causing their insertion into the postsynaptic density, which becomes larger (c). (d) EPSP elicited in response to presynaptic stimulation (see Box 12.3) prior to (black trace) and after (blue trace) LTP induction. The increase in AMPA receptors causes more cations to pass into the cell upon stimulation, thereby increasing the amplitude of the EPSP.

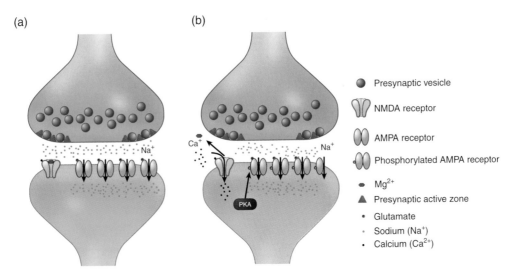

Fig. 12.14 LTP is mediated by a change in the length of time that AMPA receptors are open. (a) Schematic of a prototypical synapse that contains numerous intracellular kinases including including PKA. (b) In this scenario, LTP results from Ca^{2+} entering the postsynaptic cell through the NMDA receptor causing activation of PKA, which phosphorylates AMPA receptors already inserted in the postsynaptic density causing them to remain open for a longer period of time following glutamate binding. In consequence, more Na^+ ions pass through the AMPA receptors generating a larger EPSP.

Following stimuli that induce LTP, AMPA receptors are inserted into the postsynaptic membrane. The result is an increase in the amplitude of subsequent EPSPs (i.e. LTP). Similarly, stimulations that induce LTD result in the removal of AMPA receptors. In the case of visual system plasticity, the role of AMPA receptor movement into and out of the postsynaptic density in mediating the effects of monocular deprivation was tested using *in vivo* transfection of layer 4 cells with viruses encoding peptides that block AMPA receptor removal from the membrane. These peptides prevent the removal of AMPA receptors in the synapses that carry information from the closed eye, and this prevents the shift in ocular dominance that normally results from monocular deprivation.

(2) Postsynaptic: changes in the kinetics of AMPA receptors

In addition to increasing the number of AMPA receptors, LTP induction protocols can also change the amount of current that flows through an individual receptor (Fig. 12.14). In the case of LTP, **phosphorylation** of AMPA subunits by **kinases** such as cAMP-dependent protein kinase A (PKA) or Ca^{2+}/calmodulin kinase II (CAMKII) increases the amount of current that flows through AMPA receptors to mediate LTP. Both of these kinases regulate the shift in ocular dominance in response to monocular deprivation. However, whether these changes in AMPA receptor kinetics mediate the effects of monocular deprivation is not known, since both CAMKII and PKA are also known to regulate the trafficking of AMPA receptors into and out of the PSD.

(3) Presynaptic: changes in the release of neurotransmitter

At some synapses, LTP expression results from an increase in neurotransmitter release rather than increasing the number of

phosphorylation the addition of a phosphate group to a molecule often causing its activation or deactivation.

kinases an enzyme that transfers phosphate groups onto specific molecules, a process called phosphorylation.

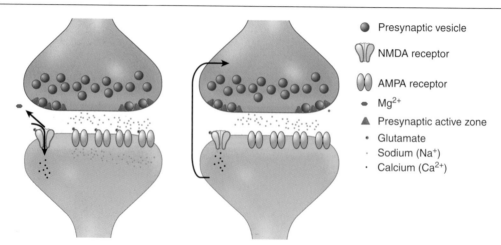

●	Presynaptic vesicle
ᴡ	NMDA receptor
ᴡ	AMPA receptor
●	Mg²⁺
▲	Presynaptic active zone
·	Glutamate
·	Sodium (Na⁺)
·	Calcium (Ca²⁺)

Fig. 12.15 LTP is mediated by an increase in presynaptic release of neurotransmitter. (a) Schematic of a prototypical synapse in which induction of LTP results in the influx of Ca²⁺ through NMDA receptors. (b) This subsequently causes the release of a retrograde factor (black arrow) that acts on the presynaptic terminal to increase subsequent neurotransmitter release. There is evidence from both visual and somatosensory cortex that **endocannabinoids** act as the retrograde factor to regulate presynaptic glutamate release in response to altered sensory experience. Similarly there is evidence from somatosensory cortex that **nitric oxide** plays a key role in the expression of experience-dependent plasticity.

nitric oxide a small gaseous molecule that acts as a local signalling molecule.

endocannabinoids naturally occurring lipids in the body that bind and activate cannabinoid receptors.

postsynaptic receptors (Fig. 12.15). The spread of the action potential into the presynaptic terminal activates calcium channels and Ca²⁺-dependent synaptic vesicle fusion at the presynaptic active zone to release neurotransmitter. Activation of postsynaptic receptors and signalling pathways then stimulates the release of molecules from the postsynaptic cell, called **retrograde messengers**. These act on the presynaptic terminal to increase subsequent neurotransmitter release. There is evidence from both visual and somatosensory cortex that **endocannabinoids** act as a retrograde factor to mediate certain forms of experience-dependent plasticity. In fact, pharmacological inhibition of receptors for endocannabinoids during monocular deprivation prevents the shift in ocular dominance in layer 3, but not in layer 4. This finding indicates that multiple mechanisms of synaptic depression and potentiation combine to mediate the effects of visual experience in the developing visual cortex.

12.2.6 Metaplasticity

A key feature of synaptic plasticity is that synapses have the ability to undergo both LTP and LTD. In other words, plasticity is **bidirectional** (Fig. 12.16). In Box 12.3 we saw that by varying the frequency of an electrical stimulus used to activate presynaptic axons, we can induce either LTP or LTD. The graph in Fig. 12.16(a) illustrates this point by plotting the magnitude of LTP or LTD induced by a range of stimulation frequencies. As the stimulation frequency is increased, there is a switch

(a)

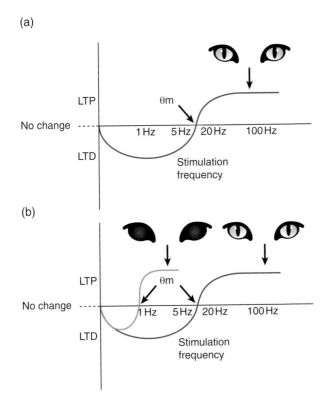

(b)

Fig. 12.16 Metaplasticity. Experience alters the stimulation frequencies necessary to induce LTP and LTD. Graph showing data for a neuron in the developing visual cortex of a normal animal (blue trace) and a dark-reared animal (orange trace). By conducting a range of experiments like those described in Box 12.3, and systematically changing the frequency of presynaptic stimulation, the change in the amplitude of the EPSP can be plotted to generate a frequency-response curve. Electrophysiological monitoring of layer 3 neurons in thin slices through the visual cortex of normally-reared animals show that low frequency presynaptic stimulation (e.g. in the example shown around 1 Hz) induces LTD and high frequency stimulation (e.g. in the example shown between 10 and 100 Hz) stimulation induces LTP of presynaptic inputs. The stimulation frequency between 1 Hz and 100 Hz at which there is a switch from LTD to LTP is referred to as the modification threshold (θm). During the sensitive period, dark-rearing for 48 hours dramatically reduces θm.

from LTD induction to LTP induction. The stimulation frequency at which this switch occurs (when neither LTD nor LTP is induced) is referred to as the **modification threshold**.

We now know that for many neurons in the developing visual cortex, the relationship between the frequency of presynaptic stimulation and the resulting change in EPSP amplitude is not fixed; a stimulation frequency that at one point in time elicits LTP, may at another point in time elicit LTD. The ability of a neuron to alter the presynaptic stimulation frequencies that induce LTD and LTP, as represented by a change in the modification threshold, is known as **metaplasticity**. Changes in the modification threshold occur in a predictable manner that is dictated by the activity history of the neuron. For example, dark-rearing removes all visual stimulation and dramatically reduces the average firing rates of visual cortical neurons; dark-rearing also causes a dramatic reduction in the modification threshold (Fig. 12.16 (b)). Metaplasticity is a key feature of developing neurons as it allows them to monitor and modify the total activity levels. Neurons that have gone through a period of low activation levels can reduce the threshold at which LTP is elicited so that they become more amenable to synaptic strengthening. Neurons that have undergone a period of high activation can increase the threshold at which LTP is initiated, thereby promoting LTD.

12.2.7 Spike-timing dependent plasticity

Hebb's postulate (Section 12.2.2) relies on the synchronous activation of presynaptic axons and postsynaptic cells. *In vivo*, experiences that induce lasting increases in synaptic strength almost certainly cause the coincident activation of many synapses; even small EPSPs can contribute to the generation of an action potential through spatial summation and hence contribute to LTP. However, to induce LTP experimentally requires intense stimulation of presynaptic axons (see Box 12.3) in order to activate a sufficient number of synapses on a given neuron to elicit axon potentials. Such intense stimulation rarely, if ever, occurs under natural conditions. This has raised the question of whether LTP and LTD are important mechanisms of neuronal plasticity *in vivo*. More recently another method for inducing LTP and LTD has been developed that allows greater control over the timing of presynaptic and post-synaptic activation and utilizes levels of presynaptic stimulation that more closely reflect activity levels found naturally. This form of synaptic plasticity is called **spike-timing dependent plasticity (STDP)**. STDP is a specialized form of LTP and LTD (referred to as **tLTP** and **tLTD** for 'timing LTP/LTD') and is another physiological manifestation of Hebb's postulate.

The key difference between STDP and standard LTP/LTD induction is that the experimenter controls the level of postsynaptic cell activation in addition to presynaptic stimulation. Using a physiological technique known as patch clamping, an experimenter is able to keep the post-synaptic neuron relatively depolarized, thereby mimicking the activation of a large number of synapses (Bert Sakmann and Erwin Neher were awarded the Nobel Prize in Physiology or Medicine in 1991 for the development of this technique and their work on ion channel function).[5] Under these conditions, the activation of even small numbers of synapses can reach the cell's threshold for the generation of action potentials. The experimenter can also control the timing of pre-synaptic stimulation and postsynaptic cell depolarization. Whether a synapse undergoes tLTP, tLTD or no change is dependent upon the precise timing of the presynaptic action potential and the occurrence of a postsynaptic action potential. In the simplest example of STDP (represented diagrammatically in Fig. 12.17(a)), if presynaptic stimulation is generated immediately prior to postsynaptic depolarization, the active synapses are strengthened (tLTP). However, if the presynaptic activation occurs a longer time before or after postsynaptic depolarization, the active synapses are weakened (tLTD). If the time difference between pre- and postsynaptic activation is great there will be no change in synaptic weight.

So how can a synapse know whether its EPSP coincided with the generation of a postsynaptic action potential? In other words, how is coincidence detection achieved? Insight into the mechanism of STDP came from the discovery that dendrites are not simply passive conductors of electrical current. In fact, action potentials generated at the axon initial segment are not only transmitted down the axon, but are also prop-agated back into the dendrites. The spread of an action potential into dendrites is called a **back-propagating action potential** (bAP) (Fig. 12.17(b)). Unlike action potentials in axons that are mediated by

---

[5] http://nobelprize.org/nobel_prizes/medicine/laureates/1991/sakmann-lecture.html [20 November 2010]. http://nobelprize.org/nobel_prizes/medicine/laureates/1991/neher-lecture.html [20 November 2010].

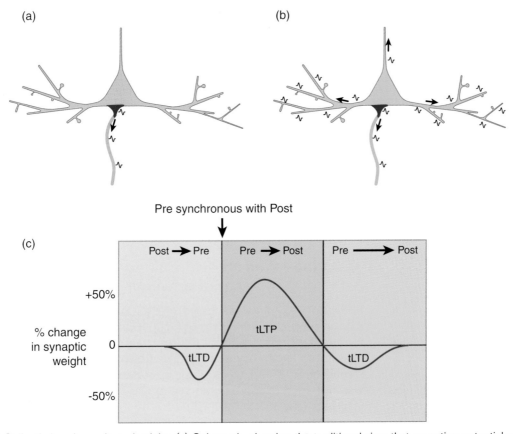

Fig. 12.17 Spike-timing dependent plasticity. (a) Schematic showing the traditional view that an action potential generated at the axon hillock (green) is propagated down the axon (arrow). (b) Schematic showing that action potentials that initiate at the axon hillock also spread back into the dendrites where they are called back-propagating action potentials or bAPs. (c) Graph demonstrating that the timing of presynaptic activation relative to the generation of a back propagating action potential determines whether there is a change in synaptic weight, i.e. whether LTP, LTD or no change occurs. When the bAP occurs just prior to presynaptic activation (blue shaded area) tLTD results. When the bAP occurs during a narrow time window after presynaptic activation, the result is tLTP (green shaded area). However, if the bAP occurs too long after presynaptic activation, the result is tLTD (pink shaded area). If presynaptic activation and the bAP occur too far apart in time, no change in synaptic strength results. The length of time between pre- and postsynaptic stimulation is indicated by the length of the arrow.

voltage-gated sodium channels (see Chapter 10), bAPs are mediated by a range of membrane proteins including both voltage-gated calcium and sodium channels. bAPs signal to recently active synapses, telling them that they have contributed to a postsynaptic signal that generated an action potential.

Evidence for STDP in developmental plasticity during cortical development is difficult to demonstrate since the mechanisms of induction (i.e. NMDA receptors and Ca^{2+} entry) and expression (trafficking of AMPA receptors) are the same as those for LTP and LTD. However, numerous researchers have provided good evidence that these mechanisms play a key role in synaptic plasticity within individual cortical cells during the sensitive period.[6]

---

[6] For further reading see Feldman, D. E. (2009) Synaptic mechanisms for plasticity in neocortex. *Annu Rev Neurosci.*, **32**, 33–55.

12.3 Cellular basis of plasticity: development of inhibitory networks

Up to this point we have focused solely on the how plasticity at excitatory synapses mediates changes in ocular dominance plasticity. However, the brain is a complex neural network that consists of many inhibitory synapses that are crucial to normal brain processing and plasticity. A role for inhibition in ocular dominance plasticity was suggested over 30 years ago, but it is only relatively recently that some details of how inhibition may regulate plasticity have emerged. Inhibition has been implicated in two main aspects of plasticity: (1) in regulating the *expression* of the effects of monocular deprivation (as opposed to *inducing* the effects) and (2) in determining the time-course of the sensitive period.

12.3.1 Inhibition mediates expression of the effects of monocular deprivation

In Section 12.2.3 we discussed several mechanisms by which synaptic strengthening and weakening (i.e. LTD and LTP) mediate the effects of monocular deprivation. These mechanisms related to excitatory synapses onto excitatory neurons. An alternative hypothesis relies on the strengthening and weakening of synapses onto inhibitory neurons without such dramatic changes in the synaptic weights at excitatory synapses (Fig. 12.18). According to the inhibition hypothesis, the non-deprived eye would activate inhibitory circuits that interfere with the ability of the deprived eye to activate excitatory cortical cells. Support for a role of inhibitory circuitry came from experiments using pharmacological blockade of **GABA** receptors in monocularly deprived animals. As discussed above, neurons in monocularly deprived animals show little if any response to stimulation of the deprived eye. However, when inhibition was removed by blocking $GABA_A$ receptors, responses to deprived-eye stimulation reappeared indicating that functional synapses were still present, but inhibitory circuits were preventing them from activating the cortical neurons. It is important to note that a role for changes in inhibition and changes in synaptic strength at excitatory synapses are not mutually exclusive and it is likely that both play a role in the myriad of anatomical and physiological effects that result from monocular deprivation.[7]

GABA the most common inhibitory neurotransmitter in the brain.

12.3.2 Development of inhibitory circuits regulates the time-course of the sensitive period for monocular deprivation

As we saw in Chapter 10, in the cerebral cortex of adult mice **GABA** signalling is generally inhibitory, but during embryonic and **perinatal** development, such signalling is excitatory instead. During this time

---

[7] For further reading on the role of inhibition in regulating ocular dominance plasticity see Hensch, T. K. (2005) Critical period plasticity in local cortical circuits. *Nat. Rev. Neurosci.*, **6**, 877–88.

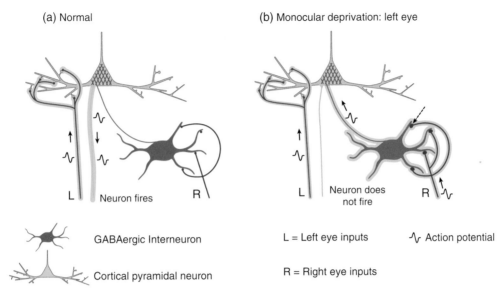

(a) Normal

(b) Monocular deprivation: left eye

L   Neuron fires   R

L   Neuron does not fire   R

GABAergic Interneuron

Cortical pyramidal neuron

L = Left eye inputs

R = Right eye inputs

Action potential

Fig. 12.18 Inhibitory regulation of ocular dominance plasticity. This is a highly simplified diagram of how inhibition could regulate the loss of functional connectivity from the deprived eye.[7] (a) Schematic of a cortical pyramidal neuron (orange) making synaptic contacts with axons carrying information from the left eye (L, blue axons) and a GABAergic interneuron (red) receiving inputs from the right eye (R, green axons). The pyramidal neuron receives synaptic contacts onto its cell body (red cross-hatch). (For the sake of simplicity, the inputs from the right eye onto the pyramidal cell are not shown as they remain unchanged by monocular deprivation.) In a normal animal, activity in the left-eye axons (indicated by yellow highlighting) causes action potentials in the pyramidal neuron. (b) In a monocularly deprived animal in which the left eye was deprived of vision, the input from the open right eye onto the GABAergic interneuron is strengthened (as shown schematically by an increase in presynaptic size – dotted arrow). It is important to remember that, unlike what was described in Fig. 12.9 for LTP and LTD, excitatory input to cortical pyramidal neurons is not altered. Therefore, following monocular deprivation, the deprived (left) eye synapses are still active, but there is strong synchronous activity at GABAergic synapses onto the cortical neuron that prevents the generation of action potentials. This mechanism could explain the silencing of input carrying information from the deprived eye that results from monocular deprivation.

frame, the visual cortex is not responsive to alterations in the visual environment. This raised the possibility that the switch to inhibition was important for determining the onset of the sensitive period for monocular deprivation. It is now clear that the development of inhibitory circuits is essential for determining the onset and termination of the sensitive period for monocular deprivation. Manipulations that either enhance or inhibit GABAergic function cause the premature initiation or delay the initiation of the sensitive period for monocular deprivation, respectively (Fig. 12.19). For example, pharmacological enhancement of GABA_A receptor activity using **benzodiazepines** or premature development of a particular subset of GABAergic neurons in the visual cortex (as identified by their expression of a calcium binding protein, parvalbumin), resulted in the ability to induce a shift in ocular dominance in response to monocular deprivation at younger ages than would be possible in a non-treated animal. Similarly, inhibiting GABAergic function through genetically deleting an enzyme needed for GABA synthesis leads to a delay in the initiation of the sensitive period, as does delaying development of GABAergic systems by rearing animals in complete darkness.

benzodiazepines a group of pharmacological agents that act as sedatives by increasing GABA receptor activity and therefore increase inhibition in neuronal networks.

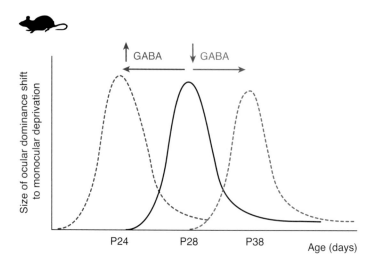

Fig. 12.19 GABA regulates the timing of the sensitive period for monocular deprivation. Graph showing the magnitude of the ocular dominance shift following a period of monocular deprivation as a function of the animal's age. In normal mice, the critical period begins around postnatal day (P) 24, peaks around P28 and is over by P32 (solid black line). In mice in which GABAergic neurotransmission is prematurely increased (blue dashed line) using GABA$_A$ receptor agonists such as benzodiazepines, there is a shift in the sensitive period to earlier ages (dashed blue line). In contrast, when the development of GABAergic function is delayed by dark-rearing or genetic deletion of enzymes that produce GABA (e.g. *Gad65*) there is a shift in the sensitive period to later ages (dashed red line).

12.4 Homeostatic plasticity

In the preceding sections we have seen how monocular deprivation causes a loss of functional connectivity between the deprived eye and neurons in the visual cortex. A recent study using mice found the surprising result that, while this was true for the vast majority of neurons in the visual cortex, a small percentage of neurons actually showed an increase in their responsiveness following monocular deprivation. Traditional Hebbian models of plasticity cannot explain this paradoxical finding, nor can it be easily explained by changes in inhibitory networks. Instead another form of synaptic plasticity, known as **homeostatic plasticity**, is needed to understand these findings.

Homeostasis is a key concept throughout the discipline of physiology and is defined as the ability of a physiological system to maintain internal stability, especially in response to external stimuli that alter the physiological state of the system. Over the last decade or so, scientists have shown that the general excitability of neurons is stabilized by homeostatic regulation. Neurons regulate their general excitability to ensure that overall firing rates do not become too high and potentially induce epileptic activity in brain circuits, or too low and hamper the fidelity of a neuronal circuit by becoming similar to levels of spontaneous activity.

So is there a specific population of cells that increase their firing rates during monocular deprivation? Recall that the majority of neurons in the visual cortex are binocular. Therefore, monocular deprivation only removes part of their functional input; the remaining input from the open eye continues to excite these cells and eventually the levels of input from the open eye will increase (Section 12.2.3). However, a small percentage of cells in the visual cortex receive input from only one eye; if they receive input solely from the deprived eye then all visually-evoked activity will be removed creating a situation similar to dark-rearing. It is these cells that appear to increase their excitability during monocular deprivation. The cellular mechanisms that mediate

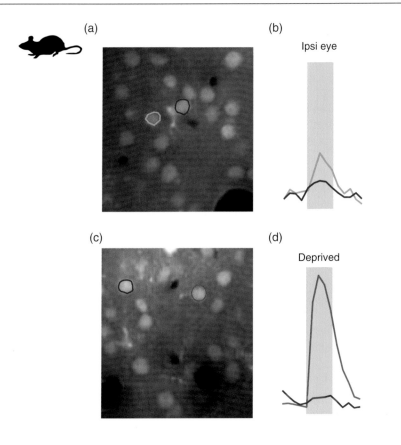

(a)

(b) Ipsi eye

(c)

(d) Deprived

Fig. 12.20 Homeostatic plasticity in mouse visual cortex in response to monocular deprivation. (a) and (b) Images of mouse visual cortex using two-photon imaging of cells filled with Ca^{2+} sensitive dyes (see Box 10.1) Cells in the visual cortex are filled with a Ca^{2+}-sensitive dye that transiently fluoresces upon an increase in intracellular Ca^{2+} levels (a,c). The amount of fluorescence reflects the magnitude of the rise in intracellular Ca^{2+}, which can be measured and plotted as an increase in fluorescence as a function of time (colour traces in (b and d). In visual cortex of a normal mouse, neurons respond to visual stimulation as shown by an increase in the level of intracellular Ca^{2+} (b). In monocularly deprived animals, some neurons show a large Ca^{2+} influx in response to visual stimulation of the deprived eye (d) (it is reopened to conduct the experiment). These data illustrate a homeostatic increase in excitability in a small portion of cells as a result of monocular deprivation. Reprinted from Neuron, **54**, Mrsic-Flogel T. D., Hofer S. B., Ohki K., Reid R. C., Bonhoeffer T., Hubener M., Homeostatic Regulation of Eye-Specific Responses in Visual Cortex during Ocular Dominance Plasticity, 961–72, 2007, with permission from Elsevier.

the induction and expression of homeostatic plasticity are a subject of intense interest (Fig. 12.20).[8]

12.5 Structural plasticity and the role of the extracellular matrix

In Section 12.1.4 we learned that monocular deprivation causes a complete shift in ocular dominance prior to the visible loss or gain of synapses. However, monocular deprivation does cause some profound changes in the shape and dynamics of **dendritic spines**. In Chapter 10 we examined how different spine morphologies reflect different stages of spine development. Spine morphology is also closely linked to synaptic weight, such that mushroom spines with large heads have more AMPA receptors in their postsynaptic density than do spines with smaller heads. Similarly spine shape has also been closely linked to spine dynamics with large mushroom-shaped spines being less dynamic than thin spines or filopodia. Recently, monocular deprivation has been shown to increase spine dynamics on certain populations of neurons in the primary visual cortex.

---

[8] For more information see Turrigiano, G. G. (2008) The self-tuning neuron: synaptic scaling of excitatory synapses. *Cell*, **135**, 422–35.

How do neurons regulate the dynamics and shape of dendritic spines? While alteration of the cytoskeleton is critical to this process (see Chapter 7), there is also a clear role for the extracellular matrix (ECM) (see Chapter 7, Box 7.2, for a recap of the ECM). During monocular deprivation there is an increase in the expression of tissue plasminogen activator (tPA), a protease that is released locally from dendrites and acts to degrade key elements of the extracellular matrix. The ECM normally acts to restrict spine dynamics and so its local disruption by tPA allows spines to change their shape more readily. This suggests that tPA is a *permissive* factor for regulating developmental plasticity, a suggestion that is supported by the finding that mice unable to produce tPA (*Tpa* knock-out mice) show reduced ocular dominance plasticity in response to monocular deprivation.

Other evidence suggests a role of the ECM in regulating the *termination* of sensitive periods. This comes from studies examining the role of **chondroitin sulphate proteoglycans** (CSPGs). In Chapter 7 we saw how CSPGs inhibit **neurite** extension in cultured neurons. It turns out that CSPGs also appear to play a critical role in restricting ocular dominance plasticity and hence terminating the sensitive period. CSPGs are present in **perineuronal nets** – ECM structures that form around subpopulations of neurons and are believed to regulate synaptogenesis and plasticity. This hypothesis was directly tested by infusing an enzyme that cleaves CSPGs into the visual cortex of *adult* rats during monocular deprivation for 7 or 14 days. In the adult animals receiving chondroitinase treatment, a clear shift in ocular dominance in response to monocular deprivation was seen. No shift was seen in uninjected animals indicating the CSPGs themselves, or molecules that are regulated by CSPGs, restrict plasticity in response to monocular deprivation in adult animals.

Although beyond the scope of this book, it is important to note that other signals in the extracellular environment have also been shown to regulate developmental plasticity. Of particular interest are observations that myelin may also serve to inhibit ocular dominance plasticity.[9] Mice that lack a key protein in myelin show an extended sensitive period well into adulthood.

In summary, it is clear that many different mechanisms regulate cortical plasticity including neurotransmitter receptor signalling pathways and extracellular signals. Some of the mechanisms *instruct* the changes determining which synapses strengthen and which weaken, while others act as *permissive* factors, determining when a neuron or group of synapses are able to respond to such instruction (i.e. are plastic). Importantly, none of these mechanisms are mutually exclusive. Rather, the complex changes in anatomical and physiological properties that occur in response to experience almost certainly result from a combination of several of these mechanisms.

chondroitin sulphate proteoglycans diverse components of the extracellular matrix (ECM).

neurite a collective term for axons and dendrites, especially applied to the immature stages during outgrowth.

---

[9] McGee, A. W., Yang, Y., Fischer, Q. S., Daw, N. W. and Strittmatter, S. M. (2005) Experience-driven plasticity of visual cortex limited by myelin and Nogo receptor. *Science*, **309**, 2222–6.

12.6 Summary

- Visual experience regulates the anatomical and physiological development of the visual cortex.
- There are critical time-windows called *sensitive periods* during which alterations of visual experience such as monocular deprivation can modify the functional features of sensory systems (i.e. neurons are plastic).
- During these sensitive periods in the visual cortex, altering visual experience can induce both competitive and associative interactions between the inputs from the two eyes.
- There is a range of cellular mechanisms that mediate the *induction* and *expression* of ocular dominance plasticity. They include long-term changes in synaptic strength, the regulation of inhibitory circuits and homeostatic plasticity.
- There are numerous mechanisms that regulate the timing of the sensitive periods.

Suggestions for Further Reading

General

In this introductory textbook we have asserted many things without extensive reference to literature which would provide the evidence for those assertions. We hope that we have succeeded in stimulating the reader to want to know more about the subjects we have discussed, including evidence on which our understanding is based. As a step up to a higher level, we suggest the textbook by Sanes, D.H., Reh, T.A. and Harris, W.A. (2006) *Development of the Nervous System*, Elsevier Academic Press, which covers many of the topics included here and more, in greater depth and with extensive referencing. An alternative containing more detail and references is by Brown, M., Keynes, R. and Lumsden, A (2001) *The Developing Brain*, Oxford University Press. With regards to brain development in mammals, the monograph by Price, D.J. and Willshaw, D.A. (2000) *Mechanisms of Cortical Development*, Oxford University Press, is also extensively referenced.

The following are some books and reviews with content relevant to specific chapters: some were referenced in the chapters themselves.

Chapter 1

Kile, B. T. and Hilton, D. J. (2005) The art and design of genetic screens: mouse. *Nature Reviews Genetics*, **6**, 557–567.

St Johnston, D. (2002) The art and design of genetic screens: *Drosophila melanogaster*. *Nature Reviews Genetics*, **3**, 176–188.

Strachan, T. and Read, A. P. (2004) *Human Molecular Genetics, Part 3*, Garland Science.

Chapter 2

Cohen, S. M. (1993). Imaginal disc development, in *The Development of Drosophila melanogaster, Vol. 2*, (eds M. Bate and A. Martinez Arias), Cold Spring Harbor Laboratory Press, New York, Pp. 747–842.

Copp, A. J. and Greene, N. D. (2010) Genetics and development of neural tube defects. *J. Pathol.*, **220**, 217–30.

Building Brains: An Introduction to Neural Development, First Edition.
David Price, Andrew Jarman, John Mason and Peter Kind.
© 2011 John Wiley & Sons, Ltd. Published 2011 by John Wiley & Sons, Ltd.

Ladher, R. K., O'Neill, P. and Begbie, J. (2010) From shared lineage to distinct functions: the development of the inner ear and epibranchial placodes. *Development*, **137**, 1777–85.

With regards to the detailed anatomy of neural development, for most organisms there are excellent websites. For example, for mouse the emap project website is http://genex.hgu.mrc.ac.uk/ [20 November 2010]; for *Drosophila*, there is the interactive fly website at http://www.sdbonline.org/fly/aimain/1aahome.htm [20 November 2010]. There are also printed atlases, such as Schambra, U. (2008) *Prenatal Mouse Brain Atlas*, Springer, that are very detailed.

Chapter 3

De Robertis, E. M. and Kuroda, H. (2004) Dorsal-ventral patterning and neural induction in Xenopus embryos. *Ann. Rev. Cell Dev. Biol.*, **20**, 285–308.

De Robertis, E. M. (2006) Spemann's organizer and self-regulation in amphibian embryos. *Nat. Rev. Mol. Cell Biol.*, **7**, 296–302.

Hemmati-Brivanlou, A. and Melton, D. (1997) Vertebrate neural induction. *Annual Reviews of Neuroscience*, **20**, 43–60.

Stern, C.D. (2005) Neural induction: old problem, new findings, yet more questions. *Development*, **132**, 2007–2021.

Wilson, V., Olivera-Martinez, I. and Storey, K. (2009) Stem cells, signals and vertebrate body axis extension. *Development*, **136**, 1591–1604.

Chapter 4

Myers, P. Z. (2008) Hox genes in development: the Hox code. *Nature Education* 1(1) (http://www.nature.com/scitable/topicpage/hox-genes-in-development-the-hox-code-41402).

Wilson, V., Olivera-Martinez, I. and Storey, K. G. (2009) Stem cells, signals, and vertebrate body axis extension. *Development*, **136**, 1591–1604.

Ingham, P. W. and Placzek, M. (2006) Orchestrating ontogenesis: variations on a theme by sonic hedgehog. *Nature Reviews Genetics*, **7**, 841–850.

Kiecker, C. and Lumsden, A. (2005) Compartments and their boundaries in vertebrate brain development. *Nature Reviews Neuroscience*, **6**, 553–564.

Mizutani, C. M. and Bier, E. (2008) EvoD/Vo: the origins of BMP signalling in the neuroectoderm. *Nature Reviews Genetics*, **9**, 663–677.

Chapter 5

Götz, M. and Huttner, W. B. (2005) The cell biology of neurogenesis. *Nature Reviews Molecular Cell Biology*, **6**, 777–788.

Guillemot, F. (2007) Spatial and temporal specification of neural fates by transcription factor codes. *Development*, **134**, 3771–3780.

Livesey, F.J. and Cepko, C.L. (2001) Vertebrate neural cell-fate determination: lessons from the retina. *Nature Reviews Neuroscience*, **2**, 109–118.

Mizutani, K-I. and Gaiano, N. (2006) Chalk one up for 'nature' during neocortical neurogenesis. *Nature Neuroscience*, **9**, 717–718.

Wu, P. S., Egger, B. and Brand, A. H. (2008) Asymmetric stem cell division: lessons from *Drosophila*. *Semin. Cell Dev. Biol.*, **19**, 283–293.

Zhong, W. and Chia, W. (2008) Neurogenesis and asymmetric cell division. *Curr. Op. Neurobiol.*, **18**, 4–11.

Chapter 6

Ghashghaei, H. T., Lai, C. and Anton, E. S. (2007) Neuronal migration in the adult brain: are we there yet? *Nat. Rev. Neurosci.*, **8**, 141–51.

Marín, O. and Rubenstein, J. L. (2001) A long, remarkable journey: tangential migration in the telencephalon. *Nat. Rev. Neurosci.*, **2**, 780–90.

Marín, O. and Rubenstein, J. L. (2003) Cell migration in the forebrain. *Annu. Rev. Neurosci.*, **26**, 441–83.

Sauka-Spengler, T. and Bronner-Fraser, M. (2008) A gene regulatory network orchestrates neural crest formation. *Nat. Rev. Mol. Cell Biol.*, **9**, 557–68.

Chapter 7

Arimura, N. and Kaibuchi, K. (2007) Neuronal polarity: from extracellular signals to intracellular mechanisms. *Nature Reviews Neuroscience*, **8**, 194–205.

Da Silva, J. S. and Dotti, C.G. (2002) Breaking the neuronal sphere: regulation of the actin cytoskeleton in neuritogenesis. *Nature Reviews Neuroscience*, **3**, 694–704.

Hall, A. and Lalli, G. (2010) Rho and Ras GTPases in axon growth, guidance, and branching. *Cold Spring Harb. Perspect Biol.*, **2**, a001818.

Hattori, D., Millard, S. S., Wojtowicz, W. M. and Zipursky, S. L. (2008). Dscam-mediated cell recognition regulates neural circuit formation. *Annu. Rev. Cell Dev. Biol.*, **24**, 597–620.

Scott, E.K. and Luo L. (2001) How do dendrites take their shape? *Nature Neuroscience*, **4**, 359–365.

Chapter 8

Dickson, B. J. (2002) Molecular mechanisms of axon guidance. *Science*, **298**,1959–64.

Evans, T. A. and Bashaw, G. J. (2010) Axon guidance at the midline: of mice and flies *Current Opinion in Neurobiology*, **20**, 79–85

Lin, A. C. and Holt, C. E. (2008) Function and regulation of local axonal translation. *Curr. Opin. Neurobiol.* **18**, 60–8

Lowery, L. A. and Van Vactor, D. (2009) The trip of the tip: understanding the growth cone machinery. *Nature Reviews Molecular Cell Biology*, **10**, 332–343.

Mortimer, D., Fothergill, T., Pujic, Z., Richards, L. J. and Goodhill, G.J. (2008) Growth cone chemotaxis. *Trends in Neurosciences*, **31**, 90–98.

Petros, T. J., Rebsam, A. and Mason, C. A. (2008) Retinal axon growth at the optic chiasm: to cross or not to cross. *Annu. Rev. Neurosci.*, **31**, 295–315.

Chapter 9

Clandinin, T. R. and Feldheim, D. A. (2009) Making a visual map: mechanisms and molecules. *Current Opinions in Neurobiology*, **19**, 174–180.

Sterratt, D., Graham, B., Gillies, A. and Willshaw, D. (2011) Principles of computational modelling in neuroscience. Cambridge University Press.

Hubermann, A. D., Feller, M. B. and Chapman, B. (2008) Mechanisms underlying development of visual maps and receptive fields. *Annual Review of Neurosciences*, **31**, 479–509.

Innocenti, G. M. and Price, D. J. (2005) Exuberance in the development of cortical networks. *Nature Reviews Neuroscience*, **6**, 955–965.

McLaughlin, T. and O'Leary, D. D. (2005) Molecular gradients and development of retinotopic maps. *Annu. Rev. Neurosci.*, **28**, 327–55.

Mombaerts, P. (2006) Axonal wiring in the mouse olfactory system. *Ann. Review of Cell and Developmental Biology,* **22**, 713–737.

Chapter 10

Boda, B., Dubos, A,. and Muller, D. (2010) Signaling mechanisms regulating synapse formation and function in mental retardation. *Curr. Opin. Neurobiol.,* **20**, 519–27.

Holtmaat, A. and Svoboda, K. (2009) Experience-dependent structural synaptic plasticity in the mammalian brain. *Nat. Rev. Neurosci.,* **10**, 647–58.

McAllister, A. K. (2007) Dynamic aspects of CNS synapse formation. *Ann. Rev. Neurosci.,* **30**, 425–450.

Spitzer, N. C. (2006) Electrical activity in early neuronal development. *Nature,* **444**, 707–12.

Waites, C. L., Craig, A. M. and Garner, C. C. (2005) Mechanisms of vertebrate synaptogenesis. *Ann. Rev. Neurosci.,* **28**, 251–274.

Wang, D. D. and Kriegstein, A. R. (2009) Defining the role of GABA in cortical development. *J. Physiol.,* **587**, 1873–9.

Yoshihara, Y., De Roo, M. and Muller, D. (2009) Dendritic spine formation and stabilization. *Curr. Opin. Neurobiol.,* **19**, 146–53.

Yuste, R. and Bonhoeffer, T. (2004) Genesis of dendritic spines: insights from ultrastructural and imaging studies. *Nat. Rev. Neurosci.,* **5**, 24–34.

Chapter 11

Conradt, B. (2009) Genetic control of programmed cell death during animal development. *Annu. Rev. Genet.,* **43**, 493–523.

De Zio, D., Giunta, L., Corvaro, M., Ferraro, E. and Cecconi, F. (2005) Expanding roles of programmed cell death in mammalian neurodevelopment. *Semin. Cell Dev. Biol.,* **16**, 281–94.

Kostović, I. and Judas, M. (2010) The development of the subplate and thalamocortical connections in the human foetal brain. *Acta Paediatr.,* **99**, 1119–27.

Reichardt, L. F. (2006) Neurotrophin-regulated signalling pathways. *Philos. Trans. R. Soc. Lond. B Biol. Sci.,* **361**, 1545–64.

Chapter 12

Berardi, N., Pizzorusso, T., Ratto, G. M. and Maffei, L. (2003) Molecular basis of plasticity in the visual cortex. *Trends Neurosci.,* **26**, 369–78.

Hensch, T. K. (2005) Critical period plasticity in local cortical circuits. *Nat. Rev. Neurosci.,* **6**, 877–88.

Hofer, S. B., Mrsic-Flogel, T. D., Bonhoeffer, T. and Hübener, M. (2006) Lifelong learning: ocular dominance plasticity in mouse visual cortex. *Curr. Opin. Neurobiol.,* **16**, 451–9.

Malenka, R. C. and Bear, M. F. (2004) LTP and LTD: an embarrassment of riches. *Neuron,* **44**, 5–21.

Sengpiel, F. and Kind, P. C. (2002) The role of activity in development of the visual system. *Curr. Biol.,* **12**, R818–26.

Smith, G. B., Heynen, A. J. and Bear, M. F. (2009) Bidirectional synaptic mechanisms of ocular dominance plasticity in visual cortex. *Philos. Trans. R. Soc. Lond. B Biol. Sci.,* **364**, 357–67.

Glossary

Actin filament – a component of the cytoskeleton; a long polymer of actin protein, also known as a microfilament.

Action potential – the self-propagating voltage change across the cell membrane as a nerve impulse is transmitted along axons and dendrites.

Activation signal – in vertebrate anteroposterior patterning, one of the signals from the mesoderm that patterns the overlying neuroectoderm.

Active transport – the ATP-dependent directed transport of molecules and organelles, particularly in axons and dendrites.

Active zone – The region of the presynaptic terminal where synaptic vesicles containing neurotransmitter fuse with the membrane to release neurotransmitter.

Acute slices – Thin sections taken from a brain (or brain region) immediately after sacrificing an animal in order to keep the cells alive, generally for physiological recording or live cell imaging.

Adaptor proteins – usually lack any enzymatic activity but mediate specific interactions between other proteins in intracellular signalling cascades by promoting the formation of protein complexes.

Adherens junction – a junction that connects the actin cytoskeleton of one cell to the cytoskeleton or extracellular matrix of a neighbouring cell.

Adrenal medulla – the inner part of the adrenal gland, containing adrenomedullary cells; the adrenal gland is situated above the kidneys and secretes several important hormones.

Adult stem cells – proliferative cells that carry on producing new cells in the adult. Good examples are in the skin and blood system, but they are also present in some parts of the brain.

Afferent – an axon passing impulses *to* a specified region of the nervous system, for example from peripheral receptors *to* central nervous system or from spinal cord *to* brain.

Allele – a version of a gene; in most species an individual inherits two alleles for each gene, one from each parent.

Amblyopia – a visual condition that is characterized by reduced visual acuity that cannot be corrected with glasses.

AMPA receptor – a type of glutamate receptor that is responsible for the majority of the initial depolarization of the excitatory postsynaptic potential following activation of an excitatory synapse.

Animal cap or **pole** – an early embryo's dorsal region, giving rise to the three germ layers, ectoderm, mesoderm and endoderm.

Anterior – the end of the embryo where the head forms; means the same as rostral.

Anterograde – forward, used to describe the direction between the cell body of a neuron and its axon terminal.

Anteroposterior axis – the axis running through an embryo from anterior to posterior; means the same as rostrocaudal axis.

Antisense RNA – a strand of RNA that is complementary to a messenger RNA.

Aortic plexuses – collections of nerve cells lying along the aorta.

Apoptosis – the process of cell death by which the triggering of a specific programme of molecular events leads to cells destroying themselves.

Apoptotic body – the name given to the remnants of a cell that has undergone apoptosis.

Ascidian – a class of marine invertebrate with saclike bodies and whose larvae possess a notochord.

Building Brains: An Introduction to Neural Development, First Edition.
David Price, Andrew Jarman, John Mason and Peter Kind.
© 2011 John Wiley & Sons, Ltd. Published 2011 by John Wiley & Sons, Ltd.

Astrocyte – a type of glial cell; they are star-shaped with many processes that enwrap neuronal synapses.

Astrocytoma – a type of brain tumour originating from proliferation of astrocytes.

Asymmetric cell division – a cell division that gives rise to two different types of daughter cell.

Asymmetric synapses – excitatory synapses identified by the fact that the postsynaptic density is more prevalent than the presynaptic active zone.

Autistic spectrum disorder – a term used to describe psychological conditions that share abnormalities in social interactions and communication as well as repetitive behaviours.

Autonomic neurons – neurons in the peripheral nervous system that control body functions below the level of consciousness, such as respiration, heart rate, digestion, and so on.

Autophosphorylation – the phosphorylation of a kinase protein by its own enzymatic activity.

Axon – the projection on a neuron that carries information away from the cell body in the form of an action potential.

Axon guidance molecules – molecules that provide cues to the growth cone of a navigating axon, instructing its direction of movement. Predominantly, they are cell surface or secreted proteins and are detected by specific receptors in the growth cone membrane.

Axon initial segment – a specialized, unmyelinated region at the start of the axon containing a high density of voltage dependent sodium channels. It is the site of axon potential initiation.

Back-propagating action potential (bAP) – the action potential that propagates into the dendrites; the bAP is a key aspect of spike-time dependent plasticity as it correlates presynaptic activity with the generation of postsynaptic action potentials.

Basal ganglia – large groups of neurons lying under the cerebral cortex responsible for the control of movements.

Basal progenitors – intermediate proliferative cells in the developing cerebral cortex that populate the subventricular zone.

Basic helix–loop– helix (**bHLH**) – a DNA-binding structure found in many developmentally important transcription factor proteins, characterized by two helices connected by a loop and usually forming dimers.

Benzodiazepines – a group of pharmacological agents that act as sedatives by increasing GABA receptor activity and therefore increasing inhibition in neuronal networks.

β-galactosidase – an enzyme encoded by the bacterial gene *lacZ*, widely used as a reporter protein.

Bidirectional plasticity – neurons can undergo both long-term depression and long-term potentiation.

Bilaterally symmetrical – most animals have bodies divided into roughly mirror-image halves (left and right).

Binocular – pertaining to both eyes.

Bipolar – a neuron with two projections emanating from the cell body or soma.

Birth-dating – the use of experimental techniques to identify the developmental time-points at which cells are generated by division of progenitors (i.e. their birth dates).

Blastocoel – a fluid-filled cavity inside a blastula or blastocyst.

Blastocyst – the mammalian embryo prior to gastrulation, comprising up to about 100 cells surrounding a fluid-filled cavity.

Blastoderm – the superficial layer of the early embryo in species whose eggs contain relatively large amounts of yolk; cell division occurs in this layer, which surrounds the yolk in insects but is a flat disc at one pole of the egg in birds.

Blastomere – any of the cells resulting from the first few cleavages of a fertilized egg during early embryonic development.

Blastopore – the opening in an early embryo formed at gastrulation by the invagination of cells to form the mesoderm and endoderm; it is the entry to the primitive gut and in some species it becomes the anus.

Blastula – a very early embryo, fluid-filled and spherical in shape.

Bone morphogenetic proteins (**BMPs**) – a family of about 20 secreted intercellular signalling molecules with functions throughout development, but particularly important in the establishment of neuroectoderm and its patterning.

Brain-derived neurotrophic factor (**BDNF**) – a member of the family of secreted proteins called neurotrophic factors with numerous functions in cellular development and survival.

Brainstem – the posterior region of the brain of vertebrates consisting of the medulla oblongata, pons and midbrain.

Branchial arches – a set of mesodermal structures on either side of the developing pharynx (the cavity at the back of the mouth) that give rise to specialized structures in the head and neck.

Brodmann maps – the representation of the human cerebral cortex as a two-dimensional map that is subdivided into discrete areas based on their cytoarchitectural differences, as characterized by Korbinian Brodmann.

Bromodeoxyuridine (BrdU) – a chemical analogue of the nucleotide thymidine, readily incorporated into newly-synthesized DNA.

Cajal–Retzius cell – a specific subtype of neuron found near the pial edge of the marginal zone of the developing cerebral cortex. Named after their co-discoverers, Santiago Ramón y Cajal and Gustaf Retzius.

Caspases – a family of cysteine-aspartic acid proteases that exist in cells as inactive forms and are cleaved to active enzymes following the induction of apoptosis.

Catabolic reactions – the metabolic breakdown of complex molecules into simpler ones, often resulting in a release of energy.

Caudal – toward the tail end of an embryo; means the same as posterior.

cDNAs – complementary DNA molecules able to generate proteins since they are copies of mRNAs.

Cell adhesion molecules (**CAM**) – cell-surface proteins that are important for mediating contact between cells.

Cell cycle – the events that occur leading to cell division, including DNA synthesis and mitosis.

Central nervous system (**CNS**) – the part of the nervous system consisting of the brain and spinal cord.

Centrosome – the intracellular organelle that organizes the microtubules of the cytoskeleton.

Cerebellum – meaning 'little brain', it is a discrete structure at the base of the brain that lies above the brain-stem. It regulates a range of functions including motor control, attention and cognition.

Cerebral cortex – in mammals, the layer of neurons covering the surface of each cerebral hemisphere.

Chain migration/collective migration – a form of cell migration in which cells migrate collectively, sliding over one another until they reach their destination

Chemoaffinity hypothesis – a hypothesis put forward by Roger Sperry postulating the existence of molecular cues known as 'chemoaffinity labels' that allow axons to make precise connections with their target cells.

Chemoattraction – see **chemotropism**.

Chemokines – chemotactic cytokines: a family of secreted proteins that attract cells by chemotaxis.

Chemorepulsion – see **chemotropism.**

Chemotaxis – directed movement of a cell in response to a chemical stimulus.

Chemotropism – describes the directed movement of a cell (or part of a cell, such as an axon) in response to a diffusible chemical cue. Such movement may be either

towards the cue (**chemoattraction**) or away from it (**chemorepulsion**).

Chiasm – see optic chiasm.

Chimera – an individual created when cells of different genotypes come together to form an embryo.

Chondroitin sulphate proteoglycans (CSPG) – components of the extracellular matrix (ECM) consisting of a protein core and large sugar side-chains (known as glycosaminoglycans).

Chordate – an animal of the phylum Chordata, comprising vertebrates and some related animals such as sea squirts. They all have a notochord at some stage of their development.

Chromatin – DNA wrapped up with histone proteins in the nucleus.

Cilia (singular cilium) – highly structured cellular outgrowths associated mostly with a variety of cellular sensory functions. Some cilia are motile (e.g. those on cells lining the trachea).

Ciliopathy – a disease whose basis is the defective structure or function of cilia.

Clone – a group of cells that are all generated by the same progenitor.

Coincidence detector – a cellular mechanism that detects whether presynaptic and postsynaptic activation occur during a defined time-window.

Colinearity – describes the fact that the order of expression domains of Hox genes corresponds to the order of the genes on the chromosome.

Columnar genes – the three homeodomain genes that give *Drosophila* neuroblasts their identity in the dorso-ventral axis.

Combinatorial – referring to the fact that molecules (often signals or transcription factors) usually act in combinations, either to affect cell behaviour or gene expression. This means that a relatively small number of such molecules can encode a large number of different outcomes.

Commissure – a bundle of axons (**commissural axons**) that extends across the midline to connect structures on either side of the nervous system. Commissures are important for coordinating neural activity on the two sides of the animal.

Commitment – a measure of how firmly a developing cell adheres to its fate.

Competence – in developmental biology, competence defines the ability of an undifferentiated cell or tissue to take on a specific fate. For instance, neuroectodermal cells are competent to make neurons, but not muscle.

Competition – an interaction that results in the strengthening or increase of one set of axonal inputs and the weakening or removal of another set of axonal inputs to the same structure.

Complementary – describes a strand of DNA or RNA that can bind to a second strand because each base on one strand can pair, in order, with the base on the opposite strand (A and T pair, C and G pair).

Confocal microscopy – a form of microscopy that uses a laser light source. This allows observation of thin optical sections of tissues and whole embryos.

Congenital – a condition present at birth.

Contact guidance – describes those mechanisms that guide a navigating axon or migrating cell and which require close physical contact to be made between the migrating cell and the cell or molecule that provides the guidance cue; it can be divided into **contact attraction** and **contact repulsion**.

Context-dependence – used to describe the fact that a regulatory molecule (e.g. signal or transcription factor) can cause different cellular responses in locations or at different times. Typically, a cell's response to a given molecule depends on its developmental history up to that point.

Contractile proteins – proteins that mediate intracellular processes causing a cell or part of a cell to contract.

Contralateral – on the opposite side.

Corpus callosum – major fibre tract composed of axons connecting the cerebral hemispheres.

Correlated activity – activity (or patterns of activity) occurring in different cells or synapses simultaneously.

Cortical plate – a sheet of neural tissue in the developing mammalian brain that gives rise to most of the layers of the cerebral cortex.

Corticospinal tract – a collection of axons that connect the cerebral cortex to the spinal cord.

Cranial nerves – the nerves emerging from the vertebrate hindbrain.

Cranial neural folds – the folds generated by the folding of the neural plate at its anterior end.

Cranial placodes – bilateral thickenings of the ectoderm of the vertebrate head that generate sensory structures.

Critical periods – time-windows during development when experience shapes brain development

Crosstalk – the phenomenon that components in signal transduction can be shared between different signal pathways.

Cytoarchitecture – the appearance of a structure in the nervous system that results from the shape or distribution of its cells or clustering of cells.

Cytodifferentiation models – a group of computational models that invoke matching molecular cues on incoming axons and target cells to explain the precise connectivity between brain regions.

Cytokines – molecules secreted by many type of cell, including cells of the nervous and immune systems, which carry signals locally between cells and operate through multicomponent receptors rather than tyrosine kinase receptors.

Cytoskeleton – the subcellular network of protein polymers within cells that gives them their shape and robustness, and underlies their ability to move or change shape. Its main components are microtubules, microfilaments and intermediate filaments.

Dark-rearing – experimentally raising an animal in complete darkness.

Defasciculation – the process in which axons leave an axon fascicle.

Default model – the name given to a hypothesis to explain neural induction, in which early embryonic cells default to a neural fate unless prevented from doing so by bone morphogenetic proteins (BMPs).

Delamination – the process in which cells in the ventral neurogenic region of insects move inside the embryo to become neuroblasts.

Dendrites – neuronal processes that are the main sites of synaptic input from other neurons.

Dendrite self-avoidance – the dendrite branches of a particular neuron do not touch or overlap each other.

Dendritic field – the volume defined by the dendrite branches of a particular neuron.

Dendritic spines – small outgrowths on the dendrites of some vertebrate neurons, including pyramidal cells of the cortex. Excitatory synapses are concentrated on dendritic spines.

Dendritic tree – a neuron's dendrites are often highly branched, morphologically resembling a tree.

Depolarization – an increase in positive charge inside a neuron relative to the outside; a response to a depolarizing stimulus.

Depolymerization – the process by which a polymer is broken into monomers.

Developmental plasticity – the ability of a neuron to alter its phenotype in response to a given stimulus during development. It is most commonly used to describe changes in the anatomical and physiological properties of neurons in response to alteration in experience.

Diencephalic vesicle or **diencephalon** – a component of the early forebrain of vertebrates, situated caudal to the telencephalic vesicle, giving rise to adult structures including the thalamus.

Differentiation – the process by which cells take on their different final forms to perform their specialized functions in the organism. Much of development is aimed at ensuring this happens correctly and in a coordinated manner throughout the body.

DiI (pronounced 'dye-eye') – abbreviation for 1,1′-diocta-decyl-3,3,3′,3′-tetramethylindocarbocyanine perchlorate, a lipophilic dye commonly used to label axon tracts.

Dimer – a molecule consisting of two structurally similar molecules.

Diploid – an organism with a pair of each type of chromosome.

Directed growth – axons growing directly into the correct region of their target.

Direction map – a two-dimensional representation of the visual cortex showing the regions that respond to a stimulus of a particular orientation(s) moving in a particular direction(s).

Dissociation – often used to describe the experimental separation of tissues into individual cells.

DNA-binding motifs – regions of transcription factor proteins that allow their binding to DNA.

Dominant – an allele of a gene (i.e. a form of a gene) is described as being dominant if its effects are observed in individuals with only one copy of the allele (i.e. in heterozygotes); a dominant mutation is a genetic change whose effect is observed in heterozygotes; dominant alleles effectively override their recessive partners.

Dorsal – the back of an organ, embryo or adult organism; where the spinal cord develops in vertebrates; opposite of ventral.

Dorsal lateral geniculate nucleus (**dLGN**) – a region of the thalamus that processes visual information; it receives input from the retina and sends information to the visual cortex.

Dorsal lip of the blastopore – the part of the rim of the blastopore that lies on the future dorsal side of the embryo; an important organizer in vertebrate embryos.

Dorsal root ganglia (**DRGs**) – collections of cell bodies of peripheral sensory neurons whose axons enter the spinal cord. DRGs are located bilaterally along the dorsolateral side of the spinal cord.

Dorsoventral axis – the axis running through an embryo from its dorsal side to its ventral side. In humans, the axis runs from our back to our front.

DSCAM – Down's Syndrome Cell Adhesion Molecule; a member of the immunoglobulin superfamily. The *Drosophila* gene can produce many thousands of isoforms, rather reminiscent of antibody variation in the immune system.

ECM – see **extracellular matrix**.

Ectoderm – the outer germ layer of the embryo whose derivatives include skin and nervous system.

Efferent – an axon passing impulses *from* a specified region of the nervous system, for example *from* brain to spinal cord or *from* spinal cord to muscle.

Electrical activity/excitability – the ability of a cell to regulate electrical current at its cell membrane.

Electrochemical gradient – the difference in electrical charge and the imbalance in ion concentrations across a membrane.

Electron-dense – describes a structure that is unable to pass electrons, therefore appearing dark on an electron micrograph.

Embryonic stem (**ES**) **cells** – pluripotent stem cells that are derived from the inner cell mass of the blastocyst.

Endocannabinoids – naturally occurring lipids in the body that bind and activate cannabinoid receptors.

Endocytosis – the process by which a cell absorbs extracellular molecules by engulfment to form intracellular vesicles. Also a way for plasma membrane and its constituents to become internalized.

Endoderm – the inner germ layer whose derivatives include the digestive and respiratory system.

Endosome – an intracellular organelle transporting material away from the plasma membrane.

Enhancer – a region of DNA that can be bound with proteins to enhance transcription levels of genes.

Enteric nervous system – a subdivision of the peripheral nervous system that controls the gastrointestinal system.

Eph receptors – transmembrane tyrosine kinase receptors that recognise ephrins.

Ephrins – a family of membrane-bound ligands for the Eph family of receptor tyrosine kinases.

Epiblast – the layer of cells in the early embryos of birds, reptiles and mammals that gives rise to the three germ layers at gastrulation.

Epidermis – the outermost layers of cells covering the exterior body surface.

Epithelium – a tissue that lines the external and internal surfaces, including internal cavities and organs and other free open surfaces of the body, of all animals and their immature developing forms.

EPSP (excitatory postsynaptic potential) – The depolarization that results in the postsynaptic cell from the activation of a given set of synapses.

Excitability – The ability of a cell to regulate the flow of electrical current across its cell membrane.

Excitable cell – a cell that can conduct action potentials.

Excitatory synapses – a synapse that, when active, causes a depolarization in the postsynaptic cell.

Experience – a stimulus or group of stimuli that changes neuronal excitation.

Experience-dependent plasticity – changes in brain function that result from alteration in neural activity induced by experience.

Explant – part of an organism that has been excised and cultured in isolation.

Extracellular matrix – the gel-like meshwork of protein and carbohydrate polymers that surrounds cells and gives structural support in most organs and tissues.

Exuberant – a term used to describe a temporary projection during development that is subsequently pruned.

Fascicle – a bundle of nerve or muscle fibres.

Fasciculation – the process by which axons become bundled together to form a fascicle.

Fate – what a cell will become as a result of its development.

Feature map – a two-dimensional representation in a brain region of a physical feature of an external stimulus.

Fibroblast growth factors (**FGFs**) – a family of growth factor proteins involved in embryonic development as well as other processes such as wound healing.

Filopodia (singular filopodium) – a finger-like cellular outgrowth associated with cell shape changes. They are important for migrating cells, growth cones and dendritic spine formation.

Floor plate – the most ventral region of the neural tube.

Fluorescent – a molecule is fluorescent if it emits light of a certain wavelength when illuminated by light of a different wavelength; for example, GFP looks green when illuminated by blue light.

FMRP – Fragile X mental retardation protein. This is absent or reduced in Fragile X Syndrome.

Forebrain (or **prosencephalon**) – the anterior portion of the brain that develops from the anterior part of the neural tube.

Forebrain-midbrain boundary – a signalling structure within the brain.

Forward genetic screen – a genetic procedure where mutants are isolated on the basis of a phenotype of interest.

Forward genetics – a traditional genetic approach in which the aim is to identify a mutated gene responsible for a phenotype of interest.

Functional connectivity – the connections between neurons that, when stimulated, contribute to the generation of action potentials in the postsynaptic neuron.

Functional properties – a general term used to describe the physiological properties of a neuron, especially those that alter the behaviour of a neuronal network or animal.

G protein – (guanine nucleotide binding protein) a large family of membrane-associated and soluble proteins involved in intracellular signalling.

G-protein-gated ion channel – an ion channel whose opening is regulated by the binding of a G protein.

GABA (γ-aminobutyric acid) – the most common inhibitory neurotransmitter in the brain.

GABAergic – a neuron or synapse that contains GABA.

Gain-of-function (mutation) – a mutation that changes the gene such that it gains a new, abnormal function.

Ganglion – a dense collection of sensory neurons and interneurons (vertebrates) or CNS neurons (*Drosophila*).

Ganglion mother cell (GMC) – the daughter cell of a neuroblast in insects; it divides only once forming two neurons or a neuron and a glial cell.

Ganglionic eminences – ventral regions of the embryonic telencephalon.

GAP (GTPase activating protein) – a regulator of small G proteins. Induces the G protein to hydrolyse its bound GTP to GDP, thereby changing the activity of the G protein.

Gap genes – a group of genes whose expression divides the early *Drosophila* embryo into large regions in the anteroposterior axis.

Gastrulation – the process in which a gastrula develops from a blastula by the movement of cells from the outer surface of the embryo to its inside, forming the primitive gut.

GEF (guanine-nucleotide exchange factor) – a regulator of small G proteins. Facilitates the binding of GTP in place of GDP, thereby changing the activity of the G protein.

Gene expression – translation of the information encoded in a gene first into mRNA and then, usually, to a protein.

Genetically tractable organism – an organism whose genetic make-up can be manipulated relatively easily.

Genotype – the genetic make-up of a cell or organism.

Germ cells – the reproductive cells, that is the eggs and sperm.

Germ layers – the three cellular layers into which the embryos of animals differentiate: ectoderm, mesoderm and endoderm.

Glia – the non-neuronal cells of the nervous system. Originally thought to provide structural support (glia derives from the Greek for 'glue') but now known to have important signalling and nutritive functions to maintain neurons.

Glutamate – An amino acid that is also the most common excitatory neurotransmitter in the vertebrate brain.

Glutamatergic – a neuron or synapse that uses the neurotransmitter glutamate.

Glycoprotein – a protein having covalently-linked carbohydrate side chains attached.

Granule cells – small neurons, with a diameter of around $10\,\mu m$, found in large numbers in the granule layer of the cerebellum.

Green fluorescent protein (GFP) – a protein derived from jellyfish that fluoresces bright green when exposed to blue light, commonly used as a marker in cell biology.

Growth cone – a specialized structure found at the leading edge of migrating axons that detects and responds to guidance cues in the environment.

Growth factor – a naturally occurring substance capable of stimulating cellular growth and differentiation and operating through a receptor on the cell surface.

Guidepost cells – cells that assist in the guidance of axonal growth by providing intermediate targets along the direction of growth.

Hebb's postulate – a theory of synaptic plasticity proposed by Donald Hebb in 1949 to explain how animals learn and store memories.

Hensen's node – a bulge at the anterior tip of the primitive streak that forms as the streak lengthens from posterior to anterior; important in organizing the embryo at gastrulation.

Hermaphrodite – an organism with both male and female sexual characteristics and organs.

Heterochronic transplant – transplantation of cells or tissue from one developing organism to another of a different age. A technique used to test how temporal events are regulated.

Heterodimer – a protein complex consisting of two different proteins.

Heterotrimeric – consisting of three different subunits.

Heterozygous – having two different alleles of a single gene.

Hindbrain (or **rhombencephalon**) – the posterior portion of the brain including the cerebellum and brainstem.

Hippocampal commissure – a large axon bundle that connects the two hippocampi across the midline of the brain.

Hippocampus – a structure of the vertebrate forebrain particularly associated with learning and memory formation.

Histones – proteins found in cell nuclei that package and order DNA into nucleosomes.

Homeobox – the DNA sequence encoding a **homeodomain.**

Homeodomain – a region in many developmentally important transcription factor proteins comprising about 60 amino acids folded into three helices, one of which interacts directly with DNA, connected by short loops.

Homeodomain code – the idea that combinations of homeodomain transcription factors specify different cell fates.

Homeostasis – the ability of a physiological system to maintain internal stability, especially in response to external stimuli that alter the physiological state of the system. Derived from the Greek, *homeo*, meaning sameness.

Homeostatic plasticity – the ability of neurons to regulate their general excitability or average firing rate.

Homeotic – typically referring to a mutation that causes the change of one body part or region to resemble another, such as leg to wing, or thoracic segment to abdominal segment.

Homodimers – a dimer derived from any two identical monomers.

Homologous recombination – a phenomenon in which nucleotide sequences are exchanged between two similar or identical strands of DNA.

Homologue – a gene or structure that is similar in different species since it was derived from their common ancestor during evolution.

Homophilic binding – binding between molecules of the same kind.

Homozygous – having both alleles of a single gene the same.

Homunculus – a representation of the human body.

Hox code – the mechanism by which the expression of combinations of Hox genes defines cellular fates.

Hox genes – a highly conserved family of related genes that confer regional identity in the anteroposterior axis. They encode transcription factors that have a related homeodomain in their structure.

HSPG (heparan sulphate proteoglycans) – cell surface and extracellular glycoproteins that possess long, complex carbohydrate side chains and are subject to extensive post-translational modifications. They act as co-factors for certain growth factors and axon guidance molecules.

Hydrolysis – the breaking of a covalent chemical bond by a water molecule.

Hyperpolarizing – an increase in negative charge inside a neuron relative to the outside; a response to a hyperpolarizing stimulus.

Hypothalamus – a neural region at the ventral base of the forebrain that regulates hormone secretion and controls many autonomic functions.

Immunocytochemistry – a laboratory technique that uses antibodies to mark cells that contain a protein of interest.

***In situ* hybridization** – a method by which a gene or messenger RNA is detected using a labelled RNA probe.

In vitro – pertaining to experiments conducted outside the organism with cells/tissue derived from it.

In vivo – pertaining to the context of the intact organism.

Individual migration – a mode of migration in which movement of cells appears to be independent of contact with other cells.

Induction – the process by which one tissue causes a change in the development of another tissue.

Induction models – a group of computational models that hypothesize that incoming axons have inherent information that specifies their orderly mapping within the target tissue to instruct the differentiation of the target tissue.

Innate – arising from the genetic programme of the animal (contrast with experience).

Inner cell mass – the cluster of pluripotent cells inside the mammalian blastocyst that gives rise to the three germ layers of the embryo.

Inner ear – the sensory part of the ear, including the cochlea, embedded in the skull and connected to the outside world via the middle ear.

Integrin – cellular receptor protein that binds laminin.

Intercellular signalling (molecules) – the process (and molecules) that mediate communication from one cell to another.

Interkinetic nuclear migration – the movement of the nucleus within an otherwise stationary cell.

Intermediate target cell – a cell that provides an intervening destination for an axon navigating from its point of origin to its final destination. Such axons commonly change their direction of movement upon reaching the intermediate target.

Interneurons – neurons within the central nervous system that function as connectors between other neurons.

Intracellular signalling (molecules) – the process (and molecules) that mediate a cell's response to an extracellular signal.

Intraflagellar transport – transport pathway that underlies growth of cilia and flagella.

Ion channel – a transmembrane protein that, when open, allows the passage of ions across membranes.

Ion pump – a transmembrane protein that actively regulates the distribution of ions across membranes.

Ionic gradient – the difference in the concentration of a particular ion or ions across a membrane.

Ipsilateral – on the same side.

Ischemia – the lack of adequate blood flow to support the normal functioning of a tissue.

Isoform – different forms of a protein often produced from the same gene by use of different combinations of exons.

Isthmic organizer – a signalling region in the developing brain.

Kinase – an enzyme that transfers phosphate groups onto specific molecules, a process called phosphorylation.

Knock-down – to reduce the levels of an mRNA or protein.

Knock-out – an organism that has been engineered to carry genes that have been made inoperative.

Labelled pathway hypothesis – suggests that axon pathways laid down by pioneer neurons express specific molecular labels that allow later-navigating axons to identify and follow specific pathways.

lacZ – a bacterial gene that encodes β-galactosidase, widely used as a reporter protein.

Lamellipodia (singular lamellipodium) – a sheet-like cellular outgrowth associated with cell shape changes. They appear on migrating cells and growth cones.

Lamina – a layer of neurons in the central nervous system.

Laminin – a protein component of the extracellular matrix.

Lateral – away from the midline of an embryo perpendicular to its rostrocaudal and dorsoventral axes; opposite of medial.

Lateral ganglionic eminence (LGE) – a lateral region of the embryonic ventral telencephalon.

Lateral inhibition – a process in which one cell inhibits neighbouring like-minded cells from acquiring the same fate.

Lateral line – a sense organ found in many species of fish and amphibians that detects water movements and allows the animal to orient itself in the water.

Lateral ventricle – a small fluid-filled cavity within the forebrain.

Leading process – a long cytoplasmic projection that protrudes in front of a migrating cell during cell migration.

Ligand – a molecule or ion that binds to a receptor molecule, for example on the cell surface, to generate a biological response.

Ligand-gated ion channel – an ion channel whose opening is regulated by the binding of an extracellular signal such as a neurotransmitter.

Lineage (of a cell) – the sequence of divisions that generated the cell, that is its cellular ancestry.

Lipophilic – having affinity for lipids.

Lissencephaly – literally means 'smooth brain'; a congenital defect in which the sulci and gyri of the cerebral cortex are absent.

Long-thin spine – a dendritic protrusion characterised by a long, thin neck and a small head. Generally believed to be an immature spine.

Long-term depression (LTD) – a long-term decrease in synaptic strength resulting from uncorrelated activity between pre- and postsynaptic elements.

Long-term potentiation (LTP) – a long-term increase in synaptic strength resulting from coordinated activity between pre- and postsynaptic elements.

Loss-of-function (mutation) – a mutation that changes the gene such that it loses its function.

Lumen – a cavity or passage in a tubular organ.

Lysosome – a membrane-bound organelle containing catabolic enzymes found in the cytoplasm of most cells.

Mantle zone – an outer layer of the neuroepithelium containing postmitotic neurons that have migrated radially away from the ventricular zone.

Map – a spatially ordered representation of a given area or physical feature of an object.

Marginal zone – a superficial layer in the cerebral cortex that is formed by the preplate splitting.

Medial – towards the midline of an embryo perpendicular to its rostrocaudal and dorsoventral axes; opposite of lateral.

Mediolateral – the axis of a bilaterally symmetrical organism from its midline to its sides.

Medulloblastoma – the most common malignant brain tumour among children; arises in the cerebellum.

Melanocytes – pigment-producing cells located in the skin, hair and eye.

Membrane potential – the imbalance of electrical charge across a membrane.

Mesencephalon (or **midbrain**) – the middle portion of the brain along its rostrocaudal axis, between the forebrain and the hindbrain.

Mesoderm – the middle germ layer of the embryo whose derivatives include muscle and bone.

Metabotropic receptor – a receptor that does not form an ion channel and hence transduces signals to the inside of the cell through the activation of intracellular signalling cascades often using heterotrimeric G proteins.

Metamorphosis – a profound change in an animal's body structure as it develops from one stage to the next, typically seen in amphibians and insects.

Metaplasticity – the ability of a neuron to change the stimulation frequencies that induce LTP and LTD.

Microfilament – a major constituent of the cytoskeleton, composed of actin protein.

Microglia – scavenger cells in the nervous system.

MicroRNA – naturally-occurring small regulatory RNAs.

Microtubule – a major component of the cytoskeleton, composed of tubulin protein.

Microtubule capture – a process by which dynamic microtubules become stabilized, triggered by interaction with other components of the cytoskeleton.

Microtubule catastrophe – the rapid dissociation of tubulin subunits from microtubules.

Microtubule-associated proteins – a heterogeneous group of proteins that bind to microtubules, usually to stabilize them and to influence their properties.

Midbrain (or **mesencephalon**) – the middle portion of the brain along its rostro-caudal axis, between the forebrain and the hindbrain.

Midbrain-hindbrain boundary – location of the isthmic organiser signalling structure within the brain.

Midline – the line dividing the left and right halves of a bilaterally symmetric animal.

Miniature excitatory postsynaptic potential (mEPSP) – An EPSP that results form the activation of a single synapse.

Mitogen – a signalling molecule that induces cells to proliferate.

Mitotic spindle – an array of microtubules that forms during cell division and serves to pull the chromosomes into each daughter cell.

Model organism – a species that is extensively studied due to its usefulness in providing insight into the structure and development of other organisms.

Modification threshold – the stimulation frequency at which there is a switch from long term depression induction to long term potentiation induction.

Monocular – pertaining to one eye.

Monocular deprivation – occlusion of vision through one eye.

Monomer – a protein consisting of one subunit.

Morphogen – a diffusible signalling molecule inducing cell responses in a concentration-dependent manner. Typically it diffuses to form a concentration gradient, thereby giving cells positional information.

Morphogenesis – differentiation and growth of tissues and organs during development.

Mosaic – organism containing two populations of cells with different genotypes in one individual that has developed from a single fertilized egg.

Motifs – specialized regions in proteins that allow them to function, for example DNA binding motifs allow transcription factors to interact with DNA.

Motogenic – an effect that stimulates the initiation of movement.

Motor protein – a protein that propels itself along intracellular filaments.

Multimeric – proteins that consist of more than one subunit.

Multipolar neuron – a type of neuron that has a single axon and several dendrites extending from its body.

Multipotent – the property of a progenitor cell that produces progeny of different types; a key property of stem cells.

Mushroom body – a structure in the insect brain that is the seat of olfactory learning and memory.

Mushroom spine – a dendritic protrusion characterised by a thin spine neck and a large spine head thereby giving the appearance of a mushroom. Generally believed to be a mature spine.

Mutual inhibition – a process in which cells inhibit each other during a competition to acquire a particular fate.

Myosin – a molecular motor protein that moves along actin filaments.

Nasal – referring to a position close to the nose in a bilaterally symmetric animal (contrast with temporal).

Necrosis – the pathological process of cell death resulting from overwhelming cellular injury.

Neighbour matching models – a group of computational models that invoke (1) the presence of signals on incoming axons that are more similar between adjacent cells than between distant ones and (2) the ability of target cells to recognize these signals, to explain the precise connectivity between brain structures.

Neocortex – the part of the cerebral cortex that has expanded massively in the evolution of higher mammals.

Nerve cord – the ventrally located CNS structure that runs the length of the insect; equivalent to the vertebrate spinal cord.

Nerve growth factor (NGF) – the first discovered member of the family of secreted proteins called neurotrophic factors with numerous functions in cellular development and survival.

Netrins – a small family of evolutionarily conserved secreted proteins that may either attract or repel growing axons, depending on the class of netrin receptor they express.

Neural cells – a general term for any cell in the nervous system, encompassing both neurons and glia.

Neural crest – part of the ectoderm located between the neural tube and the epidermis that contributes neurons and other cells throughout the body of vertebrates.

Neural induction – the process by which an inducing tissue tells a responding tissue to adopt a neural fate.

Neural networks – a group of neurons that form a circuit.

Neural plate – a sheet of neuroectoderm that rolls up to form the neural tube.

Neural precursor – defined in this book as a cell that has committed to become a neural cell, but not yet differentiated; Cf **neural progenitor**.

Neural progenitor – defined in this book as a cell that divides to give daughter cells, some of which will differentiate as neural cells. Progenitor cells are often multipotent. Cf **neural precursor**.

Neural stem cell – progenitor cells in the nervous system. Such cells typically undergo asymmetric cell division and produce a variety of progeny (they are multipotent).

Neural subtype specification – term denoting the regulatory process by which neurons become different from each other.

Neural tube – a tube of ectodermal tissue in the embryo from which the brain and spinal cord develop.

Neurite – a collective term for axons and dendrites, especially applied to the immature stages during outgrowth.

Neurite outgrowth – the process in which a new neuron grows axon and dendrites.

Neuroblastoma – a rare childhood tumour of the adrenal medulla or sympathetic nervous system.

Neuroblasts – dividing cells that will develop into neural cells; the term can be used in mammalian and non-mammalian species but is more commonly used in describing insect development.

Neuroectoderm (or **neuroepithelium**) – the neurogenic region of the ectoderm that develops into the nervous system.

Neurogenesis – the process of producing cells that will differentiate as neurons.

Neuromast – a small group of cells that will form the sensory cells of the lateral line.

Neuronal activity – see **excitability.**

Neuronal migration – the movement of neurons towards their destination in the nervous system.

Neuronal polarity – cell polarity refers to morphological asymmetries across a cell. In the case of neurons, neuronal polarity refers to the fact that neurites are differentiated into axon and dendrites.

Neuropilins – a family of receptor proteins for semaphorins.

Neuropore – the openings at one or other end of the neural tube that become progressively smaller during neurulation and eventually close.

Neurotrophic hypothesis – the hypothesis that if the neurons innervating a structure do not receive enough neurotrophic factor then they will die.

Neurotrophic molecules – secreted molecules that enhance the growth and survival of neurons.

Neurotrophins – a family of proteins including brain derived neurotrophic factor (BDNF) and nerve growth factor (NGF) that induce the survival, development and function of neurons.

Neurulation – the process by which the neural tube is formed.

Nitric oxide – a small gaseous molecule that acts as a local signalling molecule.

N-methyl-D-aspartate (NMDA) receptor – a glutamate receptor critical for synaptic plasticity and which can also be involved in the regulation of cell death.

Notochord – a mesodermally-derived rod that runs from anterior to posterior in developing chordates (including vertebrate animals). It is a transient structure that has important signalling functions.

Nuclease – a type of enzyme that breaks down nucleic acids such as DNA.

Nucleokinesis – describes the process by which the nucleus moves forward in a migrating cell.

Nucleosome – the structure responsible for the compactness of a chromosome, consisting of a sequence of DNA wrapped around a protein called histone.

Nucleus – as well as being a structure inside most cells, the term is also used to describe discrete clusters of neural cell in the nervous system, for example see **dorsal lateral geniculate nucleus (dLGN)**.

Nurse cells – cells that contribute material to a growing egg cell within the ovary.

Ocular dominance – the relative level of physiological responsiveness of a given cell in the visual cortex for stimulation of one or the other eye.

Ocular dominance bands – the overall pattern of synaptic terminals in cortical layer 4 of axons carrying information from the **dLGN**.

Ocular dominance histogram – a bar graph showing the frequency with which neurons with a particular ocular dominance classification are encountered in the visual cortex of a given animal.

Ocular dominance shift – an alteration in the distribution of the ocular dominance histogram that results from manipulation of an animal's visual experience.

Olfactory bulb – the brain region that receives input from olfactory neurons.

Olfactory interneurons – small neurons within the olfactory bulb that function as connectors between other neurons.

Oligodendrocytes – glial cells that produce processes that ensheath axons in the CNS.

Optic chiasm – structure on the ventral surface of the brain composed of the axons of retinal ganglion cells. These axons cross the midline at this point, creating the chiasm's characteristic X-shape.

Optic nerve – the bundle of axons connecting an eye to the brain.

Optic vesicles – bilateral outgrowths from the forebrain that generate the retinae and optic nerves of the eye.

Optical imaging – an imaging technique that measures local changes in oxygen metabolism. Commonly used to visualize topographic and feature maps in the cerebral cortex.

Organizer – typically a tissue or group of cells that produce signals enabling the patterned differentiation of surrounding cells (i.e. it endows them with **positional information**).

Orientation map – a two-dimensional representation of the visual cortex showing the regions that respond to a stimulus of a particular orientation.

Orientation selectivity – a physiological feature of neurons in the visual system by which they preferentially generate action potentials to stimuli of a particular orientation.

Otic placode – generates the inner ear including its sensory epithelium and the auditory and vestibular ganglia.

Otic vesicle (or **otocyst**) – the hollow chamber of the internal ear formed by the otic placode invaginating and pinching off from the surface ectoderm.

Pair-rule genes – a group of genes whose expression divides the early *Drosophila* embryo into segmental units.

PAR complex – a conserved complex of proteins that regulate cellular asymmetry in a variety of contexts, including early *C. elegans* development, neuronal polarity and asymmetric cell division of neural progenitors.

Paracrine – signalling between adjacent cells, either by contact, for example the Notch pathway, or by diffusible factors.

Parallel fibres – axons from the granule cells in the cerebellum that run parallel to the pial surface in the molecular layer where they form synapses with Purkinje cell dendrites.

Perinatal – a term meaning around the time of birth, either prenatal or postnatal.

Perineuronal net – pattern of expression of chondroitin sulphate proteoglycans and other extracellular matrix proteins on the cell soma and proximal dendrites of particular subsets of neurons.

Peripheral nervous system (PNS) – the part of the nervous system outside the brain and spinal cord linking the CNS and the rest of the body.

Pharmacological inhibition – the use of a drug to decrease the activity of a given protein, cell or neural network.

Pharynx – the passage in the front part of the neck that connects to the stomach and lungs.

Phenotype – the observable characteristics of an organism, such as its physical appearances or behaviour.

Phosphorylation – the addition of a phosphate group to a molecule, commonly causing its activation or deactivation.

Pia – a membrane that envelops the brain and spinal cord.

Pioneer neurons or **axons** – early migrating neurons or navigating axons which act as developmental cues for later developing neurons or axons.

PIP3 (phosphatidylinositol 3,4,5-trisphosphate) – a membrane-associated phospholipid second messenger involved in regulating many cellular processes, including cell shape changes, migration and neuronal polarity.

Placodes – bilateral thickenings of the ectoderm of the vertebrate head that generate sensory structures.

Plasticity – the ability to change.

Pluripotency – the ability of a cell (e.g. an embryonic stem cell) to differentiate into many of the cell types in the body.

Polymer – a molecule composed of many similar subunits.

Polymerization – the process by which monomers are assembled to generate a polymer.

Polysaccharide – a polymer of sugar (carbohydrate) subunits.

Positional information – information that an epithelial cell receives enabling it to assess its location within the epithelium and respond accordingly. Typically this information is in the form of a concentration gradient of a signalling molecule known as a morphogen.

Posterior – toward the tail end of an embryo; means the same as caudal.

Postsynaptic – pertaining to the cell or dendrite that receives a signal at a synapse.

Postsynaptic density – the **electron dense** protein complex of the postsynaptic terminal that is comprised of the neurotransmitter receptors, scaffolding molecules, signalling enzymes and cytoskeletal elements.

Postsynaptic terminal – the dendritic or somal portion of a synapse that contains the neurotransmitter receptors.

Post-translational modifications – changes that are made to a protein after it is synthesized, for example glycosylation or phosphorylation.

Prechordal plate – the mesoderm that underlies the anterior neuroectoderm; a source of signals that promote anterior regionalization of the neural tube, including cerberus.

Precursor – see **Neural precursor**.

Prepatterning – an alternative term used to describe the regionalization of the neuroectoderm.

Presynaptic – the cell generating a signal, generally in the form of a neurotransmitter, at a synapse.

Presynaptic terminal – the portion of a synapse that contains the synaptic vesicles.

Prethalamus – a subdivision of the diencephalon of the vertebrate brain.

Primary neurulation – the process by which a sheet of neuroectoderm rolls up as it grows to form the neural tube.

Primitive streak – a structure formed when epiblast cells move anteriorly along the midline of a vertebrate embryo.

Primordium – an embryological term for a region that will subsequently give rise to a particular organ or tissue.

Progenitor – see **Neural progenitor**.

Programmed cell death – the process by which cells that are no longer needed effectively commit suicide by activating an intracellular death program.

Projection neurons – a general term for neurons that project axons over a distance, rather than locally.

Proliferation – increasing cell numbers by cell division; a characteristic of progenitors and stem cells.

Promoter – a site in a DNA molecule that facilitates the transcription of a certain gene.

Proneural cluster – a contiguous group of neuroectodermal cells that express a proneural gene.

Proneural gene – a gene that controls the process by which cells commit to differentiation as neural cells.

Prosencephalon (or **forebrain**) – the anterior portion of the brain that develops from the anterior part of the neural tube.

Protease – an enzyme that breaks down proteins.

Protein kinase – an enzyme that transfers a phosphate group to a protein (usually from ATP), thereby regulating the protein's function.

Proteoglycans – extracellular matrix proteins that are heavily modified by the covalent attachment of polysaccharide groups.

Proteolytic degradation (or **cleavage**) – the breakdown of proteins into peptides and amino acids.

Protocortex – hypothesis postulating that the cortex is a 'tabula rasa' or blank slate and that identity of individual cortical areas is specified by incoming afferent axons from the thalamus.

Protomap – hypothesis postulating that the early cortex has an inherent template of the later developing cortical areas that is matched to incoming axons during development.

Proto-oncogene – a normal gene, commonly involved in controlling cell proliferation, that has the potential to promote the formation of a tumour when disregulated by mutation, overexpression or misexpression.

Protozoa – a group that includes most unicellular eukaryotic organisms, such as *Amoeba* and *Paramecium*.

Proximal dendrites – region of the dendrites that are close to the cell soma.

Purkinje cell – a major neuronal type in the cerebellum; it has a highly complex dendritic tree.

Pyramidal neuron – a major type of neuron in the vertebrate brain, characterized by a triangular-shaped cell body.

Radial glia – the neuronal progenitor cells of the vertebrate CNS.

Radial migration – a mode of migration in which newborn neurons migrate from the centre of a developing structure towards its outer edge (e.g. the cortex) or vice-versa (e.g. granule cells in the cerebellum).

Ras – the archetypal small G protein (or small GTPase).

Rearing paradigms – an experimental manipulation in which the sensory experience of an animal is altered.

Receptive field – region of sensory space that elicits a response in the cell being examined.

Receptor – a structure usually on a cell surface that binds with signalling molecules in order to control certain functions of the cell.

Receptor kinetics – features of a receptor that determine the magnitude of electrical current that it conducts. These include rate of opening and closing, permeability, and so on.

Receptor tyrosine kinases – cell surface receptors that phosphorylate tyrosine residues.

Recessive – an allele of a gene (i.e. a form of a gene) is described as being recessive if its effects are observed only in individuals with two copies of the allele (i.e. in homozygotes); a recessive mutation is a genetic change whose effect is observed in homozygotes; recessive alleles are effectively overridden by dominant partners.

Reeler – a line of mutant mice that have poor motor coordination most likely as a result of abnormal development of the cerebellum.

Regionalization – the process of dividing up the neuroectoderm into domains that will form different parts of the nervous system.

Regulatory elements – segments of DNA that regulate the expression of a gene. Examples are promoters and enhancers.

Repolarization – the restoration of the membrane resting potential following the generation of an action potential.

Reporter gene – usually a 'neutral' gene that is introduced to mark the expression pattern of an endogenous gene. Well known reporter genes are *lacZ* (a bacterial gene that encodes β-galactosidase) and green fluorescent protein.

Repression – the inhibition of a gene's expression.

Resting potential – the membrane potential when a cell is not conducting an impulse.

Retina – the light-sensitive nerve layer that lines the back of the eye.

Retinal ganglion cells (RGCs) – neurons in the retina that transmit visual information through the optic nerves, optic chiasm and optic tract to their targets in the thalamus and the superior colliculus (known as the tectum in non-mammalian vertebrates).

Retinal Waves – Periodic bursts of activity in the retina that spread locally and correlate the activity of adjacent cells.

Retinogeniculate axons – the axons of the retinal ganglion cells that project to the lateral geniculate nucleus of the thalamus.

Retinoic acid – a vitamin A derivative that is an important signalling molecule in vertebrate development.

Retinotopic map – the map of retinal ganglion cell position in a target brain structure.

Retrograde – backward, used to describe the direction between a neuron's axon terminal and its cell body.

Retrovirus – a small virus which inserts a DNA copy of its RNA genome into a chromosome of an infected cell.

Reversal potential – the membrane potential at which there is no net electrical current (i.e. the electrochemical forces are in equilibrium) across a membrane when the membrane is selectively permeable for a particular ion.

Reverse genetics – a genetic approach in which genes are selected for study, for example based on their sequence, and then manipulated to discover their function.

Reverse occlusion – a rearing regimen in which, following monocular deprivation, vision is restored to the initially deprived eye and at the same time the initially open eye is deprived of vision.

Rhombencephalon (or **hindbrain**) – the posterior portion of the brain including the cerebellum and brainstem.

Rhombomeres – anatomically distinguishable tissue blocks formed in the hindbrain (or rhombencephalon).

Ribosomes – intracellular particles, composed of RNA and protein, found in the cytoplasm of living cells and responsible for the translation of mRNAs to protein.

RNA interference – a phenomenon that occurs naturally but can be harnessed experimentally for silencing specific genes by interfering with the mRNA that they encode.

Robos – transmembrane receptors for the slit family of axon guidance molecules.

Roof plate – the cells at the dorsal apex of the neural tube.

Rostral – the end of the embryo where the head forms; means the same as anterior.

Rostral migratory stream – the path followed by olfactory neural progenitors born in the subventricular zone of the lateral ventricle to their destination in the olfactory bulb.

Rostrocaudal axis – the axis running through an embryo from rostral to caudal; means the same as anteroposterior axis.

Scaffold – a temporary cellular structure used to help guide migrating neurons to their destination.

Scaffolding proteins – types of adaptor proteins whose primary purpose is to link other proteins to create distinct signalling cascades or protein complexes.

Schwann cells – glial cells of the peripheral nervous system that produce the myelin sheath around axons.

Second messenger-gated ion channel – an ion channel whose opening is regulated by the binding of a second messenger such as cAMP or Ca^{2+}.

Second messengers – intracellular molecules that act as relays for extracellular signals bound to cell surface receptors; they include cyclic AMP, PIP3 and Ca^{2+}.

Secondary neurulation – the process by which a tube of neural tissue is formed through the hollowing out of an initially solid rod of tissue.

Segment – many animals are divided up into reiterated units called segments. In some cases this is clearly visible (e.g. the segments of an earthworm) but in many cases segments are only apparent during development. Also known as metameres.

Segmentation genes – a group of genes that confers pattern within segments in the early *Drosophila* embryo.

Selector gene – a gene that regulates an entire developmental programme (e.g. thoracic segment vs abdominal segment) rather than specifying particular cell types. Examples are Hox genes. Mutation of a selector gene tends to be homeotic.

Semaphorins – a large and diverse family of cell surface and secreted proteins with multiple roles, including guiding navigating axons.

Sense organ precursors (SOPs) (or sensory mother cells) – individual ectodermal cells from which sense organs or sensilla develop in insects. Although called precursors, they are in many respects like progenitors since they undergo cell division.

Sensilla (singular sensillum) – small, simple sense organs in insects.

Sensitive periods – distinct time-windows during development when the functional properties of neurons can be altered by experience.

Sensory bristle – the most visible type of sensillum in insects, consisting of one sensory neuron and three support cells.

Sensory receptors – the organs that transduce external stimuli into electrical signals in the nervous system.

Sensory surface – the region of a sense organ that contains the sensory receptors, for example the retina in the eye.

Sexually dimorphic – refers to structures that are of different size and organization in males and females.

Signal transduction – a process in which intercellular signalling, involving the binding of a ligand to its specific receptor, activates a set of intracellular reactions.

Slits – a small family of axon guidance molecules, evolutionarily conserved between invertebrates and mammals.

Small G proteins – a family of small cytosolic proteins that transduce signals between receptor and effector proteins to affect cell behaviour, and so on. They are regulated by the binding of GTP/GDP. Also known as small GTPases. Includes Ras, Rac, Rho and Cdc42.

Soma – the neuronal cell body (as opposed to the neurites).

Somal translocation – a mode of migration by which some newborn neurons in the cerebral cortex migrate radially. These cells are connected to the outer edge of the cortex by a long process that shortens progressively, pulling the neuron towards its destination.

Somatodendritic domain – collective term for the soma and dendrites, which together form a domain that is distinct from the axon.

Somatosensory cortex – cortical region(s) that processes touch, proprioception, temperature and pain.

Somatososensory homunculus – two-dimensional representation of the body surface in the somatosensory cortex.

Somites – segmental masses of mesoderm lying on either side of the notochord and neural tube during the development of vertebrate embryos.

Spatial summation – the adding together of nearby EPSPs and IPSPs in a dendrite.

Specification – the process by which a cell or tissue receives information directing it towards its particular fate.

Spike-timing dependent plasticity (STDP) – a mechanism of synaptic plasticity that is based on Hebb's postulate.

Spine head – the bulbous region of a dendritic spine where synapses are formed.

Spine neck – the thin region of a dendritic spine that attaches the spine head to the main shaft of the dendrite.

Spinogenesis – the formation of dendritic spines.

Spontaneous electrical activity – electrical activity that arises from the endogenous properties of a neuronal or a neural network.

Stem cell – a relatively unspecialized cell that can divide repeatedly to regenerate itself (self-renewal) and give rise to more specialized cells, such as neurons or glia.

Stochastic – random, unpredictable, occurring by chance.

Strabismus – a misalignment of the two eyes.

Stripe assay – an experimental paradigm used to examine a cell's or axon's preference for a substrate.

Stubby spines – bulbous protrusions from a dendrite that lack a spine neck.

Subplate – a deep layer of the immature cerebral cortex that is formed transiently but later disappears, having completed functions such as the direction of axons to their cortical targets.

Substantia nigra – a layer of grey matter in the midbrain that controls mobility.

Subventricular zone – the transient layer of the forebrain neural tube that contains the basal progenitor cells.

Superior colliculus – a region of the dorsal midbrain that receives visual input from the retina. Generally known as the visual tectum in non-mammalian vertebrates.

Support cells – in *Drosophila*, non-neuronal components of sensilla.

Symmetric cell division – a cell division that gives rise to identical daughter cells.

Symmetric synapse – inhibitory, GABAergic synapses characterised by the presence of postsynaptic densities of similar size to the presynaptic active zone (contrast with asymmetric synapses).

Synapse formation – see **synaptogenesis.**

Synapse specific – occurring selectively at a synapse or group of synapses.

Synapse specification and induction – the first step in synapse formation involving the correct choice of target tissue (specification) and the initiation of synapse formation (induction).

Synapse stabilization – the maintenance of a synapse.

Synapse withdrawal – the removal of a synapse.

Synapse – a specialized structure that allows communication between a neuron and another cell (such as another neuron, or a muscle fibre). The synapse is comprised of parts of both the sending (presynaptic) and receiving (postsynaptic) cell.

Synaptic cleft – the region of a synapse between the presynaptic terminal and the postsynaptic membrane.

Synaptic depression – a reduction in synaptic weight.

Synaptic efficacy – the change in membrane potential associated with a certain level of presynaptic activation.

Synaptic plasticity – the ability of a synapse to change its synaptic weight.

Synaptic potentiation – an increase in synaptic weight.

Synaptic vesicles – membrane-bound organelles in the presynaptic terminal that contain neurotransmitter.

Synaptic weight – the change in membrane potential associated with a certain level of presynaptic activation (also called synaptic efficacy).

Synaptogenesis – the process of forming a synapse.

Synaptopathy – a disease whose main symptoms are believed to arise from alterations in synaptic development and/or function.

Syncytium – having many nuclei within a common cytoplasm. The early *Drosophila* embryo is a syncytium; muscle fibres are another example.

Tandem duplication – the evolutionary process by which a section of DNA (e.g. containing one or more genes) becomes duplicated so that the chromosome now has two copies of the section in tandem. A common way in which gene families are initially formed.

Tectum – in non-mammalian vertebrates, a region of the midbrain that receives innervation from retinal ganglion cells. Known as the superior colliculus in mammals.

Telencephalic vesicles (together called the **telencephalon**) – bilateral swellings of the most anterior part of the embryonic forebrain; they generate the cerebral cortex and the basal ganglia.

Temporal – referring to the position close to the temple (beneath which sits the temporal bone) in a bilaterally symmetric animal (contrast with nasal).

Temporal summation – the adding together of coincident EPSP and IPSPs in a dendrite.

Ternary complex – a complex containing three proteins bound together.

Tetrodotoxin (**TTX**) – a toxin isolated from the pufferfish that blocks voltage-gated sodium channels and hence action potentials.

Thalamocortical axons (**TCAs**) – axons of neurons in the thalamus that synapse with cells in the cerebral cortex.

Thalamus – a structure in the centre of the vertebrate brain that transmits sensory input to the cerebral cortex, and receives reciprocal output from the cortex.

Thin spines – narrow spines with a small bulbous ending (head). These are distinct from dendritic filopodia that lack heads.

Topographic map – two-dimensional representation of the spatial position of stimuli on a sensory surface.

Transcription factors – proteins that bind to DNA to regulate gene transcription.

Transformation signal – in anteroposterior pattern, the proposed signal(s) that modulates neural induction in order to confer posterior identity on the rear part of the neuroectoderm of vertebrates.

Transgenic – describes an organism whose genetic material has been modified.

Translation – the decoding of mRNA to generate protein.

Transmembrane proteins – proteins in membranes that have both intracellular and extracellular domains.

Transport vesicles – membrane-bound organelles that transport proteins to their correct location within a cell.

Trigeminal ganglion – a sensory ganglion that transmits sensation from the face.

Trk receptors – tyrosine kinase receptors that respond to members of the neurotrophin family, comprising an extracellular domain containing the neurotrophin binding site, a transmembrane segment and an intracellular domain.

Tubulin – the protein constituent of microtubules.

Tyrosine kinase – a type of enzyme that transfers phosphate groups onto (i.e. phosphorylates) tyrosine residues in a protein.

Tyrosine kinase receptors – cell surface receptors having an intracellular tyrosine kinase domain required for their signal-transducing activity.

Uncorrelated activity – activity (or patterns of activity) occurring in cells or synapses at different times.

Unipolar neuron – one that has a single process that subsequently splits to form the dendrites and axon.

Untranslated regions, 5′ or 3′ – regions of mature RNA that do not code for proteins.

Vegetal hemisphere – an early embryo's ventral region.

Ventral – the side of an embryo or adult organism towards the chest; opposite of dorsal.

Ventral nerve cords – neural tissue running from anterior to posterior along the ventral side of many invertebrates and making up their central nervous system.

Ventricles – small fluid-filled cavities or chambers within the brain.

Ventricular zone – the inner side of the neural tube closest to its lumen in the developing vertebrate brain. This transient layer contains neuronal progenitor cells.

Ventro-temporal crescent – that part of the retina in mice that is located ventrally and temporally and projects axons to the ipsilateral side of the brain, giving a limited degree of binocular vision.

Visual acuity – a functional measure of visual capability.

Visual experience – a visual stimulus or group of stimuli that changes neuronal excitation in neurons of the visual system.

Visually-evoked potentials (VEP) – the physiological response of a small group of neurons in the visual cortex to visual stimulation.

Voltage-gated ion channel – an ion channel whose opening is regulated by a change in the distribution in electrical charge across a membrane.

Weaver – a mouse line with a naturally occurring mutation in a K^+ channel that results in altered motor function.

Whisker follicles – the sensory apparatus at the base of a facial whisker that transduces mechanical bending of the whisker into an electrical signal in the nervous system.

Wildtype – the typical form of an organism in natural conditions.

Wnt (Wnt family) – a highly evolutionarily conserved family of secreted proteins that regulate many different processes in developing and adult animals, including cell proliferation, differentiation and gene expression.

Zinc finger – a motif found in some developmentally important transcription factor proteins comprising a helix which interacts with the DNA and a sheet of amino acids stabilized and held in position relative to each other by a zinc atom.

Zona limitans intrathalamica (ZLI) – a signalling structure in the vertebrate diencephalon.

Zygote – a fertilized cell that gives rise to an embryo.

Index

Building Brains: An Introduction to Neural Development, First Edition.
David Price, Andrew Jarman, John Mason and Peter Kind.
© 2011 John Wiley & Sons, Ltd. Published 2011 by John Wiley & Sons, Ltd.

Keep up with critical fields

Would you like to receive up-to-date information on our books, journals and databases in the areas that interest you, direct to your mailbox?

Join the **Wiley e-mail service** - a convenient way to receive updates and exclusive discount offers on products from us.

Simply visit **www.wiley.com/email** and register online

We won't bombard you with emails and we'll only email you with information that's relevant to you. We will ALWAYS respect your e-mail privacy and NEVER sell, rent, or exchange your e-mail address to any outside company. Full details on our privacy policy can be found online.

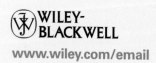

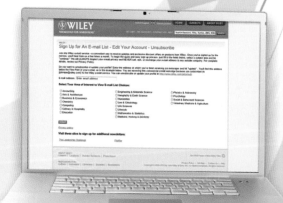

17841